Neonatology Questions and Controversies
Renal, Fluid and Electrolyte Disorders

Neonatology Questions and Controversies
Renal, Fluid and Electrolyte Disorders
Fourth Edition

Series Editor

Richard A. Polin, MD
William T. Speck Professor of Pediatrics
Executive Vice Chair Department of Pediatrics
Vagelos College of Physicians and Surgeons
Columbia University

Other Volumes in the Neonatology Questions and Controversies Series

GASTROENTEROLOGY AND NUTRITION

HEMATOLOGY AND TRANSFUSION MEDICINE

INFECTIOUS DISEASE, IMMUNOLOGY, AND PHARMACOLOGY

NEONATAL HEMODYNAMICS

NEUROLOGY

THE NEWBORN LUNG

4th Edition

Neonatology Questions and Controversies

Renal, Fluid and Electrolyte Disorders

John M. Lorenz, MD
Emeritus Professor of Pediatrics and Special
Lecturer
Vagelos College of Physicians and Surgeons
Columbia University
New York, NY

Michel G. Baum, MD
Professor of Pediatrics and Internal Medicine
Charles E. and Sara M. Seay Chair in
Pediatric Research
UT Southwestern Medical Center
Dallas, TX

Kathleen G. Brennan, MD
Assistant Professor of Pediatrics, Division of
Neonatology Associate Program Director,
Neonatal-Perinatal Fellowship
New York, NY

Consulting Editor
Richard A. Polin, MD
William T Speck Professor of Pediatrics
Executive Vice Chair Department of Pediatrics
Vagelos College of Physicians and Surgeons
Columbia University
New York, NY

ELSEVIER

Elsevier
1600 John F. Kennedy Blvd.
Ste 1800
Philadelphia, PA 19103-2899

Notice

Practitioners and researchers must always rely on their own experience and knowledge in evaluating and using any information, methods, compounds or experiments described herein. Because of rapid advances in the medical sciences, in particular, independent verification of diagnoses and drug dosages should be made. To the fullest extent of the law, no responsibility is assumed by Elsevier, authors, editors or contributors for any injury and/or damage to persons or property as a matter of products liability, negligence or otherwise, or from any use or operation of any methods, products, instructions, or ideas contained in the material herein.

Content Strategist: Sarah Barth
Senior Content Development Specialist: Vasowati Shome
Content Development Manager: Ranjana Sharma
Publishing Services Manager: Shereen Jameel
Project Manager: Haritha Dharmarajan
Design Direction: Margaret Reid

Printed in the United States of America

Last digit is the print number: 9 8 7 6 5 4 3 2

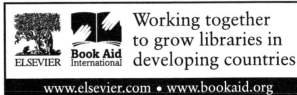

Contributors

Carolyn L. Abitbol, MD
Professor
Pediatric Nephrology
University of Miami
Miami, Florida
United States

Melvin Bonilla-Felix, MD, FAAP
Professor and Chairman
Pediatrics
University of Puerto Rico—Medical Sciences Campus
San Juan, Puerto Rico

Timothy Bunchman, MD
Professor and Director Pediatric Nephrology
Children's Hospital of Richmond
Virginia Commonwealth University School of Medicine
Richmond, Virginia
United States

James Castleman, MD, MRCOG
Consultant in Maternal and Fetal Medicine
West Midlands Fetal Medicine Centre
Birmingham Women's and Children's Hospital
Birmingham
United Kingdom

Valerie Y. Chock, MD, MS Epi
Associate Professor of Pediatrics
Neonatal and Developmental Medicine
Stanford University School of Medicine
Palo Alto, California
United States

Maria Esther Díaz González de Ferris, MD, MPH, PhD
Department of Pediatrics
The University of North Carolina Chapel Hill
North Carolina
United States

Marissa J. DeFreitas, MD
Assistant Professor of Clinical Pediatrics
Pediatric Nephrology
University of Miami
Miami, Florida
United States

Guido Filler, MD, PhD
Professor of Paediatrics
Paediatrics
Schulch School of Medicine and Dentistry
London, Ontario
Canada

Noa Fleiss, MPH, MD
Assistant Professor of Pediatrics
Department of Pediatrics
Division of Neonatology
Yale School of Medicine
New Haven, Connecticut
United States

Joseph T. Flynn, MD, MS
Chief, Division of Nephrology
Seattle Children's Hospital
Seattle, Washington
United States
Professor
Department of Pediatrics
University of Washington School of Medicine
Seattle, Washington
United States

Jean-Pierre Guignard, MD, PhD (Deceased)
Honorary Professor of Pediatric Nephrology
Department of Pediatrics
Lausanne University Medical School
Lausanne, Vaud
Switzerland

Leo Gurney, MBBS, BMedSci, MD, MRCOG
Consultant in Fetal and Maternal Medicine
Clinical Lead for Fetal Medicine
Clinical Lead for Day Assessment Unit
Birmingham Women's Hospital
Birmingham
United Kingdom

Mr Leo Gurney
Fetal Medicine Department
Birmingham Women's Hospital
Birmingham
United Kingdom

Thomas Hays, MD, PhD
Assistant Professor of Pediatrics
Department of Pediatrics
Columbia University Irving Medical Center
New York, New York
United States

C.D. Anthony Herndon, MD, FAAP, FACS
**Professor of Surgery, Director of Pediatric
   Urology, Surgeon in Chief Children's Hospital
   of Richmond**
Urology
Virginia Commonwealth University
Richmond, Virginia
United States

Silvia Iacobelli, MD, PhD
Full Professor of Pediatrics
NICU and PICU, Neonatology
Centre Hospitalier Universitaire La Réunion
Saint Pierre, France
Reunion

Mark D. Kilby, DSc, MD, FRCOG, FRCPI
Professor of Fetal Medicine
Academic Department of Obstetric and Gynaecology
Birmingham Women's Hospital
Birmingham
United Kingdom
Professor of Fetal Medicine
Lead Clinician in Fetal Medicine,
Birmingham Women's Foundation Trust
Birmingham
United Kingdom

Gina M. Lockwood, MD, MS, FAAP
Clinical Associate Professor
Urology
University of Iowa
Iowa City, Iowa
United States

Fiona L. Mackie, MBChB, MRes, PhD, MRCOG
Maternal-Fetal Medicine Subspecialty Trainee
West Midlands Fetal Medicine Centre
Birmingham Women's and Children's NHS
   Foundation Trust, Birmingham
United Kingdom

Douglas G. Matsell, MDCM
Professor
Pediatric Nephrology
University of British Columbia
Vancouver, British Columbia
Canada

Mignon Irene McCulloch, MBBCh, FCP(Paeds),
FRCPCH(UK)
Professor
Paediatric Nephrology and PICU
Red Cross War Memorial Children's Hospital
Cape Town, Western Cape
South Africa

Natalie Menassa, MD
Researcher
Pediatrics
Northeast Ohio Medical University
Rootstown, Ohio
United States

Michael G. Michalopulos, MD
Pediatric Nephrology Fellow
Pediatric Nephrology
UT Southwestern
Dallas, Texas
United States

Heather A. Morgans, DO, MS
Pediatric Nephrologist
Children's Mercy
Kansas City, Missouri
United States
Assistant Clinical Professor
Department of Pediatrics
University of Missouri-Kansas City School of
   Medicine
Kansas City, Missouri
United States

R. Katie Morris, MBChB, PhD, FRCOG
Professor
Institute of Applied Health Research
University of Birmingham
Birmingham
United Kingdom

Xamayta Negroni-Balasquide, MD, MS
Assistant Professor Pediatric Nephrology
University of Puerto Rico -Medical Science Campus
San Juan
Puerto Rico

Melissa Posner, MD
Assistant Professor of Pediatrics
Department of Pediatrics
Division of Neonatology
Yale School of Medicine
New Haven, Connecticut
United States

Raymond Quigley, MD
Professor
Department of Pediatrics
University of Texas Southwestern Medical Center
Dallas, Texas
United States

Rupesh Raina, MD
Nephrologist
Nephrology
Akron Children's
Brecksville, Ohio
United States

Steven Ringer, MD, PhD
Section Chief
Neonatology
Children's Hospital at Dartmouth Hitchcock
Lebanon, New Hampshire
United States
Professor of Pediatrics
Geisel School of Medicine
Hanover, New Hampshire
United States

Jeffrey L. Segar, MD
Professor
Department of Pediatrics
Medical College of Wisconsin
Milwaukee, Wisconsin
United States

Sidharth Sethi, MBBS, MD
Nephrologist
Pediatric Nephrology
Kidney and Urology Institute
Medanta, The Medicity
Guragon, Haryana
India

Anvitha Soundararajan, MBBS
Research Fellow
Nephrology
Cleveland Clinic Akron General
Akron, Ohio
United States

Khalid Taha, MD
Pediatric Nephrology Fellow
Pediatric Nephrology
University of British Columbia
Vancouver, British Columbia
Canada

Bradley A. Warady, MD
Professor of Pediatrics
Department of Pediatrics
University of Missouri-Kansas City School of
   Medicine
Kansas City, Missouri
United States
Director, Division of Pediatric Nephrology
Department of Pediatrics
Children's Mercy Kansas City
Kansas City, Missouri
United States
Director, Dialysis and Transplantation
Department of Pediatrics
Children's Mercy Kansas City
Kansas City, Missouri
United States

Series Foreword

Richard A. Polin, MD

*To study the phenomena of disease without books is
to sail an uncharted sea, while to study books without
patients is not to go to sea at all.*

*Medicine is learned by the bedside and not in the
classroom. Let not your conceptions of disease come
from the words heard in the lecture room or read
from the book. See and then reason and compare
and control. But see first.*

William Osler

Before the invention of the movable type by Johannes
Gutenberg in the 15th century, physicians learned
medicine by serving an apprenticeship with individuals considered experienced. There were no printed
textbooks, and medical journals were not published
until the beginning of the 19th century. By apprenticing yourself to a physician over a period of years, one
learned how to be a competent practitioner. Internships in the United States evolved from those apprenticeships in the 18th century. The term "residency"
was chosen because the physicians in training had a
"residence" at the hospital. Modern-day internships
began at Johns Hopkins Hospital in 1904. The Johns
Hopkins Hospital was founded by Osler, Halsted,
Welch, and Kelly. Halstead is credited with creating
the first surgical residency and coined the phrase "see
one, do one, teach one" (SODOTO). That educational
philosophy has been adopted by nearly every specialty
in medicine including neonatology.

Modern-day trainees in neonatology still learn how
to care for critically ill infants and how to perform
procedures by watching, assisting, and listening to
more experienced individuals at the bedside. The
SODOTO approach is considered a fundamental educational tool. However, over a 3-year period, much of
education occurs remote from the bedside during
teaching rounds and conferences. The teaching is
often more theoretical, and by design, rounds in the

nursery and conferences are passive learning exercises. In those settings, trainees listen but do not take
an active role in the educational process. Learning is
always more effective when recipients take an active
role in their own education. Ideally, they should
be questioning what they hear, reading pertinent literature, and, when the opportunity arises, teaching
others. Unfortunately, much of the information transmitted in those settings is not usually followed by
an active phase of questioning and reading by the
trainee.

Most graduates of fellowship programs turn out
to be excellent practitioners, but once they leave the
fellowship program, new information is acquired
only intermittently either at conferences or from journals and textbooks. As a source of new information,
journals provide access to the most up-to-date information. However, that information is unfiltered, and
the conclusions of a study may not be appropriate
(or perhaps risky) for a critically ill infant. Textbooks
like those in the Neonatology Questions and Controversies series offer an opportunity to hear from experts
in neonatal-perinatal medicine who have synthesized
(and filtered) the existing literature and can provide
up-to-date recommendations.

The fourth edition of the questions and controversies series will also have seven volumes. Each of them
has been extensively revised, and we have added
several new editors: Terri Inder has joined Jeffrey
Perlman for the *Neurology* volume; James Wynn joined
William Benitz and P. Brian Smith as a coeditor for
the *Infectious Disease, Immunology, and Pharmacology*
volume; and Patrick McNamara is now a coeditor
with Martin Kluckow for the *Neonatal Hemodynamics*
volume. The reader will find many completely new
chapters; however, like the last edition, each of them is
focused on day-to-day clinical decisions encountered
by neonatologists. Nothing will replace the teaching
that occurs at the bedside when confronted with a

critically ill neonate, and the SODOTO educational approach still has an important role in education. Procedures are best learned by simulations and guidance by experienced practitioners at the bedside. However, expertise as a practitioner can only be enhanced by reading and incorporating new information into daily practice, once proven safe and effective. Perhaps SODOTO should be changed to LQRT (listen, question, read, and teach). Questions and Controversies is a unique source to learn from experts in the field who have been through the LQRT process many times.

Osler's quotes at the beginning of this preface suggest that both bedside teaching and journals/textbooks have a synergistic role in physician education, and neither alone is sufficient.

As with all prior editions, I am indebted to an exceptional group of volume editors who chose the content and authors and edited the manuscripts. I also want to thank Sarah Barth (publisher), as well as Vasowati Shome and Vaishali Singh (senior content development specialists) at Elsevier, who have guided the development of this series.

Preface

Two new editors, Drs. Jack Lorenz and Kathleen Brennan, are pleased to join Dr. Michel Baum in presenting the fourth edition of *Renal, Fluid, and Electrolyte Disorders: Neonatology Questions and Controversies*. All three of us express our appreciation of Dr. William Oh's contributions to this series as editor of the first three editions, the last with Dr. Baum. We also note with sadness the passing of Professor Jean-Pierre Guignard, MD, PhD, in the spring of 2022, whose contributions to neonatal-perinatal nephrology were immense.

Readers of the third edition of *Renal, Fluid, and Electrolyte Disorders: Neonatology Questions and Controversies* will note much new material in this edition. Half the chapters cover new topics, including assessment of neonatal kidney function, pulmonary hypoplasia in the fetus with oligohydramnios, genetic causes of congenital renal malformations, effect of preterm birth on renal outcomes, dialysis and kidney transplantation, renal tubular acidosis, renal near-infrared spectroscopy, and urosepsis and uroprophylaxis. Nearly all the remaining chapters are state-of-the-art updates of chapters appearing in the last edition, and many are written by completely new authors.

The editors are grateful to all the authors of this edition for their expertise and diligence in presenting the most current information on their topics. Along with our readers, we all strive to provide the best care for our patients. It is our hope that this edition will contribute to improved care of our patients with renal, fluid, and electrolyte disorders.

John M. Lorenz
Michel G. Baum
Kathleen G. Brennan

Contents

Chapter 1

Assessment of Renal Function in Fetuses With Lower Urinary Tract Obstruction

Leo Gurney, MBBS, MRCOG, James Castleman, MD, MRCOG, Fiona L. Mackie, MBChB, MRes, PhD, MRCOG, Mark D. Kilby, DSc MD FRCOG FRCPI and R. Katie Morris, MBChB, PhD, FRCOG

Chapter Outline

Introduction

Fetal lower urinary tract obstruction (LUTO) or congenital bladder outlet obstruction has an incidence of 2.2/10,000 pregnancies and is usually diagnosed in late first or early second trimester of pregnancy with the characteristic findings of dilated fetal bladder, dilated proximal ureter, and renal hydronephrosis.[1]

LUTO represents a spectrum of congenital anomalies with the principal etiology differing according to fetal sex and additional structural anomalies. If the affected fetus is male, the principal etiology is typically posterior urethral valves (PUVs), which has accounted for approximately half of cases presenting with LUTO in some case series[2]; prune belly syndrome or urethral atresia are other important

additional causes. Female fetuses with LUTO are significantly less common and are more likely to be associated with complex etiology such as cloacal plate anomaly or monogenic megacystic microcolon syndrome.[3]

EMBRYOLOGY AND AMNIOTIC FLUID HOMEOSTASIS

Within the developing embryo, the renal tract develops from three overlapping sequential systems: the pronephros, the mesonephros, and the metanephros. These all derive from a specialized area of intermediate mesoderm: the urogenital ridge.[4] Interaction between the ureteric bud (an outpouching of the mesonephros), the metanephros, and the metanephric blastema forms the developing kidney and excretory and collecting system by 11–12 weeks' gestation, at which point fetal urine production begins.[5] Up to

20 weeks' gestation, the embryonic ureter undergoes a repeated branching process, forming the collecting system of the kidneys, renal pelvis, calyces, and collecting ducts. At this gestation, fetal urine has a low protein content and absence of glucose and phosphorus, suggesting that glomerular protein filtration is mature and tubular reabsorption is taking place.[6]

The fetal renal system continues to mature through the third trimester with further induction of the mesenchyme by epithelial ureteric structures. Renal tubular reabsorption of sodium and β_2-microglobulin and secretion of calcium increase during the second half of pregnancy.[6] Finally, from 30 weeks onward, a progressive increase is observed in fetal urinary elimination of the nitrogen compounds: urea, creatinine, and ammonia.[7]

In the first trimester, amniotic fluid is secreted by the placenta and membranes with water and solutes freely traversing fetal skin.[8] During the second trimester, the fetal skin becomes impermeable to further diffusion through keratinization. As a result, from approximately 16 weeks amniotic fluid is almost exclusively produced through fetal urination, which progressively increases until, by term, a fetus can produce on average from 750 to 1000 mL of urine per day.[8] Amniotic fluid is removed primarily through fetal swallowing, which has been seen to occur from 16 weeks' gestation and increases up to the ingestion of 200 to 450 mL of amniotic fluid per day at full term.[8] Fluid may also be eliminated via the fetal respiratory tract with term inspiratory flow rates of 200 mL/kg per day, although as alveolar phospholipid secretions can be found within the amniotic fluid, there remains uncertainty as to whether the fetal respiratory tract remains a net contributor or remover of amniotic fluid in utero. Finally, oncotic forces across the fetal membranes and placenta can also lead to reabsorption of amniotic fluid.[9]

NATURAL HISTORY OF LOWER URINARY TRACT OBSTRUCTION

The natural history of untreated LUTO is dependent upon the presence of severe oligohydramnios and associated pulmonary hypoplasia. When such features exist, cases demonstrate high mortality and morbidity rates, with up to 30% of survivors requiring renal replacement therapy.[10,11]

Prenatal Diagnosis of Lower Urinary Tract Obstruction

IMAGING

Ultrasound and the Classic Lower Urinary Tract Obstruction Triad

Suspicion of congenital LUTO (congenital bladder neck obstruction) often arises in the first trimester from ultrasound evidence of an enlarged bladder. Fetal megacystis has been defined by a longitudinal bladder diameter of greater than 7 mm, prior to 14 weeks' gestation, or a failure of bladder emptying during a 45-minute duration ultrasound scan in the second and third trimesters.[12] However, megacystis is not always associated with LUTO and may be associated with spontaneous resolution, therefore serial ultrasonography is essential to confirm the diagnosis. Diagnostic confirmation occurs with the observation on prenatal ultrasound of a "classic" triad: dilated posterior urethra (so-called keyhole sign), urinary bladder enlargement, and hydronephrosis. However, even when defining this triad using strict criteria, specificity is low with up to 23% false-positive rate reported.[13] Diagnostic accuracy can be improved with the use of clinical scoring systems. Within these scoring systems, fetal sex, ureteral size, degree of bladder distension, presence of severe oligo- or anhydramnios, and gestational age at diagnosis are key variables.[14] These systems will be described in further detail in the "Antenatal Predictors of Postnatal Renal Function" section later in this chapter.

Recently, a clinical LUTO diagnostic score has been developed to replace the classic "ultrasound triad" for prenatal diagnosis of LUTO. This clinical LUTO score was developed in a retrospective cohort study in the Netherlands, which used a multivariate analysis of a 7-year data set including 124 cases of LUTO.[14] The scoring system (Table 1.1) includes five variables—fetal sex, degree of bladder distension, ureteral size, oligo- or anhydramnios, and gestational age at referral. Using these five variables, the scoring system discriminates LUTO from nonobstructive megacystis with superior accuracy to the classic "ultrasound triad" (area under the curve [AUC] of 0.84 vs. AUC = 0.63, $P = .07$). Indeed, in this staging system, a clinical LUTO score of 9.5 predicts LUTO with 78% sensitivity and 79% specificity, which corresponds to a 96%

TABLE 1.1 Clinical Scoring System for Diagnosis of Fetal Lower Urinary Tract Obstruction

Ultrasound Features	Score
Bladder volume > 35 cm³ or urinary ascites	4
Anhydramnios or oligohydramnios (DVP < 5th centile)	4
Male sex	4
Diagnosis before 26 weeks of gestation	4
Enlarged ureter (>7 mm diameter)	1.3 per mm above 7 mm Total ≥ 9.5 has 96% positive predictive value for LUTO

LUTO, lower urinary tract obstruction, *DVP*, Deepest Vertical Pool.
Adapted from Fontanella F, Duin LK, Adama van Scheltema PN, et al. Prenatal diagnosis of LUTO: improving diagnostic accuracy. *Ultrasound Obstet Gynecol*. 2018;52(6):739–743. doi:10.1002/uog.18990

positive predictive value and 36% negative predictive value. The major strength of this study is that it mandated confirmation of the postnatal diagnosis. The authors found bladder volume showed better accuracy than longitudinal bladder diameter, which thus far has been the routine measurement for ascertaining megacystis. A bladder volume of greater than 35 cm³ is reported as the optimal predictor of LUTO diagnosis (AUC = 0.66 with 0.6–0.8 confidence interval [CI], P = .03). Fetal hydronephrosis, renal cortical appearance, and keyhole sign performed poorly in the stepwise model compared with the five variables preserved for inclusion.

Fetal Cystoscopy and MRI

Fetal cystoscopy is a tool to improve diagnostic accuracy in LUTO (simultaneous to its role in fetal intervention) that is now well recognized. This technique enables accurate prenatal diagnosis of PUV, urethral stenosis, and urethral atresia, with a high sensitivity and specificity for PUV.[15] However, it is associated with significant risks of pregnancy loss.

In utero fetal MRI may be used as a diagnostic adjunct to ultrasound for many prenatal conditions. The use of this technique to improve diagnostic accuracy in LUTO may be helpful, in selected cases, to distinguish cloacal plate anomaly and megacystic microcolon syndrome.[16] Models using imaging combination of ultrasound and MRI have been demonstrated in the literature[17]; however, these have yet to arrive in routine clinical practice.

ROLE OF GENETIC TESTING IN PRENATAL LUTO DIAGNOSIS

Fetal Sex Testing

Since PUVs occur only in boys, the prenatal diagnosis of fetal sex is necessary to inform appropriate management and counseling of parents. Female sex is associated with worse prognosis as this group includes more complex cloacal plate anomalies.[18] Ultrasound diagnosis of phenotypic sex is challenging in the first trimester, even with modern high-resolution equipment.[19–22] Fetal sex becomes easier to identify in later gestation, although factors such as reduced amniotic fluid, fetal position, and maternal obesity may adversely affect image quality and diagnostic accuracy. Positive identification of either the female labia or the male genitalia should be used to diagnose phenotypic sex.

Genetic testing now provides a more accurate means of identifying fetal sex and helping for better prognostication of LUTO. An invasive prenatal test (chorionic villus sample or amniocentesis), which would be offered in the context of a complex structural difference, is the gold standard for diagnosis of fetal sex. Cell-free fetal DNA-based testing of the maternal blood now allows a noninvasive prenatal diagnosis of fetal sex, without the procedure-related risk of miscarriage or preterm birth, which can make women reluctant to have an invasive test.[23]

Genetic Anomalies Associated With Lower Urinary Tract Obstruction

The majority of congenital bladder neck obstruction (LUTO) cases are isolated and associated with either PUVs or urethral atresia.[1] However, the differential diagnosis of fetal megacystis should also include chromosomal abnormalities, genetic syndromes and developmental anomalies, submicroscopic chromosomal anomalies, pathologic copy number variants, and other genetic variants.[3,24] The wide spectrum of etiologies and prognoses makes the counseling and management of this condition particularly challenging.[3] As with all fetal structural anomalies, suspicion of genetic syndromes or chromosomal abnormalities is raised by the presence of malformations affecting multiple systems. A careful history from the pregnant patient asking about consanguinity and the documentation of a family history (pedigree) is important.[25] Rates of genetic syndromes or chromosomal abnormalities are significant in cases of fetal megacystis and should prompt consideration of genetic counseling and evaluation.

Ultrasound finding of megacystis can represent a broad range of genetic syndromes. A recent retrospective multicenter study from the Netherlands of 541 pregnancies with fetal megacystis found an incidence of 9% of genetic abnormalities. Among these, 40 chromosomal abnormalities were diagnosed: trisomy 18 ($n = 24$), trisomy 21 ($n = 5$), monosomy X (Turner syndrome) ($n = 5$), trisomy 13 ($n = 3$), and 22q11 deletion ($n = 3$). Fetal macrosomia was detected in six cases and an "overgrowth syndrome" was suspected or detected in four cases, comprising two infants with Beckwith-Wiedemann syndrome (associated with bladder polyps or urethral valves) and two with Sotos syndrome (usually associated with urethral atresia). Megacystis microcolon intestinal hypoperistalsis syndrome was diagnosed in five (1%) cases and prenatally suspected only in one case.[3] Thus, it is important to appreciate that megacystis may also be present as a concomitant finding in miscellaneous genetic syndromes, developmental anomalies, and chromosomal abnormalities.

Genetic testing is also important in differentiating between some of the more severe etiologies of LUTO. Prune belly syndrome is a relatively rare congenital anomaly sequence characterized by severe megacystis, hydronephrosis, deficient abdominal wall musculature, and bilateral undescended testes (in males).[26] A high prevalence of nonurologic anomalies (up to 70%) are noted, and prune belly syndrome may be associated with both chromosomal abnormalities and single-gene abnormalities (*ACTA2* gene modification). Megacystis microcolon intestinal hypoperistalsis syndrome (MMIHS) almost exclusively affects female fetuses and is characterized by prenatal ultrasound dilation of both the distal bowel and bladder, with a primary abnormality of the smooth musculature. The genetic basis of MMIHS has been ascribed to a number of different mutations with a variety of inheritance patterns including: ACTG2 (a dominantly inherited variant present in a third of MMIHS cases), and MYH11, MYL9, MYLK and LMOD1 variants (relatively rare and autosomal recessively inherited).[27–29] The prognosis of both prune belly syndrome and MMIHS are very poor. Additionally, MMIHS, although usually lethal, is rarely associated with significant renal impairment, and thus any form of prenatal bladder drainage would be inappropriate.[30] Thus discriminating MMIHS and prune belly syndrome from LUTO remains crucial both to better prognosticate outcomes for families and to determine whether fetal intervention is warranted. Therefore, when diagnostic concern for either of these conditions is raised, prompt referral to genetic counseling and testing should be considered.

Antenatal Predictors of Postnatal Renal Function

This section aims to outline the current evidence supporting the prenatal assessment of fetal renal function and demonstrate how this may improve the accuracy of prenatal diagnosis to assist genetic counseling for parents and best identify fetuses that may benefit most from prenatal intervention.

ULTRASOUND
Bladder Size and Appearance

As noted previously, a bladder with a longitudinal diameter ≥ 7 mm in the third trimester is consistent with a diagnosis of megacystis; however, many of these cases will resolve if the fetal karyotype is normal.[12] The largest cohort study investigating the natural history of fetal megacystis indicated that spontaneous resolution was less likely to occur in fetuses with a longitudinal bladder diameter ≥ 15 mm. Additionally, the study found that such fetuses were more likely to suffer urologic sequelae requiring surgery after birth, particularly if the bladder size had not normalized by 23 weeks of gestation.[13]

Although the appearances of enlarged bladder and a thickened bladder wall are indicative of a diagnosis of LUTO, there are limited data correlating such ultrasonographic appearances with postnatal renal function. A retrospective review of 17 patients looked at ultrasonographic changes in fetuses with known PUV and correlated these to postnatal renal outcome; of these, only two of the eight patients (25%) with mild upper renal tract dilatation, or dilatation limited only to the bladder, had postnatal renal failure.[31] Another study aimed at producing an antenatal staging system for LUTO using a large retrospective multicenter cohort found that the risk of perinatal mortality and severely impaired postnatal renal function was greater with increased bladder volume at diagnosis (with >5.4 cm^3 characterized as severe); this effect was independent of renal appearance.[32] Thus, bladder changes may be predictive of poor postnatal renal outcome, an effect that is strengthened if prenatal renal changes are also observed on ultrasound.

Renal Appearance

Ultrasonographic changes in fetal renal appearance are observed in LUTO and include renal pyelectasis (an increase in the fetal pelvis Antero-posterior (AP) diameter ≥ 7 mm), renal cortical dysplasia (echogenic or thin appearance of renal cortex on ultrasound), or the presence of renal (macro-) cysts. The appearance of such changes can be used to stage the severity of LUTO and assist in decisions regarding the selection of appropriate candidates for intervention.[33] The presence of renal dysplasia, for example, is associated with poor perinatal survival.[33] To date the only systematic review correlating antenatal ultrasonographic features with postnatal renal function found renal cortical appearance to have the best predictive value of poor postnatal renal function with a sensitivity of 0.57 (95% CI 0.37–0.76); specificity 0.84 (95% CI 0.71–0.94), and AUC of 0.78.[34]

The renal parenchymal area (RPA), defined as the area of the kidney in maximal longitudinal length with the renal pelvis subtracted, has been suggested as a prenatal ultrasonographic marker of postnatal renal function.[35] A cohort study of fetuses who had all undergone vesicoamniotic shunting (VAS) intervention following prenatal diagnosis of LUTO found a significant association with static growth of the RPA and postnatal end-stage renal failure at 1 year of age (sensitivity, 0.714; specificity, 0.882; and positive likelihood ratio, 6.071 for RPA of 8 cm^2 in the third trimester).[35]

Cystic appearance of the fetal kidneys on prenatal ultrasound (sensitivity 0.57 and specificity 0.84) and low amniotic fluid (sensitivity 0.63 and specificity 0.76) were predictors of postnatal renal function in a meta-analysis, although studies showed considerable heterogeneity in diagnostic values and reported outcomes.[34]

Other ultrasound technologies are now emerging that may contribute to its interperformer reliability and predictive power. Ultrasound assessment of the fetal kidneys is to a certain extent subjective. Use of gray scale histograms may be an objective method for assessing renal hyperechogenicity[36] and is a promising method for predicting renal function.[37] Fetal renal vascularization has also been examined using three-dimensional power Doppler, with a high vascularization index correlating with postnatal renal impairment[38]; however, such techniques have yet to make their way into routine clinical practice.

Thus, fetal renal appearance and measurements on prenatal ultrasound can guide prognosis and further management of the pregnancy but are most useful when combined with other methods to predict outcome.

Amniotic Fluid Volume

From approximately 16 weeks' gestation, amniotic fluid is largely derived from fetal urination; therefore, the amniotic fluid volume (AFV) can be a valuable prognostic factor in the assessment of LUTO.

The presence of oligohydramnios (deepest vertical pool of amniotic fluid of <2 cm) or anhydramnios (no measurable fluid) prior to 20 weeks' gestation is correlated with pulmonary hypoplasia and fetal or neonatal mortality[39]; however, the role of AFV alone in predicting postnatal renal function remains less certain.

Historically an early prenatal ultrasound diagnosis of LUTO has been associated with worse prognosis. This relationship was due in large part to an association with oligohydramnios and subsequent pulmonary hypoplasia.[40] The presence of adequate amniotic fluid during the canicular phase of lung development between 16 and 24 weeks is important for neonatal survival as babies with pulmonary hypoplasia may die from ventilatory failure irrespective of their renal function.

Data from the North American Fetal Therapy Network highlight the relationship between earlier oligohydramnios and poor outcome. A cohort of 32 fetuses with LUTO and normal midgestational fluid volumes demonstrated 97% survival, and only 32% of babies required renal replacement therapy, indicating a favorable renal prognosis if the AFV is not low by 20 weeks.[11] Similarly, use of a combination of prenatal bladder volume and AFV to stage fetuses with LUTO also demonstrated a positive relationship between babies with normal AFV and good postnatal renal function at

20 weeks' gestation.[32] Those babies categorized as mild (normal AFV at 20 weeks) had a 90% chance of survival with good renal function, whereas those categorized as severe (bladder volume $\geq 5.4 \, cm^3$ and/or oligo- or anhydramnios before 20 weeks) had perinatal survival of 45%, and among survivors severe renal dysfunction requiring dialysis or transplantation in the first year of life was observed in 44%.[32] Hyperechogenic kidneys and reduced amniotic fluid on ultrasound were shown to be the best predictors of poor postnatal renal function in yet another study, resulting in a predictive model that requires external validation.[36] Despite this work, caution is encouraged with respect to AFV, which demonstrated poor sensitivity in univariate analysis in a recent study of 124 LUTO patients in the Netherlands.[14]

MRI

Fetal MRI can provide vital information as an adjunct to ultrasonography in the diagnosis of prenatal conditions, with a well-established clinical usage in the diagnosis of fetal neurologic problems.[41] The three areas where MRI can add value in the assessment of fetal LUTO are the improvement of diagnostic accuracy, the detection of additional abnormalities not detected on ultrasound, and the assessment of renal function.[42]

Functional renal assessment using MRI is becoming more widespread in adults; however, its use in fetal life has yet to be well investigated.[42] Diffusion-weighted imaging measurements can be used to assess direction of fluid flow within the kidney and therefore can provide an indication of glomerular filtration rate. In an MRI study of 11 fetuses with suspected PUV, diffusion-weighted imaging measurements were successfully used to predict the nadir creatinine and estimated glomerular filtration rate at 1 postnatal year of age, although numbers were small and follow-up studies are needed to confirm these findings.[43] Other functional techniques such as blood oxygen level-dependent MRI are on the horizon and have great potential to improve prenatal diagnostic accuracy in the assessment of fetal renal function.[44]

BIOCHEMICAL ANALYTES

Prenatal imaging alone is not able to accurately predict renal function, and therefore invasive sampling techniques may be used as adjuncts. Samples of fetal urine and fetal serum can be obtained in utero and the biochemical profile analyzed to gain more information to help determine which fetuses may have salvageable renal function, and thus will benefit most from in utero therapy.

Urinary Sampling Techniques and Fetal Urinary Analytes

Vesicocenteses (fetal bladder taps) are performed under ultrasound guidance using a 22-gauge spinal needle, with the needle tip inserted into the lower portion of the bladder, ideally avoiding the placenta.[45] The interpretation of the biochemical profile of the first urine specimen should be cautious as this sample will be from stagnant urine and thus is not a true representation of the current renal function. It is recommended that a second and third vesicocentesis should be performed 48 hours after each other and sent for biochemical analysis as they are thought to be more reflective of any renal damage.[46] Serial sampling also allows for examination of the trend in the biochemical profile with decreasing concentrations of electrolytes indicating a better prognosis. This is because renal dysplasia is associated with fewer glomeruli and impaired tubular function, therefore solutes that are normally reabsorbed by the tubules are excreted in higher concentrations in the urine in cases of LUTO.[47] It is important to note that the concentration of fetal urine changes during pregnancy and is more hypotonic by 20–21 weeks as the nephrons mature, thus gestation-specific cutoffs are most accurate.[48]

The most common biochemicals analyzed from fetal urine include sodium, calcium, chloride, and cystatin C, which act as markers of fetal renal tubular function, with an increase in concentration being associated with renal tubular dysfunction or damage.[48] An increased urine osmolality denotes worsening renal function and is also calculated. β_2-Microglobulin is a low-molecular-weight protein that is filtered by the glomeruli, and 99.9% is reabsorbed by the proximal renal tubule; thus higher urinary concentrations are thought to reflect worse tubular or glomerular damage and are thus associated with a worse postnatal outcome.[47] Muller et al. found a β_2-microglobulin level > 2 mg/L had a sensitivity of 80% and specificity of 83% in predicting postnatal renal failure. For reference ranges for β_2-microglobulin, sodium, calcium, ammonia and creatinine, dependent on gestation, see Figure 1.1.[49]

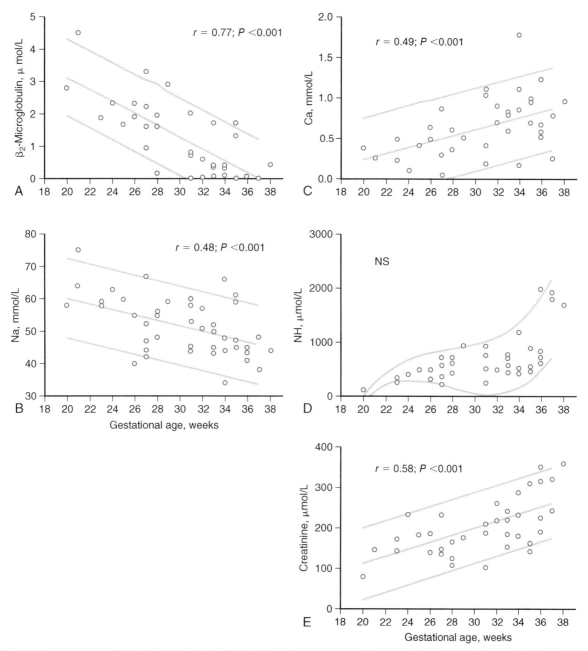

Fig. 1.1 Reference ranges of fetal urine biochemical profile in children whose serum creatinine was <50 μmol/L at 1–2 years; 5th, 50th, and 95th centiles shown. (Adapted from Muller F, Dommergues M, Bussières L, et al. Development of human renal function: reference intervals for 10 biochemical markers in fetal urine. *Clin Chem.* 1996;42(11):1855–1860.)

TABLE 1.2   Pooled Results of Studies With Similar Characteristics Included in Review of Fetal Urinalysis to Predict Poor Postnatal Outcome

Index Test	Threshold	No. of Studies	LR+ (95% CI)	LR− (95% CI)
Sodium	>95th centile	3	4.46 (1.71–11.6)	0.39 (0.17–0.88)
Sodium	>100 mEq/L or 100 mmol/L	3	3.13 (0.78–12.58)	0.37 (0.12–1.12)
Sodium	>100 mg/dL	3	3.33 (1.84–6.02)	0.44 (0.19–1.01)
β_2-microglobulin	>2/2.5 mg/dL	4	3.50 (0.37–33.5)	0.46 (0.19–1.13)
β_2-microglobulin	>10 mg/dL	2	4.61 (0.65–32.68)	0.52 (0.24–1.13)
β_2-microglobulin	>13 mg/dL	3	2.92 (1.28–6.69)	0.53 (0.24–1.17)
Calcium	>95th centile	2	6.65 (0.23–190.96)	0.19 (0.05–0.74)
Calcium > 0.95 mmol/L or > 1.25 mmol/L	>0.95 mmol/L or > 1.25 mmol/L	3	3.44 (1.78–6.65)	0.43 (0.26–0.69)
Osmolality	>200 mOsm/L or >210 mOsm/L	4	3.41 (1.88–6.19)	0.33 (0.14–0.77)
Chloride	>90 mmol/L or >90 mEq/L	3	3.09 (0.57–16.71)	0.46 (0.15–1.42)

CI, confidence interval; *LR+*, pooled positive likelihood ratio; *LR−*, pooled negative likelihood ratio.
From Nicolini U, Spelzini F. Invasive assessment of fetal renal abnormalities: urinalysis, fetal blood sampling and biopsy. *Prenat Diagn*. 2001;21(11):964–969. doi:10.1002/pd.212

A comprehensive systematic review in 2007[48] demonstrated that although sodium, calcium and β_2-microglobulin were correlated with renal function, they have poor diagnostic accuracy (Table 1.2). This may have been related to the interstudy heterogeneity and small sample sizes of the studies included. Follow-up studies have continued to include fetal urinalysis as part of their protocols, although in these studies having a "favorable urinalysis" did not differentiate between survivors and nonsurvivors at 6 months (60% vs. 50%, odds ratio = 2.34 [95% CI 0.35–16.98]).[33]

Fetal Blood Analytes

To obtain more accurate predictors of fetal renal function, fetal serum testing has been investigated. Benefits of serum analysis are the ability to assess glomerular filtration rate and to perform rapid karyotyping and permitting serial assessment of renal function after shunting has been performed.[47] The main focus of fetal serum testing has been β_2-microglobulin, with serum levels ≤ 5.6 mg/L being associated with a more stable postnatal renal function compared with those with a serum level >5.6 mg/L (odds ratio =15.00, 95% CI 0.70–709.89; $P = .1026$, $n = 14$ patients).[50] A Parisian study that performed serial serum measurements of β_2-microglobulin in 42 fetuses with lower or bilateral urinary tract obstruction found that the last serum sample was more predictive of postnatal renal function

than the first sample (sensitivity of first vs. last sample 96.4% vs. 64.3%, $P = .005$), although the specificity was not statistically significantly different (85.7% vs. 78.6%, respectively).[51] When the same researchers compared serum β_2-microglobulin with urine β_2-microglobulin, they found both to be predictive of adverse postnatal outcome but demonstrated little difference in prognostic ability of serum vs. urinary β_2-microglobulin (AUC = 0.908 vs. 0.909, respectively, $P = .96$).[52] Urea, creatinine, and uric acid have a low molecular weight and are able to cross the placenta, thus are influenced by maternal concentrations and are not useful markers in this context.[53]

OTHER PREDICTIVE FACTORS AND MODELING

Staging systems for pathology are useful in clinical practice to counsel families, develop care pathways, consider case selection for fetal therapy, and stratify risk of the full spectrum of important outcomes, for example, ventilatory and renal function at birth as well as survival. Various groups have researched the most clinically relevant variables in relation to prediction of perinatal outcomes. In evaluating these variables and creating staging systems, it is important to consider the interaction between variables and the progression throughout intrauterine life, which may not be evidenced in studies that report a "snapshot" at a particular gestational age.

TABLE 1.3	**Staging of Fetal Lower Urinary Tract Obstruction**			
	Stage 1	**Stage 2**	**Stage 3**	**Stage 4**
Description	Mild LUTO	Moderate to severe LUTO with likely preserved renal function	Severe LUTO with likely abnormal renal function	Severe LUTO with intrauterine renal failure
Amniotic fluid volume	Normal	Oligo- or anhydramnios	Oligo- or anhydramnios	Usually anhydramnios
Renal anatomy	Normal (apart from hydronephrosis)	Hyperechogenic ± bilateral hydronephrosis	Hyperechogenic, possibly cystic and dysplastic	Hyperechogenic and dysplastic with cortical cysts
Fetal urine	Favorable	Favorable	Unfavorable	Unfavorable

LUTO, lower urinary tract obstruction.

Adapted from Ruano R, Sananes N, Wilson C, et al. Fetal lower urinary tract obstruction: proposal for standardized multidisciplinary prenatal management based on disease severity. *Ultrasound Obstet Gynecol*. 2016;48(4):476–482. doi:10.1002/uog.15844

A large multicenter retrospective cohort study examined the time of oligo- or anhydramnios onset in perinatal mortality and postnatal renal function.[32] The best predictor of perinatal mortality for fetuses assessed before 26 weeks was again bladder volume. Therefore, the authors propose that cases of LUTO with bladder volume ≥ 5.4 cm^3 or reduced amniotic fluid before 20 weeks of gestation be defined as severe and those with bladder volume < 5.4 cm^3 where the AFV remains normal at 20 weeks be classed as moderate. Simply put, the larger the bladder, the more severe the obstruction and the higher chance of developing reduced amniotic fluid earlier. In this system, the risk of perinatal mortality in patients with severe LUTO is 55%, and the risk of severely impaired postnatal renal function (defined as estimated glomerular filtration rate <30 mL/min per 1.73 m^2) is 44%. This compares to 26% mortality and 31% severe renal impairment in the moderate group. In mild LUTO (bladder volume < 5.4 cm^3 and normal amniotic fluid up to 26 weeks), these data suggest parents can expect 90% survival with acceptable renal function in over 90%. All cases in this cohort with bladder volume >200 cm^3 and oligohydramnios before 18 weeks of gestation had a poor outcome. Indeed gestational age at the appearance of oligohydramnios alone was a strong predictor of perinatal mortality, with diagnosis of oligohydramnios before 26 weeks having an AUC of 0.95.

Ruano and colleagues have also developed a staging system for LUTO, which combines ultrasound appearance, AFV, and fetal urinalysis (Table 1.3).[33,54] In stage 1 LUTO (the mildest form) there is normal sonographic appearance of the renal parenchyma and AFV and nonconcerning fetal urinalysis. In stage 2 LUTO the kidneys are hyperechogenic and the amniotic fluid volume is reduced, but the fetal urinalysis remains favorable. Stage 3 LUTO is as similar to stage 2 (with perhaps developing renal cysts or dysplasia) and with a concerning fetal urinalysis. Stage 4 is the most severe LUTO, where the kidneys are dysplastic and cystic with lack of corticomedullary differentiation; stage 4 LUTO is associated with anhydramnios and fetal anuria ("intrauterine renal failure," described in next section). This staging system requires further prospective validation and longer-term follow-up of survivors.

To date, there is no single fetal urine- or serum-based prognostic factor able to accurately predict outcome or determine which fetuses would benefit from in utero therapy. This work represents the efforts of multiple groups to combine these factors in a model to improve predictive ability. Although each of these predictive models requires external validation, they represent important next steps in both prediction and counseling.

Prenatal Procedural Therapies

VESICOAMNIOTIC SHUNTING

Interventions to bypass the bladder outlet obstruction for the fetus in utero have been in development since the 1960s and involve two main methods: VAS and fetal cystoscopy and ablation of urethral valves. VAS involves the placement of a pigtail catheter through the mother's abdomen into the fetal bladder (with the distal end freely draining into the amniotic cavity). The only randomized controlled trial comparing prenatal VAS treatment with conservative management for LUTO was closed early due to slow recruitment. However, the VAS group demonstrated a trend toward improved neonatal survival after 28 days,[55] and in a subsequent systematic review VAS has been associated with improved survival with an odds ratio of 2.54 (95% Cl 1.14–5.67).[56]

Investigations are ongoing to determine if appropriately targeted intervention from specialists in fetal medicine and surgery (VAS or serial amnioinfusion; see Chapter 14) may be able alter the natural history of the condition and break the link between gestational age and adverse outcome.

FETAL CYSTOSCOPY AND POSTERIOR URETHRAL VALVE ABLATION

Fetal cystoscopy involves percutaneous in utero insertion of a cystoscope into the fetal bladder, thus allowing for simultaneous diagnostic evaluation of the fetal bladder and urethra and potential treatment with laser or physical disruption of PUVs.[57] A cohort study examining 2-year outcomes found that cystoscopy enhanced the diagnostic accuracy of the underlying causes of LUTO and that survival among fetuses receiving treatment for PUV was 56%, with normal renal function at 2 years of 73% of the surviving cohort.[15]

A multicenter cohort study comparing the efficacy of VAS and fetal cystoscopy for treatment of LUTO observed increased survival in fetuses that underwent treatment (43.8% VAS, 38.2% fetal cystoscopy) compared with the no-treatment group (19.7% survival). Although there were no statistical differences in the survival rates of the two treatment groups, it was suggested that fetuses undergoing cystoscopy and treatment for PUV demonstrated improved postnatal renal function compared with controls. However, this effect was not observed for those fetuses that underwent VAS.[58] The complication rates of both procedures are high: VAS is associated with rupture of membranes, shunt blockage, and shunt displacement in up to 40% of cases,[55] and cystoscopy is associated with fistula

formation.[58] It is also technically difficult to visualize the fetal bladder neck by fetoscopy. Given the complication rates and uncertain outlook for babies undergoing intervention, careful patient selection is vital to justify such procedures. Factors to consider when selecting patients for intervention include underlying etiology, the degree of obstruction, and a careful assessment of fetal renal function based upon renal imaging appearances, amniotic fluid levels, assessment of fetal urinary electrolytes, and the use of models or staging systems to synthesize this information. Precise prognostication in cases of LUTO is also paramount to enable clinicians to improve the accuracy of counseling to parents, thus helping parents in difficult decision making such as when termination of pregnancy is considered.

STAGING FOR PRENATAL PROCEDURAL THERAPIES

Criteria to discriminate LUTO cases amenable to treatment (e.g., PUV) from cases not amenable to treatment (e.g., complex megacystis, urethral atresia) and those likely to resolve without intervention is critical. In 142 cases of early megacystis prior to 17 weeks of gestation, an algorithm comprising normal nuchal translucency, longitudinal bladder diameter > 12 mm, and absence of umbilical cord cyst on ultrasound had a 92% sensitivity and 73% specificity for selecting the cases of isolated PUVs that would be amenable to treatment. The authors propose 12 mm as the optimal cutoff for longitudinal bladder diameter, with measurements under this threshold associated with high chance of spontaneous resolution.[13] The z scores for longitudinal bladder diameter have subsequently been published based on 1238 fetal urinary bladder measurements. A z score < 5.2 identified fetuses with PUVs from other subtypes of LUTO with a sensitivity of 74% and specificity of 85%.[59] Enlarged nuchal translucency (>95th centile) was shown to be a better predictor of complex megacystis (with chromosome difference, genetic syndrome, or multiple structural malformations) and not amenable to treatment for PUV than longitudinal bladder diameter with the established 15-mm cutoff. First-trimester identification of an umbilical cord cyst with megacystis is a strong predictor of urethral atresia and therefore is also a poor prognostic sign.

Clinical disease staging and perinatal risk stratification is important in LUTO to enable clinicians to tailor prenatal counseling and offer fetal interventions when appropriate, prior to the development of pulmonary hypoplasia or irreversible renal damage.[60] It is important that such models continue to be refined to improve the prognostic information given to parents and to deliver personalized care that avoids inappropriate invasive therapy.

Intrauterine Renal Failure Concept

Intrauterine renal failure was introduced as a concept by Ruano and colleagues to describe the most severe forms of LUTO where perinatal mortality is high (almost universal) due to pulmonary hypoplasia or need for renal replacement therapy.[61] Reduced bladder refilling and a reduction in liquor even after vesicocentesis demonstrate intrauterine renal failure and are characteristic of those fetuses with the poorest prognosis. In a fetus with renal failure the urine output is so poor that the bladder will not refill in the 48 hours following drainage. Ruano et al. suggested that intrauterine renal failure is predicted by a bladder refilling volume <27% over 2 days. The expected prenatal ultrasound phenotype in renal failure includes kidneys that are cystic and echogenic, lacking corticomedullary differentiation, and a bladder that is distended and thick walled (unless already ruptured).

Conclusion

Once the diagnosis of LUTO is suspected, the use of a variety of imaging modalities should be considered including ultrasound, MRI, and fetal cystoscopy, in combination with genetic testing, to improve diagnostic accuracy and to rule out any underlying severe genetic etiology. In addition, a comprehensive assessment of the fetus should be undertaken to help refine the etiology and prognosis for the fetus and allow individualized counseling for the parents that may include discussion of prenatal intervention in some cases.

The evaluation of antenatal fetal renal function forms a vital part of this process. It is clear that one modality alone is insufficient to accurately assess prenatal renal function; however, a combination of techniques including ultrasound and invasive techniques to sample fetal analytes, together with the use of staging models, appear to offer the best predictive value.

It is hoped that modern imaging techniques, such as the use of functional MRI, may further refine the future ability of clinicians to investigate antenatal fetal renal function and to accurately predict postnatal outcome.

REFERENCES

1. Malin G, Tonks AM, Morris RK, Gardosi J, Kilby MD. Congenital lower urinary tract obstruction: a population-based epidemiological study. *BJOG.* 2012;119(12):1455–1464. doi:10.1111/j.1471-0528.2012.03476.x
2. Anumba DO, Scott JE, Plant ND, Robson SC. Diagnosis and outcome of fetal lower urinary tract obstruction in the northern region of England. *Prenat Diagn.* 2005;25(1):7–13. doi:10.1002/pd.1074
3. Fontanella F, Maggio L, Verheij JBGM, et al. Fetal megacystis: a lot more than LUTO. *Ultrasound Obstet Gynecol.* 2019;53(6): 779–787. doi:10.1002/uog.19182
4. Bard JB, Woolf AS. Nephrogenesis and the development of renal disease. *Nephrol Dial Transplant.* 1992;7(7):563–572. doi:10.1093/ndt/7.7.563
5. Campbell S, Wladimiroff JW, Dewhurst CJ. The antenatal measurement of fetal urine production. *J Obstet Gynaecol Br Commonw.* 1973;80(8):680–686. doi:10.1111/j.1471-0528.1973. tb16049.x
6. Nicolaides KH, Cheng HH, Snijders RJ, Moniz CF. Fetal urine biochemistry in the assessment of obstructive uropathy. *Am J Obstet Gynecol.* 1992;166(3):932–937.
7. Muller F, Dommergues M, Bussieres L, et al. Development of human renal function: reference intervals for 10 biochemical markers in fetal urine. *Clin Chem.* 1996;42(11):1855–1860.
8. Gilbert WM, Brace RA. Amniotic fluid volume and normal flows to and from the amniotic cavity. *Semin Perinatol.* 1993; 17(3):150–157.
9. Gilbert WM, Brace RA. The missing link in amniotic fluid volume regulation: intramembranous absorption. *Obstet Gynecol.* 1989;74(5):748–754.
10. Holmes N, Harrison MR, Baskin LS. Fetal surgery for posterior urethral valves: long-term postnatal outcomes. *Pediatrics.* 2001;108:E7.
11. Johnson MP, Danzer E, Koh J, et al. Natural history of fetal lower urinary tract obstruction with normal amniotic fluid volume at initial diagnosis. *Fetal Diagn Ther.* 2018;44(1):10–17. doi:10.1159/000478011
12. Liao AW, Sebire NJ, Geerts L, Cicero S, Nicolaides KH. Megacystis at 10-14 weeks of gestation: chromosomal defects and outcome according to bladder length. *Ultrasound Obstet Gynecol.* 2003;21(4):338–341. doi:10.1002/uog.81
13. Fontanella F, Duin L, Adama van Scheltema PN, et al. Fetal megacystis: prediction of spontaneous resolution and outcome. *Ultrasound Obstet Gynecol.* 2017;50(4):458–463. doi:10.1002/uog.17422
14. Fontanella F, Duin LK, Adama van Scheltema PN, et al. Prenatal diagnosis of LUTO: improving diagnostic accuracy. *Ultrasound Obstet Gynecol.* 2018;52(6):739–743. doi:10.1002/uog.18990
15. Sananes N, Cruz-Martinez R, Favre R, et al. Two-year outcomes after diagnostic and therapeutic fetal cystoscopy for lower urinary tract obstruction. *Prenat Diagn.* 2016;36(4):297–303. doi:10.1002/pd.4771

16. Chauvin NA, Epelman M, Victoria T, Johnson AM. Complex genitourinary abnormalities on fetal MRI: imaging findings and approach to diagnosis. *AJR Am J Roentgenol.* 2012;199(2): W222–W231. doi:10.2214/AJR.11.7761

17. Werner H, Lopes J, Ribeiro G, et al. Three-dimensional virtual cystoscopy: noninvasive approach for the assessment of urinary tract in fetuses with lower urinary tract obstruction. *Prenat Diagn.* 2017;37(13):1350–1352. doi:10.1002/pd.5188

18. Oliveira EA, Rabelo EA, Pereira AK, et al. Prognostic factors in prenatally-detected posterior urethral valves: a multivariate analysis. *Pediatr Surg Int.* 2002;18(8):662–667.

19. Emerson DS, Felker RE, Brown DL. The sagittal sign—an early second trimester sonographic indicator of fetal gender. *J Ultrasound Med.* 1989;8:293–297.

20. Reece EA, Winn HN, Wan M, Burdine C, Green J, Hobbins JC. Can ultrasonography replace amniocentesis in fetal gender determination during the early second trimester? *Am J Obstet Gynecol.* 1987;156:579–581.

21. Mazza V, Di Monte I, Pati M, et al. Sonographic biometrical range of external genitalia differentiation in the first trimester of pregnancy: analysis of 2593 cases. *Prenat Diagn.* 2004;24:677–684.

22. Efrat Z, Akinfenwa OO, Nicolaides KH. First-trimester determination of fetal gender by ultrasound. *Ultrasound Obstet Gynecol.* 1999;13(5):305–307.

23. Shaw J, Scotchman E, Chandler N, Chitty LS. Preimplantation genetic testing: non-invasive prenatal testing for aneuploidy, copy-number variants and single-gene disorders. *Reproduction.* 2020;160(5):A1–A11. doi:10.1530/REP-19-0591

24. Boghossian NS, Sicko RJ, Kay DM, et al. Rare copy number variants implicated in posterior urethral valves. *Am J Med Genet A.* 2016;170(3):622–633. doi:10.1002/ajmg.a.37493

25. Cheung KW, Morris RK, Kilby MD. Congenital urinary tract obstruction. *Best Pract Res Clin Obstet Gynaecol.* 2019;58:78–92. doi:10.1016/j.bpobgyn.2019.01.003

26. Tonni G, Ida V, Alessandro V, Bonasoni MP. Prune-belly syndrome: case series and review of the literature regarding early prenatal diagnosis, epidemiology, genetic factors, treatment, and prognosis. *Fetal Pediatr Pathol.* 2013;31(1):13–24. doi:10.3109/15513815.2012.659411

27. Tuzovic L, Tang S, Miller RS, et al. New insights into the genetics of fetal megacystis: ACTG2 mutations, encoding γ-2 smooth muscle actin in megacystis microcolon intestinal hypoperistalsis syndrome (Berdon syndrome). *Fetal Diagn Ther.* 2015; 38(4):296–306. doi:10.1159/000381638

28. Gauthier J, Ouled Amar Bencheikh B, Hamdan FF, et al. A homozygous loss-of-function variant in MYH11 in a case with megacystis-microcolon-intestinal hypoperistalsis syndrome. *Eur J Hum Genet.* 2015;23(9):1266–1268. doi:10.1038/ejhg.2014.256

29. Halim D, Wilson MP, Oliver D, et al. Loss of LMOD1 impairs smooth muscle cytocontractility and causes megacystis microcolon intestinal hypoperistalsis syndrome in humans and mice. *Proc Natl Acad Sci U S A.* 2017;114(13):E2739–E2747. doi:10.1073/pnas.1620507114

30. Tuzovic L, Anyane-Yeboa K, Mills A, Glassberg K, Miller R. Megacystis-microcolon-intestinal hypoperistalsis syndrome: case report and review of prenatal ultrasonographic findings. *Fetal Diagn Ther.* 2014;36(1):74–80. doi:10.1159/000357703

31. Hutton KA, Thomas DF, Davies BW. Prenatally detected posterior urethral valves: qualitative assessment of second trimester scans and prediction of outcome. *J Urol.* 1997;158(3 Pt 2): 1022–1025.

32. Fontanella F, van Scheltema PNA, Duin L, et al. Antenatal staging of congenital lower urinary tract obstruction. *Ultrasound Obstet Gynecol.* 2019;53(4):520–524. doi:10.1002/uog.19172

33. Ruano R, Sananes N, Wilson C, et al. Fetal lower urinary tract obstruction: proposal for standardized multidisciplinary prenatal management based on disease severity. *Ultrasound Obstet Gynecol.* 2016;48(4):476–482. doi:10.1002/uog.15844

34. Morris RK, Malin GL, Khan KS, Kilby MD. Antenatal ultrasound to predict postnatal renal function in congenital lower urinary tract obstruction: systematic review of test accuracy. *BJOG.* 2009;116(10):1290–1299. doi:10.1111/j.1471-0528. 2009.02194.x

35. Moscardi PRM, Katsoufis CP, Jahromi M, et al. Prenatal renal parenchymal area as a predictor of early end-stage renal disease in children with vesicoamniotic shunting for lower urinary tract obstruction. *J Pediatr Urol.* 2018;14(4):320.e1-320.e6. doi:10.1016/j.jpurol.2018.07.004

36. Duin LK, Fontanella F, Groen H, et al. Prediction model of postnatal renal function in fetuses with lower urinary tract obstruction (LUTO)—development and internal validation. *Prenat Diagn.* 2019;39(13):1235–1241. doi:10.1002/pd.5573

37. Murata S, Sugiyama N, Maemura K, Otsuki Y. Quantified kidney echogenicity in mice with renal ischemia reperfusion injury: evaluation as a noninvasive biomarker of acute kidney injury. *Med Mol Morphol.* 2017;50(3):161–169.

38. Bernardes LS, Francisco RP, Saada J, et al. Quantitative analysis of renal vascularization in fetuses with urinary tract obstruction by three-dimensional power-Doppler. *Am J Obstet Gynecol.* 2011;205(6):572.e1–7. doi:10.1016/j.ajog.2011.06.063

39. Shipp TD, Bromley B, Pauker S, et al. Outcome of singleton pregnancies with severe oligohydramnios in the second and third trimesters. *Ultrasound Obstet Gynecol.* 1996;7(2):108–113. doi:10.1046/j.1469-0705.1996.07020108.x

40. Hutton KA, Thomas DF, Arthur RJ, Irving HC, Smith SE. Prenatally detected posterior urethral valves: is gestational age at detection a predictor of outcome? *J Urol.* 1994;152(2 Pt 2): 698–701. doi:10.1016/s0022-5347(17)32684-8

41. Griffiths PD, Bradburn M, Campbell MJ, et al. Use of MRI in the diagnosis of fetal brain abnormalities in utero (MERIDIAN): a multicentre, prospective cohort study. *Lancet.* 2017;389(10068): 538–546. doi:10.1016/S0140-6736(16)31723-8

42. Chalouhi GE, Millischer AÉ, Mahallati H, et al. The use of fetal MRI for renal and urogenital tract anomalies. *Prenat Diagn.* 2020;40(1):100–109. doi:10.1002/pd.5610

43. Faure A, Panait N, Panuel M, et al. Predicting postnatal renal function of prenatally detected posterior urethral valves using fetal diffusion-weighted magnetic resonance imaging with apparent diffusion coefficient determination. *Prenat Diagn.* 2017;37(7):666–672. doi:10.1002/pd.5063

44. Avni R, Golani O, Akselrod-Ballin A, et al. MR imaging-derived oxygen-hemoglobin dissociation curves and fetal-placental oxygen-hemoglobin affinities. *Radiology.* 2016;280(1):68–77. doi:10.1148/radiol.2015150721

45. Haeri S. Fetal lower urinary tract obstruction (LUTO): a practical review for providers. *Matern Health Neonatol Perinatol.* 2015;1:26.

46. Johnson MP, Corsi P, Bradfield W, et al. Sequential urinalysis improves evaluation of fetal renal function in obstructive uropathy. *Am J Obstet Gynecol.* 1995;173:59–65.

47. Nicolini U, Spelzini F. Invasive assessment of fetal renal abnormalities: urinalysis, fetal blood sampling and biopsy. *Prenat Diagn.* 2001;21(11):964–969. doi:10.1002/pd.212

48. Morris RK, Quinlan-Jones E, Kilby MD, Khan KS. Systematic review of accuracy of fetal urine analysis to predict poor postnatal renal function in cases of congenital urinary tract obstruction. *Prenat Diagn.* 2007;27(10):900–911.

49. Muller F, Dommergues M, Bussières L, et al. Development of human renal function: reference intervals for 10 biochemical markers in fetal urine. *Clin Chem.* 1996;42(11):1855–1860.

50. Chon AH, de Oliveira GH, Lemley KV, Korst LM, Assaf RD, Chmait RH. Fetal serum β2-microglobulin and postnatal renal function in lower urinary tract obstruction treated with vesicoamniotic shunt. *Fetal Diagn Ther.* 2017;42(1):17–27.

51. Spaggiari E, Faure G, Dreux S, et al. Sequential fetal serum β2-microglobulin to predict postnatal renal function in bilateral or low urinary tract obstruction. *Ultrasound Obstet Gynecol.* 2017;49(5):617–622. doi:10.1002/uog.15968

52. Spaggiari E, Stirnemann JJ, Benedetti S, et al. Comparison of biochemical analysis of fetal serum and fetal urine in the prediction of postnatal renal outcome in lower urinary tract obstruction. *Prenat Diagn.* 2018;38(8):555–560.

53. Nava S, Bocconi L, Zuliani G, Kustermann A, Nicolini U. Aspects of fetal physiology from 18 to 37 weeks' gestation as assessed by blood sampling. *Obstet Gynecol.* 1996;87(6):975–980. doi:10.1016/0029-7844(96)00056-7

54. Ruano R, Dunn T, Braun MC, Angelo JR, Safdar A. Lower urinary tract obstruction: fetal intervention based on prenatal staging. *Pediatr Nephrol.* 2017;32(10):1871–1878.

55. Morris RK, Malin GL, Quinlan-Jones E, et al. Percutaneous vesicoamniotic shunting versus conservative management for fetal lower urinary tract obstruction (PLUTO): a randomised trial. *Lancet.* 2013;382(9903):1496–1506.

56. Saccone G, D'Alessandro P, Escolino M, et al. Antenatal intervention for congenital fetal lower urinary tract obstruction (LUTO): a systematic review and meta-analysis. *J Matern Fetal Neonatal Med.* 2020;33(15):2664–2670. doi:10.1080/14767058.2018.1555704

57. Quintero RA, Johnson MP, Romero R, et al. In-utero percutaneous cystoscopy in the management of fetal lower obstructive uropathy. *Lancet.* 1995;26;346(8974):537–540. doi:10.1016/s0140-6736(95)91381-5

58. Ruano R, Sananes N, Sangi-Haghpeykar H, et al. Fetal intervention for severe lower urinary tract obstruction: a multicenter case-control study comparing fetal cystoscopy with vesicoamniotic shunting. *Ultrasound Obstet Gynecol.* 2015;45(4):452–458. doi:10.1002/uog.14652

59. Fontanella F, Duin LK, Suresh S, Bilardo CM. Z-scores of fetal bladder size for antenatal differential diagnosis between posterior urethral valves and urethral atresia. *Ultrasound Obstet Gynecol.* 2021;58(6):875–881. doi:10.1002/uog.23647

60. Fontanella F, Duin L, Adama van Scheltema PN, et al. Antenatal workup of early megacystis and selection of candidates for fetal therapy. *Fetal Diagn Ther.* 2019;45(3):155–161.

61. Ruano R, Safdar A, Au J, et al. Defining and predicting "intrauterine fetal renal failure" in congenital lower urinary tract obstruction. *Pediatr Nephrol.* 2016;31(4):605–612. doi:10.1007/s00467-015-3246-8

Chapter 2

Assessment of Neonatal Kidney Function

Guido Filler, MD, PhD, and Maria Esther Díaz-González de Ferris, MD, MPH, PhD

Chapter Outline

Background

Two thirds of drugs are eliminated by the kidneys,[1] and their function levels must be taken into account for diagnostic and treatment plans. Kidney function level identifies acute kidney injury (AKI), or chronic kidney disease (CKD) but it cannot be measured directly,[2] so clinicians have to calculate the clearance of a marker (for instance, inulin) over a given time period. A comprehensive review on measuring kidney function is in our extensive book chapter in *Pediatric Nephrology*.[3] Briefly: In the late 1920s, Moller introduced urea clearance as a measure of kidney function and defined it as "the volume of blood that a one minute's excretion of urine suffices to completely clear of urea."[4–7] In the 1930s, investigators searched for a biomarker that would not be reabsorbed or secreted after introduction into the tubules. The ideal glomerular filtration rate (GFR)

marker must be physiologically inert, cleared only by the kidney, freely filtered at the glomerulus, and stable in terms of plasma concentration,[8] without reabsorption or secretion by the tubules. In 1934, Richards introduced inulin because of its high molecular weight and its resistance to enzymes,[9] and its clearance was described by Shannon in 1935.[10] Subsequently, inulin, which is only eliminated by glomerular filtration (without undergoing any tubular absorption or secretion), became the standard for measuring kidney function. Smith introduced the inulin clearance for renal function measurement in 1956, but it is clinically impractical.[11]

Kidney clearance describes the volume of plasma that is completely cleared of a substance by the kidneys per unit of time. The kidney clearance of a substance x (C_x) is calculated as:

$$C_x = U_x \cdot V/P_x$$

where V is the urine flow rate (mL/min), U_x is the urine concentration of the substance x, and P_x is the plasma concentration of substance x. Typically, C_x is expressed in mL/min per 1.73 m² body surface area (BSA).[2] C_x is equal to the GFR only when a substance is freely permeable across the glomerular capillary and not synthesized, transported, or metabolized by the kidney.[12] The only marker that truly fulfills these requirements is inulin,[2,3] but its availability is very limited and prohibitively expensive. Inulin clearance was replaced in the 1970s by exogenous substances such as ⁵¹Cr-ethylenediamine tetraacetic acid (EDTA), ⁹⁹Tc-diethylenetriamine pentaacetic acid (DTPA), ¹²⁵I-iothalamate, and iohexol. Most of these substances are labeled with a radioisotope. Iohexol can be used both hot and cold. Although now serving as the new standard, these methods are impractical for daily clinical use, especially in neonates.

Importantly, GFR only accounts for a fraction of the removal of toxins or drugs from the body, as most toxic substances are highly bound to plasma protein and require tubular secretion rather than glomerular filtration. Homer W. Smith clearly demonstrated that para-aminohippuric (PAH) acid was the most suitable agent for the evaluation of kidney plasma flow and introduced the PAH clearance, which is still used in some centers today.[13] In the past, inulin and PAH clearance studies were performed concurrently. PAH clearance more closely reflects nephron endowment when compared with GFR.[2] Due to the autoregulation of the kidney, GFR can be maintained across a wider range of nephron endowment. Only when the filtration fraction is normal (the ratio of GFR/PAH clearance is ~16%) and there is no hyperfiltration will GFR accurately reflect PAH clearance.[14] Hyperfiltration may result in inappropriately high GFR.[14] Glomerular hyperfiltration can be caused by vasodilation of the afferent arterioles, as in patients with diabetes or after a high-protein meal and/or by efferent arteriolar vasoconstriction owing to activation of the renin-angiotensin-aldosterone system, leading to glomerular hypertension.[15]

We take for granted that kidney function should be indexed to BSA. However, does this make sense when (1) gaining body weight increases BSA, which would automatically increase GFR, and (2) the body fat does not participate in renal clearance? The biological principle of a finite number of nephrons at 36 weeks of gestation and with subsequent slow attrition[16] is not reflected in the life course of GFR. Bird et al. questioned indexing GFR to BSA for some time and proposed to use the extracellular volume (ECV) instead.[17,18] Indexing GFR to ECV reflects this biological principle, whereas GFR indexed to BSA remains the same until young adulthood.[17–19] Peters et al. published a robust formula for the calculation of ECV,[20] but indexing GFR to ECV rather than BSA is rarely utilized.

Nephron Development In Utero

The development of the kidneys and urinary tract is complex as we relive evolution during embryogenesis. Three different embryonic stages are reported and the first two involute: pronephros,[21,22] mesonephros,[22] and metanephros.[23] Each time, arteries, veins, and ureters are formed, which could be the explanation for the high rate of congenital anomalies of the kidney and urinary tract. Importantly, the ureteric bud invades the mass of metanephric mesenchyme, which induces multiple generations of dichotomous branching of the bud and the formation of layers of nephrons at the ureteric bud tips. The majority of the nephrons of the final kidney, the metanephros, form between weeks 20 and 36 of gestation.[24] Previously it was thought that nephrogenesis stops with preterm birth, but a recent study shows that some reduced and altered nephrogenesis continues for a maximum of 4–6 weeks post-delivery but results in abnormal glomeruli.[25]

Urine production occurs at mesonephros and metanephros stages, beginning at approximately 9 weeks of gestational age. The kidneys produce a significant proportion of the amniotic fluid.[26] The fetal metanephros produces dilute urine, which slowly increases from approximately 15 mL/h at 20 weeks of gestation to about 50 mL/h at term.[27] The large volume of hypotonic urine is essential for normal fetal fluid maintenance and amniotic fluid amount.[28]

Only 3% of the cardiac output in fetal lambs (weighing 80–450 g) accounts for the renal blood flow and GFR is low, and the adult lamb has 25% of the cardiac output going to the kidneys.[29] Studies in humans do not exist, but the principle is the same for all mammals. An adult human also distributes 25% of the cardiac output to the kidneys.[29]

Hereditary and In Utero Factors Affecting Nephron Endowment

According to the hyperfiltration theory,[30] the number of functioning nephrons determines kidney function at all life stages.[31] Other factors such as hereditary disease, maternal/congenital conditions, in utero exposures, and prematurity play a significant role in nephron endowment and lifelong renal function.

Nephron endowment is affected by maternal health conditions and even diet. Maternal diabetes has been associated with congenital anomalies of the kidney and urinary tract.[32] Pregnant women with CKD or nephrotic syndrome are at risk to develop maternal (e.g., preeclampsia, AKI, cellulitis, and premature rupture of membranes) and/or neonatal morbidity (e.g., low birth weight, intrauterine growth retardation).[33] Maternal CKD is a risk factor for preterm deliveries or intrauterine growth retardation, especially if the mothers have hypertension.[34] Maternal protein restriction[35] and famine in animal models[36] have also been associated with reduced nephron endowment. Rodent models suggest that maternal obesity may be related to CKD later in life.[37] Also, leptin deficiency impairs kidney development in animal models.[38] In other words, both famine and feast during pregnancy affect the nephron endowment.

In utero exposure to medications such as immunosuppressants (mycophenolate mofetil and cyclosporine), antihypertensives (e.g., angiotensin converting enzyme inhibitors or angiotensin receptor blockers), aminoglycosides, prostaglandin synthetase inhibitors, dexamethasone, furosemide, antiepileptics, Adriamycin], and cyclophosphamide are known to cause fetopathies, kidney dysfunction, or even end-stage kidney disease in the neonate.[39] Substance use during pregnancy such as alcohol,[40] nicotine,[41] and illicit drugs[42] have also been associated with abnormal kidney development.

Multiple risk factors may also affect nephron endowment after birth including prematurity, neonatal sepsis, AKI, drugs, and therapeutic interventions.[43] In a multivariate analysis, Cuzzolin et al. determined that maternal use of nonsteroidal antiinflammatory drugs (NSAIDs) and/or neonatal intubation, respiratory distress syndrome, low Apgar score, and use of NSAIDs were associated with reduced nephron endowment.[43]

Prematurity and Nephrogenesis

The incidence of prematurity has increased and remains the second largest direct cause of child mortality. Premature deliveries occur in 11% of pregnancies.[44] In prematurity, nephrogenesis is incomplete and responsible for adult kidney pathologies.[45] It was believed that the stress of premature delivery induced apoptosis and termination of nephrogenesis,[46] but this may not uphold. In a baboon model, Gubhaju et al. demonstrated modified nephrogenesis after preterm delivery. The glomeruli were abnormal with a cystic Bowman space and shrunken glomerular tuft, especially in the superficial renal cortex, where the latest generation of nephrons would form.[23] Extreme prematurity especially alters nephrogenesis.[47] Metabolic factors complicating preterm birth also have additional consequences for the nephrogenesis. In a baboon model, Callaway et al. demonstrated that hyperglycemia alone has a significant impact on normal nephrogenesis and did not find increased apoptosis in that animal model.[45] In summary, prematurity affects normal nephrogenesis, reduces nephron endowment, and is a risk factor for reduced longevity/abnormal kidney function later in life, sometimes manifesting as early as 11 years of age with CKD and hypertension.[48] Finally, nephron endowment can be reduced with in utero growth.[49]

Adaptation of Renal Function in Infancy in the First Year of Life

When indexed to BSA, GFR remains constant from 18 months to 18 years of age,[2] which is substantially different during the neonatal and infancy periods. During pregnancy and in the first 18 months of life, kidney function undergoes substantial developmental changes from 3% blood flow to 25% blood flow. After birth, there is a delicate balance between vasoconstrictive and vasodilatory renal forces, resulting in ongoing high vascular resistance in renal vessels. The low GFR of the neonate limits the postnatal adaptation of kidney function to endogenous and exogenous stress.[50] Systemic vascular resistance decreases markedly in the first 7 days of life, resulting in a redistribution of blood flow to the kidneys. The low effective renal blood flow and GFR are responsible for altered pharmacokinetics of drugs excreted by the kidney in the neonate,[51] and significant tubular reabsorption in the distal nephron blunts the neonate's ability to excrete an acute saline load.[52] Therefore 5% or 10% dextrose solutions without any sodium or low saline concentrations are utilized in neonates.

The measured GFR[53] and estimated GFR (eGFR)[51] in full-term neonates is 30%–40% of adult values, and it is even lower in preterm neonates when factored for body surface area. Tubular function is also immature. Tubular secretion is immature at birth (even for full-term neonates) and approaches adult values by 7 months of age.[54] Tubular secretion capacity in children and adolescents can exceed that of adults.[54] Tubular reabsorption can be both an active or passive process.[55] In preterm infants (<34 weeks of gestation), the glucose transport system is immature, resulting in tubular glycosuria.[55]

Kidney Function Measurement in Clinical Practice

Kidney function measurement allows AKI recognition, drug dosing, and research, particularly since two-thirds of drugs are cleared by the kidney.[1] Kidney function determines the progression of CKD[56] and predicts outcomes in heart failure.[57,58] Clinicians must be familiar with the methods of assessing kidney function, be aware of the strengths and limitations of the various techniques, and be mindful about technical aspects when using either endogenous or exogenous markers.[2,59] Although exogenous markers can determine the clearance of the substance over time through the kidneys, these have rarely been used in the neonatal period; therefore, we will start with endogenous biomarkers of GFR next.

Endogenous Kidney Function Markers

SERUM CREATININE

Creatinine, 2-imido-5-keto-3-methyl-tetrahydroimidazole, is the internal anhydride of creatine and originates from spontaneous nonenzymatic, nonreversible degradation of creatine and phosphocreatine in the muscle. Approximately 2% of muscle creatine is converted to creatinine daily. Kidney, liver, pancreas, and testes also contribute to creatine synthesis. Creatine is taken up by the muscle against its concentration gradient. In the muscle, the ratio of creatine to phosphocreatine is approximately 1:2. Creatinine in humans under physiological conditions is considered an inert substance with some exceptions. Creatinine has a low molecular weight (113 Daltons), is not protein-bound, is freely filtered at the glomerulus, and is secreted by the tubule.[60]

The history of creatinine is discussed in detail in our recent book chapter in *Pediatric Nephrology*.[3] The most common measurement method is the Jaffe reaction. It has been modified by many investigators over the years, but noncreatinine substances (noncreatinine chromogens) in the serum react in the presence of picric acid, which substantially affects the accuracy, especially bilirubin. Miller and Dubos introduced two bacterial enzymes to decompose creatinine in blood and used the Jaffe reaction to measure total creatinine equivalent before and after the addition of these enzymes.[61,62] These are preferable for neonates, but rarely used due to cost. Unfortunately, creatinine has many limitations:

- **Tubular secretion:** Creatinine is secreted by the tubules and therefore does not even meet the requirements of a GFR marker, especially in CKD.[2,63–65] Secreted creatinine leads to overestimation of GFR in CKD.[66] Tubular secretion of creatinine divided by inulin clearance increases progressively from 0.16 in adult patients with normal GFR to 0.92 in patients with GFR less than 40 mL/min.[67] In addition to secretion, creatinine may undergo reabsorption as well, especially in neonates.[68]

- **Dependency on muscle mass:** As outlined previously, creatinine is formed from creatine, which reflects the muscle mass of the individual. Males have higher muscle mass than females, and children have a lower muscle mass than adults.[69,70] Whereas this is not a major problem in neonates, there still needs to be an adjustment for height and muscle mass.

- **Dependency on nutrition:** Dietary intake of protein also affects GFR. Uncooked meat contains creatine and increasing meat intake increases creatine, thus increasing creatinine production and excretion. Furthermore, the cooking process converts creatine to creatinine, which is easily absorbed and increases serum concentrations of creatinine.[71]

- **Nonrenal clearance:** Extrarenal clearance of creatinine is 1.7 to 2 mL/min by the gastrointestinal tract,[72] which is negligible in a healthy adult with normal GFR, but in a patient with CKD who has a low GFR, this becomes relevant, including neonates.
- **Analytical method:** There used to be considerable variability in the reference range for serum creatinine based on the laboratory method.[73,74] Proficiency testing surveys by the College of American Pathologists demonstrated substantial variability.[75] The traceability of the creatinine measurements to higher-order reference methods (isotope dilution mass spectrometry [IDMS] reference method) improved the accuracy of creatinine measurements.[76] However, creatinine levels are quite low in neonates, sometimes as low as 10 μmol/L. Although both Jaffe and enzymatic creatinine methods have the same limit of detection of 10 μmol/L, the older Jaffe method measures creatinine higher in low levels and has more limitations than the enzymatic method at 20 μmol/L vs. 30 μmol/L.[77] Many neonates may have normal values below 20 μmol/L. Despite IDMS traceability, the original Jaffe method remains influenced by chromogens such as bilirubin, ketones, some proteins, and drugs like cephalosporins.[78,79]
- There are four methods for the measurement of creatinine: Jaffe, compensated Jaffe, enzymatic liquid, and dry chemistry methods. In 2015, Hoste et al. compared 26 routine instruments representing 13 different creatinine methods and found that CKD stage classification differed in 47% of cases. Hoste et al. wrote: "Although most creatinine assays claim to be traceable to the gold standard (ID-GC/MS), large inter-assay differences still exist. The inaccuracy in the lower concentration range is of particular concern and may lead to clinical misinterpretation for CKD staging when the creatinine-based eGFR is used. Further research to improve harmonization between methods is required."[80]
- **Timed urine sampling:** Creatinine clearance determinations involving timed urine collections (i.e., 24-hour creatinine clearance)[81,82] can improve the accuracy of GFR estimation; however, this is impractical and highly inaccurate in neonates.[81]

Small-Molecular-Weight Proteins

Small-molecular-mass proteins such as cystatin C (CysC), beta-trace proteins (BTPs), and β_2-microglobulin (B2M), have been proposed GFR measures since they are almost freely filtered through the normal glomerular basement membrane, are not affected by muscle mass or diet, and are reabsorbed or degraded by proximal tubular cells.[83–85] Of these, CysC is the best studied small-molecular-weight protein and is superior for the detection of mildly impaired GFR as proven in metaanalyses.[86,87] A downside of plasma or serum proteins is the fact that they can be influenced by circumstances in which protein synthesis is increased, as in hyperthyroidism,[88] or decreased, as in prolonged low-protein diets.[89] The clinician must be aware that hyperthyroidism or cachexia can influence the serum or plasma concentration of CysC, BTP, and B2M. Hypertriglyceridemia can also affect CysC.[90] B2M concentrations are associated with inflammation, as it is an acute phase protein.[91] Nonetheless, B2M estimates fetal GFR in unborn children with obstructive uropathy with good results.[92]

CYSTATIN C

CysC is a low-molecular-weight protein (13.3 kDa) produced in all nucleated human cells.[93] It is freely filtered through the glomeruli, and unlike creatinine, is less affected by nonrenal factors.[60,85,93–95] Studies in large patient cohorts confirmed that serum CysC levels are only affected by measured GFR as this low-molecular-weight protein features stable secretion from most human tissues and has no nonrenal elimination.[96] Very large doses of glucocorticoids can increase the production of CysC[97,98] but not low and medium doses of glucocorticoids.[99] The literature about the impact on CysC levels altered by thyroid dysfunction is inconsistent, with one study showing an effect on CysC levels,[100] whereas other studies found no association with thyroid function markers.[101,102]

There are robust reference intervals, albeit somewhat biased to mostly Caucasian European population: 0.75 ± 0.09 mg/L for children aged 4–19 years; 0.74 ± 0.10 mg/L for males and 0.65 ± 0.09 mg/L for females aged 20–59 years, and 0.83 ± 0.10 mg/L for individuals older than 60 years of age.[103] Given the substantial developmental changes of kidney function after birth, much higher CysC values (up to 2.8 mg/L) were found at birth, followed by a rapid postnatal decline, reflecting maturation of kidney function.[104–106] CysC concentrations fall after birth, whereas the eGFR using the Filler formula[107] slowly increases until 18 months of life.[16]

The reciprocal of CysC correlates better with a gold standard GFR measurement than the reciprocal of serum creatinine.[108–110] CysC is independent of body composition.[111–113] Current automated and rapid particle-enhanced immunoturbidimetric and immunonephelometric methods (more precise than the original radioimmuno- or enzyme-linked immunosorbent assays)[114,115] allow for low-cost, rapid-turnaround, and large-scale use of serum CysC as a clinically useful GFR marker.[115]

In a metaanalysis of 46 studies CysC was superior to creatinine in both adults and children for the detection of impaired measured GFR.[116] Pooled data analysis of 3703 individuals compared correlation coefficients between GFR and the reciprocals of serum creatinine and CysC. The correlations for CysC (mean $r = 0.816$ [95% confidence interval: 0.804–0.826]) were significantly better than for creatinine (mean $r = 0.742$ [95% confidence interval: 0.726–0.758]). Receiver operating characteristic plots for a pooled sample of 997 individuals showed a significantly better area under the receiver operating characteristic curve (mean $= 0.926$ [95% confidence interval: 0.892–0.960]) for CysC compared with creatinine (mean $r = 0.837$ [95% confidence interval: 0.796–0.878]). This metaanalysis from 2002 was followed by another metaanalysis of 24 studies (pooled number of participants: 2007), which confirmed the findings.[87]

Moreover, there are certified standardized reference material for CysC,[117] and most commercial suppliers of CysC are now using these certified reference materials for calibration, thereby having a similar worldwide standardization as we have for creatinine with IDMS traceability.[76] When the results of the CKiD study were reanalyzed using PENIA and certified reference materials, this rendered better results.[118]

Unfortunately, CysC is still not widely available in many parts of the world. This is despite the fact that for the best accuracy of estimation of GFR from endogenous biomarkers, a combination of creatinine and CysC is recommended, both for children[118] and adults.[119] There are problems with knowledge translation, although solutions can be found through intense collaboration with the clinical biochemists to implement a cost-effective solution on the existing multianalyzer platform with a turnaround time of 1 hour.[120]

BETA TRACE PROTEIN

BTP is another surrogate marker for estimation of GFR.[121–123] Like CysC, it is a low-molecular-weight protein (molecular weight 20–31 kDa). Representing 3% of the proteins in the cerebrospinal fluid, BTP has traditionally been used as a marker for cerebrospinal fluid leakage[124,125]; however, the isoform in blood is from the coronaries. The availability of serum BTP for the measurement of eGFR is limited.[125–127] Although both brain and serum BTP are composed of an identical amino acid sequence, they vary in molecular size due to differences in oligosaccharide structure and N-glycosylation. Compared with BTP in cerebrospinal fluid, serum and urine BTPs have longer sugar chains and higher sialylation.[128]

BTP as a marker of GFR shares many of the features of CysC.[129] Its use as a GFR marker was first described by Priem et al. in 1999.[130] We have previously described the history, indications, benefits, and limitations of BTP as a marker of GFR.[125] BTP has some advantages over CysC as it does not have a significant relationship with C-reactive protein, it is unaffected by body composition, it adequately reflects GFR during the third trimester, and its concentration is independent of thyroid function.[131] In the pediatric realm, the reciprocal of BTP correlates strongly with both ^{51}Cr EDTA and ^{99}Tc DTPA measurements of kidney function. Unlike CysC, which is strongly positively charged, BTP has an isoelectric point of 5.5 or lower.[132,133] BTP may be a more favorable GFR estimate in pregnancy[134] and in neonates[135] as it does not cross the placenta. Neonatal and pediatric reference intervals have been published,[136] and formulae for eGFR based on BTP have been developed and validated for children[122] and adults.[127] Using both BTP and another endogenous small-molecular-weight protein, B2M, Inker et al. published a study from the CKD-EPI data set, which, unlike creatinine or CysC, did not show any differences due to sex.[137] However, this formula is not applicable to children.[138]

Availability of BTP is limited and costly. There is also no higher-order reference material available to standardize the measurement. There are two main assays available: Cayman Chemicals (an ELISA method) and Siemens Healthcare (a particle-enhanced nephelometric immunoassay using polyclonal rabbit antibodies against human urinary BTP). The techniques and antibodies differ, which may recognize different glycoprotein epitopes and therefore may not bind to all BTP isoforms.

Taken together, CysC and BTP are the most suitable eGFR markers in the neonate for the first 72 hours of life, and arguably up to 1 week of chronological age,[106] as creatinine is not as accurate during this period.[19] Since bilirubin affects Jaffe method for the measurement of creatinine, CysC is also preferred. Whereas the best way to estimate GFR in older children is through a combination of CysC and creatinine, this has not been established in neonates and infants.

Exogenous Methods

There are significant limitations to the inulin clearance, including limited availability and methodological aspects for the quantitation of inulin in the blood and urine samples with substantial inter- and intrapatient variability.[2] However, if inulin clearance is employed, we would recommend a bolus injection of 5000 mg of inulin per 1.73 m^2, with a maximum dose of 5000 mg. Inulin must be infused at a constant rate, over 30 seconds. Extravasation must be avoided, as this would result in an overestimation of GFR. Sampling times must be four or more, with an ideal extension to 240 minutes. For the evaluation, a two-compartmental model (intra- and extravascular volume) using the concentrations at the actual time points must be utilized, ideally with NonMem or other appropriate pharmacokinetic software programs like WinNonLin.[139] It is unclear if any centers are still utilizing inulin clearance. There is only one supplier left in the world who provides it at a high cost. Inulin clearance measurements were gradually replaced by nuclear medicine methods in the 1970s and 1980s. These methods typically involve the injection of a radiolabeled pharmaceutical with features like inulin, although none of them have zero plasma protein binding, which would be essential for pure glomerular filtration measurement.

^{99}Tc DTPA[67] is available worldwide, but requires relatively high doses, especially with concomitant imaging,[140] and has 11.0% plasma protein binding.[141]

^{51}Cr EDTA clearance[142] is widely used in Europe and features tight binding of chromium to pharmaceutical, radiation dose 0.074 MBq/kg to 3.7 MBq/kg. Its plasma protein binding is 12.2%.[141]

^{125}I-iothalamate[143–145] is widely used in the United States and can be combined with dimercaptosuccinic acid or mercaptoacetyltriglycine imaging.[140] It may allow for the simultaneous assessment of extracellular fluid volume and GFR.[146] It can be combined with ^{131}I-hippuran for simultaneous determination of effective renal plasma flow.[146] Unfortunately, there may be up to 38% overestimation when compared with inulin in healthy people.[147] Its plasma protein binding is 9.6%.[144] Montreal Children's Hospital uses it with a subcutaneous injection.[148]

Cold iohexol[149,150] is used in North America and Scandinavia. It does not pose any radiation exposure and has only 2.0% plasma protein binding, and therefore forms the second-best exogenous GFR marker after inulin.[151]

The quantitation of the pharmaceutical through the simple nuclear medicine method of simply counting the disappearance of the isotope counts over time allows for faster and more accurate GFR measurement. Each center will have experience with one method and will have reasons for choosing one method over the other. For instance, at the University Medical Centre Groningen, Netherlands, ^{125}I-iothalamate is used combined with ^{131}I-hippuran for the simultaneous determination of effective renal plasma flow.[146] ^{131}Iodine emits radiation in the form of medium-energy gamma rays and mostly beta particles, whereas ^{125}iodine emits soft gamma radiation with a maximum energy of 35 KeV, so that both isotopes can be identified with different cameras.

COMPARISON OF EXOGENOUS GLOMERULAR FILTRATION RATE METHODS: TECHNICAL ASPECTS

Theoretically, the most attractive exogenous biomarker is iohexol because of its low plasma protein binding and the fact that it can be used without radiolabeling. A higher plasma protein binding will result in a larger proportion of clearance through tubular secretion, leading to the overestimation of GFR. However, iohexol GFR estimates demonstrate considerable scatter in clinical studies.[152] The least bias and the best agreement between inulin clearance and nuclear medicine scans are with ^{51}Cr EDTA, in both transplant and nontransplant pediatric patients.[2,3,140] In a study of 40 pediatric renal transplant patients, the error ranged from +2.2 to +2.8 mL/min per 1.73 m^2 when comparing ^{51}Cr EDTA and inulin clearance, which is an exceptional agreement.[153] Unfortunately, ^{51}Cr EDTA is not available in the United States or Canada.

There are important technical aspects to be considered when employing exogenous methods, which can result in substantial errors. The most important issue is extravasation of the radiopharmaceutical, which results in overestimation of GFR. Nuclear medicine methods should always assess for extravasation by taking a gamma (or beta) camera picture of the injection site.[2,3] Furthermore, sampling is often started too early. Samples must not be drawn before the infused substance reaches equilibrium with the entire extracellular volume, which can be as long as 90 minutes in the nephrotic state.[2,3] Also, many centers do not use a proper nonlinear two-compartmental model but rather just determine the slope of the log-transformed pixel counts of two time point measurements instead of three, making it impossible to reveal altered equilibration of the pharmaceutical between both the intravascular and extravascular compartments.[2] Furthermore, most centers employ a single-shot plasma disappearance method, even though inulin clearance uses timed urine collections. The major disadvantage of plasma clearance is the duration of testing needed to calculate the clearance curve accurately, which can be as long as 8 hours.[154]

GOLD STANDARD MEASURED GLOMERULAR FILTRATION RATE IN NEONATES

Nori Smeets et al. summarized the findings of 944 term neonates based on measured GFR.[53] Smeets' team analyzed 50 studies from 1947 to 2014 that included 1041 measured GFR values from 944 neonates. Of these, individual participant data were available for 367, and the other 577 neonates were represented by 44 aggregated data points. The authors included exogenous GFR markers such as inulin (44% of studies, 28.4% of patients), mannitol (6% of studies, 6.3% of patients), or ^{51}Cr-EDTA (2% of studies, 0.6% of patients), and 48% of studies with 64.7% of patients having creatinine clearance, potentially skewing findings. Most of the studies were small (median number of participants were 8 for inulin, 21 for creatinine clearance, and 11 for

mannitol). The authors included 268 individual or aggregated inulin clearance studies. Their main finding was that measured GFR doubled within the first 5 days of life from 19.6 (95% confidence interval 14.7–24.6) mL/min per 1.73 m^2 to 40.6 (36.7–44.5) mL/min per 1.73 m^2 and then slowly rose to 59.4 (45.9–72.9) mL/min per 1.73 m^2 at 4 weeks of age.

IMPRACTICAL ASPECTS OF EXOGENOUS GLOMULAR FILTRATION RATE MEASUREMENT

Many centers routinely perform annual GFR measurements in their patients with CKD. As stated earlier, inulin clearance became impractical in the 1980s, and nuclear medicine methods or cold iohexol clearance replaced inulin clearance. Noninulin methods to measure GFR have inherent challenges. From the institution's perspective, these are the challenges: Technician and/or nurse need to be trained in the handling of radioisotopes for nuclear medicine scans and equipment and they need proficiency safe disposal of isotopes. Both accurate bookkeeping and a special license to hold and use radioactive isotopes are required. Based on the frequency of the test being administered, the timely delivery of the radioisotope is important, as well as the appropriate usage of the radioisotope before its decay. To ensure that the patient is safe to receive the isotope, there is a need for a pregnancy test for females of reproductive age and documentation of past allergic reactions. From the patient's stance, these are the following drawbacks: the need to be in the hospital for an extended period, large-bore intravenous access for frequent blood draws, intravenous administration of radioisotope, in some instances the need for iodine prior to the procedure.

IMAGING FOR THE MEASUREMENT OF KIDNEY FUNCTION

Imaging, especially when calculating kidney volume z scores, has been proposed as an alternative for the assessment of kidney function.[155] MRI can serve as a tool to assess interstitial fibrosis in kidney allografts.[156] Several authors, especially Abitbol et al., have been using ultrasound-based renal volumes and renal volume z scores for the assessment of kidney function.[157] This may work well for neonates in whom there is no hyperfiltration; however, later in life, there may be glomerular hypertrophy and an increase of the renal cortex, which masks decreased nephron endowment. Renal length z score by ultrasound measurement in children with solitary functioning kidneys does not predict kidney function at 7 years of age (mean follow-up of 5 years).[158] The investigators obtained ultrasound images at 32 weeks, 37 weeks, and 6 months of age. Kidney volume, length, kidney cortex, and medulla thickness were measured and compared between preterm and term babies.[159]

It is difficult to get renal volumes from radiologists. Mostly only kidney length is reported. Kidney length or kidney volume z scores are rarely reported, and the authors are unaware of any center that differentiates the volumes of medulla and cortex. Our group has recently studied the relationship between kidney length and kidney volume z scores and found poor agreement.[160] On the other hand, special CT scans may become a tool for measuring both kidney cortex and kidney medulla blood flow.[161] At this point in time, the role of imaging as a tool for the measurement of kidney function remains to be established.

Neonate-Related Issues of Kidney Function Measurement

Measuring serum creatinine in the first 3 days of life reflects maternal levels in all neonates, regardless of gestational age.[106] The placenta primarily handles creatinine in the fetus, which is transported across the placenta in a bidirectional fashion, mostly by simple diffusion.[162] Transport is passive from mother to fetus across the placenta.[163] Nava et al. obtained fetal blood sampling from 157 fetuses (18–37 weeks of gestation) and 134 mothers and reported that maternal and fetal concentrations of glucose ($r = 0.79$, $P < .001$), urea ($r = 0.96$, $P < .001$), creatinine ($r = 0.83$, $P < .001$), and uric acid ($r = 0.94$, $P < .001$) correlated significantly.[164] Our group has also observed a tight correlation between maternal renal function and the serum creatinine of a neonate for at least 72 hours, which renders creatinine inaccurate in this age group when aiming at precisely assessing renal function.[106] We also have reviewed this topic in detail in a previous publication, and based on this body of evidence, it appears that CysC is a reasonably available biomarker for the assessment of neonatal renal function.[19] CysC[135,158] or

BTP[162] offers more accurate estimates of neonatal kidney function.

Another indirect measure of kidney function in this age group includes renal length by ultrasound images. In the preterm neonate, nephron endowment is compromised,[16] and muscle mass is decreased so the creatinine levels are lower. Full-term healthy neonates will begin to recruit nephrons, and serum creatinine will be reflective of actual levels by day 3 of life. If the neonate was exposed to adverse circumstances in utero, such as maternal malnutrition (as in the Dutch cohort that formed the basis for the Barker hypothesis/thrifty phenotype), and/or medications (i.e., angiotensin-converting enzyme inhibitors), alcohol, and other substances, then the neonate's baseline level of renal function may not be accurate or represent steady-state levels.

If creatinine is used to assess GFR, a constant must be factored into the equation. The constant is dependent on the age of the child. For neonatal serum creatinine–based GFR estimation in clinical care, a new constant for the Schwartz bedside formula (constant * height/serum creatinine ratio) of 0.31 using imperial units or 26.5 using SI units was introduced,[53] thereby replacing the constant of 0.45 from 1987.

Conclusions

Kidney function cannot be assessed directly, and GFR is the best surrogate of renal function. The gold standard for GFR measurement is inulin clearance (ideally combined with simultaneous PAH clearance); however, it is not practical in the clinical setting. There is good agreement with nuclear medicine methods such as ^{99}Tc iohexol, ^{99}Tc DTPA, ^{51}Cr EDTA, iothalamate. Iohexol and iothalamate can also be performed without radiolabeling. In the neonatal setting, these methods have rarely been employed.

Creatinine, albeit a marker afflicted with many technical problems, is the most used endogenous biomarker of kidney function. CysC is a superior biomarker to measure kidney function and can be used even at 1 day of life, but its availability is limited. Currently, the best tool for estimation of GFR is the combination of CysC and creatinine measurements. However, in the immediate postnatal period, only CysC should be used. The role of imaging for the assessment of kidney function requires additional research.

Acknowledgments

We thank our patients and their parents and caregivers for participating in research projects to help optimize the care of children with kidney disease. We thank our families for the patience that was required to prepare this manuscript.

REFERENCES

1. Filler G, Kirpalani A, Urquhart BL. Handling of drugs in children with abnormal renal function. In: Avner ED, Harmon WE, Niaudet P, Yoshikawa N, Emma F, Goldstein S, eds. *Pediatric Nephrology*. Springer Berlin Heidelberg; 2015:1-28.
2. Filler G, Yasin A, Medeiros M. Methods of assessing renal function. *Pediatr Nephrol*. 2014;29(2):183-192.
3. Filler G, Ferris M, Gattineni J. Assessment of kidney function in children, adolescents, and young adults. In: Emma F, Goldstein S, Bagga A, Bates CM, Shroff R, eds. *Pediatric Nephrology*. Springer Berlin Heidelberg; 2021. Available at: https://doi.org/10.1007/978-3-642-27843-3_87-1.
4. Moller E, McIntosh JF, Van Slyke DD. Studies of urea excretion. IV: relationship between urine volume and rate of urea excretion by patients with Bright's disease. *J Clin Invest*. 1928;6(3):485-504.
5. McIntosh JF, Moller E, Van Slyke DD. Studies of urea excretion. III: the influence of body size on urea output. *J Clin Invest*. 1928;6(3):467-483.
6. Moller E, McIntosh JF, Van Slyke DD. Studies of urea excretion. II: relationship between urine volume and the rate of urea excretion by normal adults. *J Clin Invest*. 1928;6(3):427-465.
7. Van Slyke DD, McIntosh JF, Moller E, Hannon RR, Johnston C. Studies of urea excretion: VI. Comparison of the blood urea clearance with certain other measures of renal function. *J Clin Invest*. 1930;8(3):357-374.
8. Filler G, Sharma AP. How to monitor renal function in pediatric solid organ transplant recipients. *Pediatr Transplant*. 2008;12(4):393-401.
9. Richards AN, Westfall BB, Bott PA. Renal excretion of inulin, creatinine and xylose in normal dogs. *Exp Biol Med*. 1934;32(1):73-75.
10. Shannon JA, Smith HW. The excretion of inulin, xylose and urea by normal and phlorizinized man. *J Clin Invest*. 1935;14(4):393-401.
11. Smith HW. *Principles of Renal Physiology*. Oxford University Press; 1956.
12. Filler G, Bökenkamp A, Hofmann W, et al. Cystatin C as a marker of GFR—history, indications, and future research. *Clin Biochem*. 2005;38(1):1-8.
13. Navar LG. The legacy of Homer W. Smith: mechanistic insights into renal physiology. *J Clin Invest*. 2004;114(8):1048-1050.
14. Huang SH, Sharma AP, Yasin A, Lindsay RM, Clark WF, Filler G. Hyperfiltration affects accuracy of creatinine eGFR measurement. *Clin J Am Soc Nephrol*. 2011;6(2):274-280.
15. Bokenkamp A. Kidney function itself, and not cystatin C, is correlated with height and weight. *Kidney Int*. 2005;67(2):777-778; author reply 8-9.
16. Filler G, Bhayana V, Schott C, Diaz-Gonzalez de Ferris ME. How should we assess renal function in neonates and infants? *Acta Paediatr*. 2021;110(3):773-780.
17. Bird NJ, Henderson BL, Lui D, Ballinger JR, Peters AM. Indexing glomerular filtration rate to suit children. *J Nucl Med*. 2003;44(7):1037-1043.
18. Peters AM, Snelling HL, Glass DM, Love S, Bird NJ. Estimated lean body mass is more appropriate than body surface area for scaling glomerular filtration rate and extracellular fluid volume. *Nephron Clin Pract*. 2010;116(1):c75-c80.
19. Filler G, Guerrero-Kanan R, Alvarez-Elias AC. Assessment of glomerular filtration rate in the neonate: is creatinine the best tool? *Curr Opin Pediatr*. 2016;28(2):173-179.
20. Peters AM. The kinetic basis of glomerular filtration rate measurement and new concepts of indexation to body size. *Eur J Nucl Med Mol Imaging*. 2004;31(1):137-149.
21. Peters AM, Snelling HL, Glass DM, Bird NJ. Estimation of lean body mass in children. *Br J Anaesth*. 2011;106(5):719-723.
22. Harrison MR, Golbus MS, Filly RA, et al. Management of the fetus with congenital hydronephrosis. *J Pediatr Surg*. 1982;17(6):728-742.
23. Moritz KM, Wintour EM. Functional development of the meso- and metanephros. *Pediatr Nephrol*. 1999;13(2):171-178.
24. Gubhaju L, Sutherland MR, Horne RS, et al. Assessment of renal functional maturation and injury in preterm neonates during the first month of life. *Am J Physiol Renal Physiol*. 2014;307(2):F149-F158.
25. Moritz KM, Wintour EM, Black MJ, Bertram JF, Caruana G. Factors influencing mammalian kidney development: implications for health in adult life. *Adv Anat Embryol Cell Biol*. 2008;196:1-78.
26. Black MJ, Sutherland MR, Gubhaju L, Kent AL, Dahlstrom JE, Moore L. When birth comes early: effects on nephrogenesis. *Nephrology (Carlton)*. 2013;18(3):180-182.
27. Jahnukainen T, Chen M, Berg U, Celsi G. Antenatal glucocorticoids and renal function after birth. *Semin Neonatol*. 2001;6(4):351-355.
28. Rabinowitz R, Peters MT, Vyas S, Campbell S, Nicolaides KH. Measurement of fetal urine production in normal pregnancy by real-time ultrasonography. *Am J Obstet Gynecol*. 1989;161(5):1264-1266.
29. Gulbis B, Jauniaux E, Jurkovic D, Gervy C, Ooms HA. Biochemical investigation of fetal renal maturation in early pregnancy. *Pediatr Res*. 1996;39(4 Pt 1):731-735.
30. Brenner BM, Lawler EV, Mackenzie HS. The hyperfiltration theory: a paradigm shift in nephrology. *Kidney Int*. 1996;49(6):1774-1777.
31. Bertram JF, Douglas-Denton RN, Diouf B, Hughson MD, Hoy WE. Human nephron number: implications for health and disease. *Pediatr Nephrol*. 2011;26(9):1529-1233.
32. Davis EM, Peck JD, Thompson D, Wild RA, Langlois P. Maternal diabetes and renal agenesis/dysgenesis. *Birth Defects Res A Clin Mol Teratol*. 2010;88(9):722-727.
33. De Castro I, Easterling TR, Bansal N, Jefferson JA. Nephrotic syndrome in pregnancy poses risks with both maternal and fetal complications. *Kidney Int*. 2017;91(6):1464-1472.
34. Bateman BT, Bansil P, Hernandez-Diaz S, Mhyre JM, Callaghan WM, Kuklina EV. Prevalence, trends, and outcomes of chronic hypertension: a nationwide sample of delivery admissions. *Am J Obstet Gynecol*. 2012;206(2):134.e1-8.
35. Fanos V, Puddu M, Reali A, Atzei A, Zaffanello M. Perinatal nutrient restriction reduces nephron endowment increasing

renal morbidity in adulthood: a review. *Early Hum Dev.* 2010;86(suppl 1):37-42.

36. Rabadi MM, Abdulmahdi W, Nesi L, et al. Maternal malnourishment induced upregulation of fetuin-B blunts nephrogenesis in the low birth weight neonate. *Dev Biol.* 2018;443(1):78-91.

37. Glastras SJ, Chen H, Pollock CA, Saad S. Maternal obesity increases the risk of metabolic disease and impacts renal health in offspring. *Biosci Rep.* 2018;38(2).

38. Briffa JF, McAinch AJ, Romano T, Wlodek ME, Hryciw DH. Leptin in pregnancy and development: a contributor to adulthood disease? *Am J Physiol Endocrinol Metab.* 2015;308(5):E335-E350.

39. Schreuder MF, Bueters RR, Huigen MC, Russel FG, Masereeuw R, van den Heuvel LP. Effect of drugs on renal development. *Clin J Am Soc Nephrol.* 2011;6(1):212-217.

40. Gray SP, Cullen-McEwen LA, Bertram JF, Moritz KM. Mechanism of alcohol-induced impairment in renal development: could it be reduced by retinoic acid? *Clin Exp Pharmacol Physiol.* 2012;39(9):807-813.

41. Mao C, Wu J, Xiao D, et al. The effect of fetal and neonatal nicotine exposure on renal development of AT(1) and AT(2) receptors. *Reprod Toxicol.* 2009;27(2):149-154.

42. Hunter ES III, Kotch LE, Cefalo RC, Sadler TW. Effects of cocaine administration during early organogenesis on prenatal development and postnatal growth in mice. *Fundam Appl Toxicol.* 1995;28(2):177-186.

43. Cuzzolin L, Fanos V, Pinna B, et al. Postnatal renal function in preterm newborns: a role of diseases, drugs and therapeutic interventions. *Pediatr Nephrol.* 2006;21(7):931-938.

44. Blencowe H, Cousens S, Oestergaard MZ, et al. National, regional, and worldwide estimates of preterm birth rates in the year 2010 with time trends since 1990 for selected countries: a systematic analysis and implications. *Lancet.* 2012;379(9832):2162-2172.

45. Callaway DA, McGill-Vargas LL, Quinn A, et al. Prematurity disrupts glomeruli development, whereas prematurity and hyperglycemia lead to altered nephron maturation and increased oxidative stress in newborn baboons. *Pediatr Res.* 2018;83(3):702-711.

46. Hargitai B, Szabo V, Hajdu J, et al. Apoptosis in various organs of preterm infants: histopathologic study of lung, kidney, liver, and brain of ventilated infants. *Pediatr Res.* 2001;50(1):110-114.

47. Hinchliffe SA, Sargent PH, Howard CV, Chan YF, van Velzen D. Human intrauterine renal growth expressed in absolute number of glomeruli assessed by the disector method and Cavalieri principle. *Lab Invest.* 1991;64(6):777-784.

48. Vollsaeter M, Halvorsen T, Markestad T, et al. Renal function and blood pressure in 11 year old children born extremely preterm or small for gestational age. *PLoS One.* 2018;13(10):e0205558.

49. Boubred F, Daniel L, Buffat C, et al. The magnitude of nephron number reduction mediates intrauterine growth-restriction-induced long term chronic renal disease in the rat. A comparative study in two experimental models. *J Transl Med.* 2016;14(1):331.

50. Toth-Heyn P, Drukker A, Guignard JP. The stressed neonatal kidney: from pathophysiology to clinical management of neonatal vasomotor nephropathy. *Pediatr Nephrol.* 2000;14(3):227-239.

51. Loebstein R, Koren G. Clinical pharmacology and therapeutic drug monitoring in neonates and children. *Pediatr Rev.* 1998;19(12):423-428.

52. Solhaug MJ, Wallace MR, Granger JP. Role of renal interstitial hydrostatic pressure in the blunted natriuretic response to saline loading in the piglet. *Pediatr Res.* 1990;28(5):460-463.

53. Smeets N, IntHout J, van der Burgh M, Schwartz G, Schreuder MF, de Wildt SN. Maturation of glomerular filtration rate in term-born neonates: an individual participant data meta-analysis. *J Am Soc Nephrol.* 2022;33(7):1277-1292.

54. Arant Jr BS. Developmental patterns of renal functional maturation compared in the human neonate. *J Pediatr.* 1978;92(5):705-712.

55. Jones DP, Chesney RW. Development of tubular function. *Clin Perinatol.* 1992;19(1):33-57.

56. Furth S, Pierce C, Hui WF, et al. Estimating time to end stage renal disease in children with CKD. *Am J Kidney Dis.* 2018.

57. Waldum-Grevbo B. What physicians need to know about renal function in outpatients with heart failure. *Cardiology.* 2015;131(2):130-138.

58. Kurishima C, Masutani S, Kuwata S, et al. Cystatin C and body surface area are major determinants of the ratio of N-terminal pro-brain natriuretic peptide to brain natriuretic peptide levels in children. *J Cardiol.* 2015;66(2):175-180.

59. Filler G, Lee M. Educational review: measurement of GFR in special populations. *Pediatr Nephrol.* 2018;33(11):2037-2046.

60. Schwartz GJ, Furth SL. Glomerular filtration rate measurement and estimation in chronic kidney disease. *Pediatr Nephrol.* 2007;22(11):1839-1848.

61. Miller BF, Dubos R. Studies on the presence of creatinine in human blood. *J Biol Chem.* 1937;121.

62. Dubos R, Miller BF. The production of bacterial enzymes capable of decomposing creatinine. *J Biol Chem.* 1937;121.

63. Shemesh O, Golbetz H, Kriss JP, Myers BD. Limitations of creatinine as a filtration marker in glomerulopathic patients. *Kidney Int.* 1985;28(5):830-838.

64. Shannon JA. The renal excretion of creatinine in man. *J Clin Invest.* 1935;14(4):403-410.

65. Seikaly MG, Browne R, Bajaj G, Arant Jr BS. Limitations to body length/serum creatinine ratio as an estimate of glomerular filtration in children. *Pediatr Nephrol.* 1996;10(6):709-711.

66. Herrera J, Rodriguez-Iturbe B. Stimulation of tubular secretion of creatinine in health and in conditions associated with reduced nephron mass. Evidence for a tubular functional reserve. *Nephrol Dial Transplant.* 1998;13(3):623-629.

67. Ferens WA, Hovde CJ. Escherichia coli O157:H7: animal reservoir and sources of human infection. *Foodborne Pathog Dis.* 2011;8(4):465-487.

68. Berglund F. Urinary excretion patterns for substances with simultaneous secretion and reabsorption by active transport. *Acta Physiol Scand.* 1961;52:276-290.

69. Heymsfield SB, Arteaga C, McManus C, Smith J, Moffitt S. Measurement of muscle mass in humans: validity of the 24-hour urinary creatinine method. *Am J Clin Nutr.* 1983;37(3):478-494.

70. Schwartz GJ, Gauthier B. A simple estimate of glomerular filtration rate in adolescent boys. *J Pediatr.* 1985;106(3):522-526.

71. Narayanan S, Appleton HD. Creatinine: a review. *Clin Chem.* 1980;26(8):1119-1126.

72. Shafi T, Levey AS. Measurement and estimation of residual kidney function in patients on dialysis. *Adv Chronic Kidney Dis.* 2018;25(1):93-104.

73. Horio M, Orita Y. Comparison of Jaffe rate assay and enzymatic method for the measurement of creatinine clearance. *Nihon Jinzo Gakkai Shi.* 1996;38(7):296-299.

74. Arant Jr BS. Estimating glomerular filtration rate in infants. *J Pediatr.* 1984;104(6):890-893.

75. Proficiency testing survey, creatinine. Northfield Il: College of American Pathologists; 1995:29-30.

76. Ceriotti F, Boyd JC, Klein G, et al. Reference intervals for serum creatinine concentrations: assessment of available data for global application. *Clin Chem.* 2008;54(3):559-566.

77. Kume T, Saglam B, Ergon C, Sisman AR. Evaluation and comparison of Abbott Jaffe and enzymatic creatinine methods: could the old method meet the new requirements? *J Clin Lab Anal.* 2018;32(1):e22168.

78. Delanaye P, Cavalier E, Cristol JP, Delanghe JR. Calibration and precision of serum creatinine and plasma cystatin C measurement: impact on the estimation of glomerular filtration rate. *J Nephrol.* 2014;27(5):467-475.

79. Perrone RD, Madias NE, Levey AS. Serum creatinine as an index of renal function: new insights into old concepts. *Clin Chem.* 1992;38(10):1933-1953.

80. Hoste L, Deiteren K, Pottel H, Callewaert N, Martens F. Routine serum creatinine measurements: how well do we perform? *BMC Nephrol.* 2015;16:21.

81. Hellerstein S, Simon SD, Berenbom M, Erwin P, Nickell E. Creatinine excretion rates for renal clearance studies. *Pediatr Nephrol.* 2001;16(8):637-643.

82. Dodge WF, Travis LB, Daeschner CW. Comparison of endogenous creatinine clearance with inulin clearance. *Am J Dis Child.* 1967;113(6):683-692.

83. Jung K, Schulze BD, Sydow K, Pergande M, Precht K, Schreiber G. Diagnostic value of low-molecular mass proteins in serum for the detection of reduced glomerular filtration rate. *J Clin Chem Biochem.* 1987;25(8):499-503.

84. Jung K. Low-molecular-mass proteins in serum and their relationship to the glomerular filtration rate. *Nephron.* 1987; 47(2):160.

85. Filler G, Huang SH, Yasin A. The usefulness of cystatin C and related formulae in pediatrics. *Clin Chem Lab Med.* 2012; 50(12):2081-2091.

86. Dharnidharka VR, Kwon C, Stevens G. Serum cystatin C is superior to serum creatinine as a marker of kidney function: a meta-analysis. *Am J Kidney Dis.* 2002;40(2):221-226.

87. Roos JF, Doust J, Tett SE, Kirkpatrick CM. Diagnostic accuracy of cystatin C compared to serum creatinine for the estimation of renal dysfunction in adults and children—a meta-analysis. *Clin Biochem.* 2007;40(5-6):383-391.

88. Graninger W, Pirich KR, Speiser W, Deutsch E, Waldhausl WK. Effect of thyroid hormones on plasma protein concentrations in man. *J Clin Endocrinol Metab.* 1986;63(2):407-411.

89. Deng D, Yao K, Chu W, et al. Impaired translation initiation activation and reduced protein synthesis in weaned piglets fed a low-protein diet. *J Nutr Biochem.* 2009;20(7):544-552.

90. Witzel SH, Butts K, Filler G. Elevated triglycerides may affect cystatin C recovery. *Clin Biochem.* 2014;47(7-8):676-678.

91. Revillard JP, Vincent C, Clot J, Sany J. beta 2-Microglobulin and beta 2-microglobulin-binding proteins in inflammatory diseases. *Eur J Rheumatol Inflamm.* 1982;5(4):398-405.

92. Spaggiari E, Faure G, Dreux S, et al. Sequential fetal serum beta2-microglobulin to predict postnatal renal function in bilateral or low urinary tract obstruction. *Ultrasound Obstet Gynecol.* 2017;49(5):617-622.

93. Filler G, Bokenkamp A, Hofmann W, Le Bricon T, Martinez-Bru C, Grubb A. Cystatin C as a marker of GFR—history, indications, and future research. *Clin Biochem.* 2005;38(1):1-8.

94. Andersen TB, Eskild-Jensen A, Frokiaer J, Brochner-Mortensen J. Measuring glomerular filtration rate in children; can cystatin C replace established methods? A review. *Pediatr Nephrol.* 2009;24(5):929-941.

95. Bokenkamp A, Herget-Rosenthal S, Bokenkamp R. Cystatin C, kidney function and cardiovascular disease. *Pediatr Nephrol.* 2006;21(9):1223-1230.

96. Grubb AO. Cystatin C—properties and use as diagnostic marker. *Adv Clin Chem.* 2000;35:63-99.

97. Jungers P, Skhiri H, Zingraff J, et al. [Benefits of early nephrological management in chronic renal failure]. *Presse Med.* 1997;26(28):1325-1329.

98. Holden RM, Beseau D, Booth SL, et al. FGF-23 is associated with cardiac troponin T and mortality in hemodialysis patients. *Hemodial Int.* 2012;16(1):53-58.

99. Foster J, Reisman W, Lepage N, Filler G. Influence of commonly used drugs on the accuracy of cystatin C-derived glomerular filtration rate. *Pediatr Nephrol.* 2006;21(2):235-238.

100. Stevens LA, Schmid CH, Greene T, et al. Factors other than glomerular filtration rate affect serum cystatin C levels. *Kidney Int.* 2009;75(6):652-660.

101. Al-Malki N, Heidenheim PA, Filler G, Yasin A, Lindsay RM. Cystatin C levels in functionally anephric patients undergoing dialysis: the effect of different methods and intensities. *Clin J Am Soc Nephrol.* 2009;4(10):1606-1610.

102. Huang SH, Filler G, Yasin A, Lindsay RM. Cystatin C reduction ratio depends on normalized blood liters processed and fluid removal during hemodialysis. *Clin J Am Soc Nephrol.* 2011;6(2):319-325.

103. Galteau MM, Guyon M, Gueguen R, Siest G. Determination of serum cystatin C: biological variation and reference values. *Clin Chem Lab Med.* 2001;39(9):850-857.

104. Fischbach M, Graff V, Terzic J, Bergere V, Oudet M, Hamel G. Impact of age on reference values for serum concentration of cystatin C in children. *Pediatr Nephrol.* 2002;17(2):104-106.

105. Filler GM. The challenges of assessing acute kidney injury in infants. *Kidney Int.* 2011;80(6):567-568.

106. Bariciak E, Yasin A, Harrold J, Walker M, Lepage N, Filler G. Preliminary reference intervals for cystatin C and beta-trace protein in preterm and term neonates. *Clin Biochem.* 2011;44(13):1156-1159.

107. Filler G, Lepage N. Should the Schwartz formula for estimation of GFR be replaced by cystatin C formula? *Pediatr Nephrol.* 2003;18(10):981-985.

108. Bokenkamp A, Domanetzki M, Zinck R, Schumann G, Byrd D, Brodehl J. Cystatin C—a new marker of glomerular filtration rate in children independent of age and height. *Pediatrics.* 1998;101(5):875-881.

109. Filler G, Priem F, Vollmer I, Gellermann J, Jung K. Diagnostic sensitivity of serum cystatin for impaired glomerular filtration rate. *Pediatr Nephrol.* 1999;13(6):501-505.

110. Ylinen EA, Ala-Houhala M, Harmoinen AP, Knip M. Cystatin C as a marker for glomerular filtration rate in pediatric patients. *Pediatr Nephrol.* 1999;13(6):506-509.

111. Bokenkamp A, Domanetzki M, Zinck R, Schumann G, Brodehl J. Reference values for cystatin C serum concentrations in children. *Pediatr Nephrol.* 1998;12(2):125-129.

112. Vinge E, Lindergard B, Nilsson-Ehle P, Grubb A. Relationships among serum cystatin C, serum creatinine, lean tissue mass and glomerular filtration rate in healthy adults. *Scand J Clin Lab Invest.* 1999;59(8):587-592.

113. Sharma AP, Kathiravelu A, Nadarajah R, Yasin A, Filler G. Body mass does not have a clinically relevant effect on cystatin C eGFR in children. *Nephrol Dial Transplant.* 2009;24(2):470-474.

114. Kyhse-Andersen J, Schmidt C, Nordin G, et al. Serum cystatin C, determined by a rapid, automated particle-enhanced turbidimetric method, is a better marker than serum creatinine for glomerular filtration rate. *Clin Chem.* 1994;40(10):1921-1926.

115. Li J, Dunn W, Breaud A, Elliott D, Sokoll LJ, Clarke W. Analytical performance of 4 automated assays for measurement of cystatin C. *Clin Chem.* 2010;56(8):1336-1339.

116. Filler G, Huang SH, Yasin A. The usefulness of cystatin C and related formulae in pediatrics. *Clin Chem Lab Med.* 2012;50(12):2081-2091.

117. Grubb A, Blirup-Jensen S, Lindstrom V, Schmidt C, Althaus H, Zegers I. First certified reference material for cystatin C in human serum ERM-DA471/IFCC. *Clin Chem Lab Med.* 2010;48(11):1619-1621.

118. Schwartz GJ, Schneider MF, Maier PS, et al. Improved equations estimating GFR in children with chronic kidney disease using an immunonephelometric determination of cystatin C. *Kidney Int.* 2012;82(4):445-453.

119. Inker LA, Schmid CH, Tighiouart H, et al. Estimating glomerular filtration rate from serum creatinine and cystatin C. *N Engl J Med.* 2012;367(1):20-29.

120. Ismail OZ, Bhayana V, Kadour M, Lepage N, Gowrishankar M, Filler G. Improving the translation of novel biomarkers to clinical practice: the story of cystatin C implementation in Canada: a professional practice column. *Clin Biochem.* 2017;50(7-8):380-384.

121. Huang SH, Sharma AP, Yasin A, Lindsay RM, Clark WF, Filler G. Hyperfiltration affects accuracy of creatinine eGFR measurement. *Clin J Am Soc Nephrol.* 2011;6(2):274-280.

122. Benlamri A, Nadarajah R, Yasin A, Lepage N, Sharma AP, Filler G. Development of a beta-trace protein based formula for estimation of glomerular filtration rate. *Pediatr Nephrol.* 2010;25(3):485-490.

123. White CA, Akbari A, Doucette S, et al. Estimating GFR using serum beta trace protein: accuracy and validation in kidney transplant and pediatric populations. *Kidney Int.* 2009;76(7):784-791.

124. Hochwald GM, Pepe AJ, Thorbecke GJ. Trace proteins in biological fluids. IV. Physicochemical properties and sites of formation of gamma-trace and beta-trace proteins. *Proc Soc Exp Biol Med.* 1967;124(3):961-966.

125. Filler G, Kusserow C, Lopes L, Kobrzynski M. Beta-trace protein as a marker of GFR—history, indications, and future research. *Clin Biochem.* 2014;47(13-14):1188-1194.

126. Witzel SH, Huang SH, Braam B, Filler G. Estimation of GFR using beta-trace protein in children. *Clin J Am Soc Nephrol.* 2015;10(3):401-409.

127. White CA, Akbari A, Doucette S, et al. A novel equation to estimate glomerular filtration rate using beta-trace protein. *Clin Chem.* 2007;53(11):1965-1968.

128. Hoffmann A, Nimtz M, Conradt HS. Molecular characterization of beta-trace protein in human serum and urine: a potential diagnostic marker for renal diseases. *Glycobiology.* 1997;7(4):499-506.

129. Filler G, Priem F, Lepage N, et al. Beta-trace protein, cystatin C, beta(2)-microglobulin, and creatinine compared for detecting impaired glomerular filtration rates in children. *Clin Chem.* 2002;48(5):729-736.

130. Priem F, Althaus H, Birnbaum M, Sinha P, Conradt HS, Jung K. Beta-trace protein in serum: a new marker of glomerular filtration rate in the creatinine-blind range. *Clin Chem.* 1999;45(4):567-568.

131. Chen HH. beta-trace protein versus cystatin C: which is a better surrogate marker of renal function versus prognostic indicator in cardiovascular diseases? *J Am Coll Cardiol.* 2011;57(7):859-860.

132. Harrington MG, Aebersold R, Martin BM, Merril CR, Hood L. Identification of a brain-specific human cerebrospinal fluid glycoprotein, beta-trace protein. *Appl Theor Electrophor.* 1993;3(5):229-234.

133. Hiraoka A, Seiki K, Oda H, et al. Charge microheterogeneity of the beta-trace proteins (lipocalin-type prostaglandin D synthase) in the cerebrospinal fluid of patients with neurological disorders analyzed by capillary isoelectrofocusing. *Electrophoresis.* 2001;22(16):3433-3437.

134. Akbari A, Lepage N, Keely E, et al. Cystatin-C and beta trace protein as markers of renal function in pregnancy. *BJOG.* 2005;112(5):575-578.

135. Filler G, Grimmer J, Huang SH, Bariciak E. Cystatin C for the assessment of GFR in neonates with congenital renal anomalies. *Nephrol Dial Transplant.* 2012;27(9):3382-3384.

136. Zwiers AJ, Cransberg K, de Rijke YB, et al. Reference ranges for serum beta-trace protein in neonates and children younger than 1 year of age. *Clin Chem Lab Med.* 2014;52(12):1815-1821.

137. Inker LA, Tighiouart H, Coresh J, et al. GFR Estimation using beta-trace protein and beta2-microglobulin in CKD. *Am J Kidney Dis.* 2016;67(1):40-48.

138. Filler G, Alvarez-Elias AC, Westreich KD, Huang SS, Lindsay RM. Can the new CKD-EPI BTP-B2M formula be applied in children? *Pediatr Nephrol.* 2016;31(12):2175-2177.

139. Bokenkamp A, Herget-Rosenthal S. Urinary cystatin C as a marker of GFR? A word of caution. *Pediatr Nephrol.* 2004;19(12):1429.

140. Piepsz A, Colarinha P, Gordon I, et al. Guidelines for glomerular filtration rate determination in children. *Eur J Nucl Med.* 2001;28(3):BP31-BP36.

141. Rehling M, Nielsen LE, Marqversen J. Protein binding of 99Tcm-DTPA compared with other GFR tracers. *Nucl Med Commun.* 2001;22(6):617-623.

142. Hermos CR, Janineh M, Han LL, McAdam AJ. Shiga toxin-producing Escherichia coli in children: diagnosis and clinical manifestations of O157:H7 and non-O157:H7 infection. *J Clin Microbiol.* 2011;49(3):955-959.

143. Barbour GL, Crumb CK, Boyd CM, Reeves RD, Rastogi SP, Patterson RM. Comparison of inulin, iothalamate, and 99mTc-DTPA for measurement of glomerular filtration rate. *J Nucl Med.* 1976;17(4):317-320.

144. Brouhard BH, Travis LB, Cunningham RJ III, Berger M, Carvajal HF. Simultaneous iothalamate, creatinine, and urea clearances in children with renal disease. *Pediatrics.* 1977;59(2):219-223.

145. Bajaj G, Alexander SR, Browne R, Sakarcan A, Seikaly MG. 125Iodine-iothalamate clearance in children. A simple method to measure glomerular filtration. *Pediatr Nephrol.* 1996; 10(1):25-28.

146. Visser FW, Muntinga JH, Dierckx RA, Navis G. Feasibility and impact of the measurement of extracellular fluid volume simultaneous with GFR by 125I-iothalamate. *Clin J Am Soc Nephrol.* 2008;3(5):1308-1315.

147. Odlind B, Hallgren R, Sohtell M, Lindstrom B. Is 125I iothalamate an ideal marker for glomerular filtration? *Kidney Int.* 1985;27(1):9-16.

148. Sharma AK, Mills MS, Grey VL, Drummond KN. Infusion clearance of subcutaneous iothalamate versus standard renal clearance. *Pediatr Nephrol.* 1997;11(6):711-713.

149. Canfield RL, Henderson Jr CR, Cory-Slechta DA, Cox C, Jusko TA, Lanphear BP. Intellectual impairment in children with blood lead concentrations below 10 microg per deciliter. *N Engl J Med.* 2003;348(16):1517-1526.

150. Krutzen E, Back SE, Nilsson-Ehle P. Determination of glomerular filtration rate using iohexol clearance and capillary sampling. *Scand J Clin Lab Invest.* 1990;50(3):279-283.

151. Zhang P, Kim W, Zhou L, et al. Dietary fish oil inhibits antigen-specific murine Th1 cell development by suppression of clonal expansion. *J Nutr.* 2006;136(9):2391-2398.

152. Seegmiller JC, Burns BE, Schinstock CA, Lieske JC, Larson TS. Discordance between iothalamate and iohexol urinary clearances. *Am J Kidney Dis.* 2016;67(1):49-55.

153. Medeiros FS, Sapienza MT, Prado ES, et al. Validation of plasma clearance of 51Cr-EDTA in adult renal transplant recipients: comparison with inulin renal clearance. *Transpl Int.* 2009;22(3):323-331.

154. Bjornstad P, Cherney DZ, Maahs DM. Update on estimation of kidney function in diabetic kidney disease. *Curr Diab Rep.* 2015;15(9):57.

155. DeFreitas MJ, Katsoufis CP, Infante JC, Granda ML, Abitbol CL, Fornoni A. The old becomes new: advances in imaging techniques to assess nephron mass in children. *Pediatr Nephrol.* 2021;36(3):517-525.

156. Beck-Tolly A, Eder M, Beitzke D, et al. Magnetic resonance imaging for evaluation of interstitial fibrosis in kidney allografts. *Transplant Direct.* 2020;6(8):e577.

157. Abitbol CL, Seeherunvong W, Galarza MG, et al. Neonatal kidney size and function in preterm infants: what is a true estimate of glomerular filtration rate? *J Pediatr.* 2014;164(5): 1026-1031.e2.

158. Restrepo JM, Torres-Canchala L, Viafara LM, Agredo MA, Quintero AM, Filler G. Renal length z-score for the detection of dysfunction in children with solitary functioning kidney. *Acta Paediatr.* 2021;110(2):652-658.

159. Li J, Guandalini M, McInnes H, Kandasamy Y, Trnka P, Moritz K. The impact of prematurity on postnatal growth of different renal compartments. *Nephrology (Carlton).* 2020;25(2):116-124.

160. Torres-Canchala L, Rengifo M, Filler G, Arias JC, Ramirez O, Restrepo JM. Low agreement between renal volume and renal length z-scores. *Pediatr Nephrol.* 2020;in press.

161. Filler G, Ramsaroop A, Stein R, et al. Is testosterone detrimental to renal function? *Kidney Int Rep.* 2016;1(4):306-310.

162. Filler G, Lopes L, Harrold J, Bariciak E. beta-trace protein may be a more suitable marker of neonatal renal function. *Clin Nephrol.* 2014;81(4):269-276.

163. Davis BM, Miller RK, Brent RL, Koszalka TR. Materno-fetal transport of creatine in the rat. *Biol Neonate.* 1978;33(1-2):43-54.

164. Nava S, Bocconi L, Zuliani G, Kustermann A, Nicolini U. Aspects of fetal physiology from 18 to 37 weeks' gestation as assessed by blood sampling. *Obstet Gynecol.* 1996;87(6): 975-980.

Chapter 3

Diagnosis and Management of Neonatal Acute Kidney Injury

Natalie Menassa, Anvitha Soundararajan, MBBS, Sidharth Sethi, Mignon Irene McCulloch, MBBCh, FCP(Paeds), FRCPCH(UK), Timothy Bunchman, MD, and Rupesh Raina MD

Chapter Outline

Introduction

Acute kidney injury (AKI) is defined as a decrease in overall kidney function, resulting in reduction of glomerular filtration rate (GFR) and subsequent retention of waste products such as urea. As a result, there is a loss of established electrolyte, acid-base, and fluid balance regulation. AKI is a serious, underrecognized yet common complication that occurs in neonates who receive intensive medical care, and there is a well-documented association with increases in mortality (20%–50%) in the neonate.[1] The loss of vital kidney-mediated compensatory mechanisms prevents critically ill neonates from responding to any number of insults that occur within the prenatal, perinatal, or postnatal periods.

Previously, the characterization of AKI in existing literature was highly variable and lacking in clearly defined standardized practices. This changed upon the publication of defining guidelines set forth by Kidney Disease: Improving Global Outcomes (KDIGO) in 2012, who consider the official definition of AKI to include any one of the following: an increase in serum creatinine (SCr) ≥ 0.3 mg/dL (≥26.5 μmol/L) within 48 hours, increase in SCr to ≥ 1.5 times baseline (known or presumed to have occurred within the prior 7 days), or urine volume < 0.5 mL/kg per hour for 6 hours.[2] The modified neonatal KDIGO criteria is summarized in Table 3.1. Utilization of these criteria have changed perceptions of AKI in the literature, with many newer studies disproving previously held beliefs regarding the reversibility of AKI and challenging the use of renal replacement therapy as the sole gold standard for treatment.[3] As the field of AKI continues to evolve with newly standardized practices, the question of whether these findings can be applied to neonates has remained largely unclear. AKI is one of the most prevalent disease processes that occurs in critically ill neonates, with the reported incidence of AKI in neonatal intensive care unit (NICU) admissions reported to be 56% by Shalaby et al.[4] In this chapter, we aim to present the latest knowledge of the epidemiology, pertinent risk factors, clinical outcomes, assessment, preventative measures, and treatments associated with neonatal AKI.

AKI Stage	SCr Criteria	Urine Output Criteria (Hourly Rate)
0	No change in SCr or SCr rise < 0.3 mg/dL	≥0.5 mL/kg per h
1	SCr rise ≥ 0.3mg/dL rise within 48 h or SCr rise ≥ 1.5–1.9 × baseline SCr[a]	<0.5 mL/kg per h × 6–12 h
2	SCr rise ≥ 2.0–2.9 × baseline SCr[a]	< 0.5 mL/kg per h for >12 h
3	SCr rise ≥ 3 X baseline SCr[a] or SCr ≥ 2.5 mg/dL[b] or kidney support therapy utilization	<0.3 mL/kg per h for ≥24 h or anuria for ≥12 h

TABLE 3.1   Modified Neonatal KDIGO Criteria

AKI, acute kidney injury; *KDIGO*, Kidney Disease: Improving Global Outcomes; *ScR*, serum creatinine.
[a]Reference SCr is the lowest prior SCr measurement.
[b]This is lower than the original KDIGO definition as an SCr of 2.5 mg/dL in neonates suggests a glomerular filtration rate <10 mL/min per 1.73 m².

Epidemiology and Risk Factors

Fetal kidney development begins with formation of the nephron around 5 weeks of gestation, followed by urine production at 9–10 weeks. Passage of urine in the fetal period is essential for lung development and contributes to production and composition of amniotic fluid.[3] Nephrogenesis continues until anywhere from 34 to 36 weeks of gestation, with up to 60% estimated to be completed within the third trimester.[5] Previous literature has found that each additional kilogram of fetal weight produces about 200,000 nephrons, which further demonstrates the detrimental effects of compromised fetal growth.[3] For these reasons, extremely low birth weight (ELBW) (classified as any neonate < 1000 g) is one of the most significant predisposing conditions to developmentally immature kidney formation, AKI, and chronic kidney disease (CKD). The causes of ELBW are multifactorial, but most often go hand in hand with prematurity and low gestational age. Other pertinent risk factors include low APGAR score, intubation, asphyxia, and hypoxia secondary to neonatal respiratory distress syndrome.[6]

In 2017, a large multicenter, multinational observational cohort study known as the AWAKEN study sought to strengthen the findings of multiple smaller-sample, single-center research analyses that associated neonatal AKI with worsened clinical outcomes. In this work, the incidence of AKI among varying gestational age demonstrated a U-shaped distribution, with the highest rates occurring in neonates aged > 36 weeks (37%) and those between 22 and < 29 weeks (48%).

Neonates within the middle group (29–36 weeks' gestation) had a rate of 18%. These data suggest that infants at either extreme of gestational age, due to the various prenatal and perinatal complications associated with each end, are more likely to become critically ill with subsequent organ dysfunction. Common insults to these neonates include respiratory failure, sepsis, necrotizing enterocolitis, and hypoxic ischemic encephalopathy (HIE) in the preterm group and maternal infection, meconium-stained fluid, and HIE in those over 36 weeks.[7]

When evaluating an AKI, the underlying cause may fall within any one of the following categories: prerenal, intrinsic, and postrenal. In a study by Timovska et al. seeking to evaluate the most prevalent of these etiologies in a group of 50 patients, 78.5% were prerenal, 19.5% intrinsic renal, and 2.0% postrenal.[5] Causes of neonatal prerenal AKI are those that compromise the perfusion of kidney parenchyma, most commonly due to hemodynamic instability, poor volume status, shunt-forming congenital heart defects such as patent ductus arteriosus, and ischemic injury. Other neonates who are at risk for prerenal insults are those who require central vascular access for nutrition, medication delivery, and clinical monitoring due to significantly increased risk for renal vein and artery thrombosis.[6] Another mechanism of injury is the vicious cycle created by polyuria that results from functionally immature kidneys that cannot properly concentrate urine. As increased free water losses create a hypovolemic state, subsequent hypotension prevents adequate perfusion and further weakens the ability of the kidneys to effectively compensate for volume losses.

Intrinsic renal injury is a frequent complication of nephrotoxic medication administration, which are often necessary for lifesaving medical treatment. An investigation by Rhone et al. showed 87% of all neonates included in the study were exposed to nephrotoxic medications for 14 days on average.[8] Some of the most common offenders in the prenatal and perinatal period include maternal use of angiotensin-converting enzyme inhibitors, indomethacin for tocolysis, and antenatal steroids used for respiratory maturation. Neonates with infections requiring antibiotics, antivirals, and antifungal medications are also predisposed to intrinsic insults. This is especially true in those administered vancomycin, aminoglycosides, amphotericin, and acyclovir. Nonsteroidal antiinflammatory drugs are another well-known nephrotoxic therapy used for patent ductus arteriosus closure or intraventricular hemorrhage prophylaxis.[9] Sepsis, acquired congenital kidney malformations, and acute tubular necrosis are other processes implicated in intrinsic renal injury. Obstructive uropathy due to lesions such as posterior urethral valves can cause prenatal and postnatal renal injury. Risk factors associated with AKI according to various studies are summarized in Table 3.2.

Clinical Outcomes

Sepsis is one of the most prevalent complications seen in AKI, and there exists a proven significant association in a cross-sectional study by Momtaz et al.[1] Of the 49 neonates with AKI included in this work, there was a mortality rate of 36.7% with sepsis as the most prominent cause of mortality in 30.5% of cases. According to the AWAKEN study, infants with AKI had a fourfold higher independent odds of death and longer hospital length of stay than those without AKI (median 23 days versus 19 days). They also touched on the link between AKI and respiratory complications, such as length of mechanical ventilation and incidence of bronchopulmonary dysplasia. In neonates 29–32 weeks' gestation, AKI was more likely to have poor composite outcomes of moderate to severe bronchopulmonary dysplasia (BPD) compared to infants without BPD.[6]

Advances in research surrounding AKI have shifted the ideas surrounding the mechanism of its disease process. The concept of AKI being a dysfunction of one organ has evolved, and it is now considered to be a systemic pathology with multiorgan involvement. There have been documented associations in AKI with intraventricular hemorrhage and abnormal findings on brain MRI in multiple studies. In addition, AKI that occurs during HIE has been shown to increase the odds of abnormal MRI at 7–10 postnatal days.[3] These data demonstrate the importance of early diagnosis and management of AKI.

Assessment

Consideration should be given to the clinical history and physical examination as crucial components of the assessment of patients with AKI. Assessment of gestational age and prenatal (ultrasounds), maternal (nephrotoxic drug), birth (fetal heart rate monitoring and resuscitation), and postnatal (nephrotoxic medications, hypotension) events should all be included in a thorough clinical history. Vital signs and volume status should be the main focus of the physical examination. Evaluation of serum electrolytes, fluid balance, and body weight is also necessary for a full assessment of the patient. Although this metric may not be as useful in premature newborns, measuring fractional sodium excretion can assist in differentiating prerenal (hypovolemia) from intrinsic (acute tubular necrosis) causes of AKI. Finally, an ultrasound should be performed to assess any potential postrenal (obstruction) causes of AKI.[10]

The ways in which AKI is clinically diagnosed and assessed have been variable between studies. Although the KDIGO guidelines have allowed for significant improvements in classification of AKI, there are complications to consider when applying these criteria to neonates. SCr is known to be the most reliable laboratory measure of GFR due to its resistance to change with variables such as diet and hydration. KDIGO guidelines do not account for the lack of a reliable and consistent baseline SCr in the neonatal period, especially within the first days of life. At this time, SCr levels are known to be elevated due to residual transfer of maternal creatinine through the placenta, which serves as an inaccurate reflection of

TABLE 3.2   Risk Factors Associated With Acute Kidney Injury According to Various Studies

Study	Population	Size	Risk Factors Associated With AKI
Cataldi et al. (2005)[47]	Preterms	172	Low APGAR scores, exposure to ampicillin, ceftazidime, ibuprofen
Cuzzolin et al. (2006)[48]	Preterms	246	Maternal NSAIDs, intubation at birth, low APGAR scores, ibuprofen
Mathur et al. (2006)[49]	Sepsis	200	Lower birth weight, meningitis, DIC, and shock
Koralkar et al. (2011)[50]	VLBW	229	Lower birth weight, gestational age, APGAR scores, UAC
Gadepalli et al. (2011)[51]	Congenital diaphragmatic hernia	68	Lower 5-min Apgar score, AKI correlated with left-sided CDH
Türker et al. (2011)[52]	Newborns	78	PDA, DIC, SNAPPE-II
Viswanathan et al. (2012)[53]	ELBW	472	High mean airway pressures, lower MAP, cefotaxime
Selewski et al. (2013)[54]	Asphyxia therapeutic hypothermia	96	Asystole at the time of birth, clinical seizures before cooling, persistent pulmonary hypertension, elevated gentamicin or vancomycin levels, pressor support, transfusions
Bruel et al. (2013)[55]	<33 weeks	1461	Serum sodium variation, PDA, catecholamine treatment, nosocomial infections, BPD, cerebral lesions, surgery
Bolat et al. (2013)[56]	General NICU	1992	PIH, PPROM, Antenatal steroids, SGA, birthweight < 1500 g, intubation, UVC, ibuprofen therapy for PDA closure, sepsis
Askenazi et al. (2013)[57]	Birth weight >2000 g, gestational age >34 weeks, 5-min Apgar < 7	58	Lower birth weight, male, lower Apgar scores at 5 min, lower cord pH, mechanical ventilation
El-Badawy et al. (2015)[58]	NICU	100	Sepsis, nephrotoxic drug administration, shock
Zhang et al. (2016)[59]	NICU	215	Bacteremia, lower baseline eGFR, maximum sodium concentration
Kriplani et al. (2016)[60]	NICU	80	Younger age, bacteremia, maximum sodium concentration
Bansal et al. (2017)[61]	NICU	1745	Male sex, sepsis
Ghobrial et al. (2018)[62]	NICU	90	History of maternal illness, low body temperature, sepsis, prematurity, and respiratory distress
El-sadek et al. (2019)[63]	NICU	60	Higher plasma cystatin C and lower estimated glomerular filtration rate cystatin
Mazaheri and Rambod (2019)[64]	Preterm	206	Prematurity, low birth weight, low 1- and 5-min Apgar scores, and the need for mechanical ventilation, sepsis
Askenazi et al. (2020)[65]	Extremely low gestational age neonates	923	Lower gestational age, lower birth weight
Mwamanenge et al. (2020)[66]	Critically ill neonates	378	Neonatal sepsis, severe pneumonia, use of gentamicin.
Hamsa et al. (2020)[67]	NICU	163	Hypernatremic dehydration, etc.

AKI, acute kidney injury; *BPD*, bronchopulmonary dysplasia; *CDH*, congenital diaphragmatic hernia; *DIC*, disseminated intravascular coagulation; *eGFR*, estimated glomerular filtration rate; *ELBW*, extremely low birth weight; *MAP*, mean arterial pressure; *NICU*, neonatal intensive care unit; *NSAID*, nonsteroidal antiinflammatory drug; *PDA*, patent ductus arteriosus; *PIH*, pregnancy-induced hypertension; *PPROM*, preterm premature rupture of the membranes; *SGA*, small for gestational age; *SNAPPE-II*, score for neonatal acute physiology and perinatal extension II; *UAC*, umbilical artery catheter; *UVC*, umbilical venous catheter; *VLBW*, very low birth weight.

true intrinsic renal function in the neonate. In patients with sepsis and hemodynamic abnormalities, the innate values of SCr may be even less clear. Another consideration in utilization of SCr is its 42- to 72-hour delay in reflecting kidney dysfunction, at which time 25%–50% of kidney function may have already been compromised.[6]

Urine output is known to serve as a highly sensitive and early indicator of kidney dysfunction, but there are multiple factors that complicate the use of this measure in the neonate. The use of bladder catheterization can pose risks of infection and structural deformation to an already vulnerable patient population. Measuring output via diaper weight is also confounded by presence of stool and evaporation secondary to humidified incubators. Diuretics can invalidate the use of urine output to assess renal function.[4]

Due to these presented limitations in AKI classification criteria, some investigators have advocated for creation of percentile charts that compare renal function across a wide range of existing gestational norms. Accounting for the additional variables that exist within the neonatal patient population, rather than applying the established AKI criteria set for children and adults, may help to improve the accuracy of diagnosis. In addition, clinical imaging with ultrasound is recommended in any neonate that presents with kidney dysfunction to assess for congenital malformation or intrinsic renal defects.

As a result of the difficulties seen in neonatal SCr values, recent studies have explored the use of novel biomarkers to determine if a patient has AKI. There exists a vast array of biomarkers under current analysis, with serum cystatin C and neutrophil gelatinase-associated lipocalin (NGAL) proving themselves to be two of the most favorable. NGAL has been one of the most promising markers presented in the literature thus far, with a study by Sweetman et al. directly comparing its efficacy in diagnosing AKI against previously set KDIGO guidelines. NGAL is found within neutrophils that are released from the renal distal tubules as initial proinflammatory activity begins, which allows it to be an early indicator of kidney injury.[11] An elevation in NGAL also occurs at a significantly earlier time than SCr.[7] An analysis by Demirel et al. revealed that serum cystatin C has shown great potential in ELBW infants, as it was found to have no association

with birth weight, gestational age, or hydration status, in contrast to creatinine, which has a negative correlation with gestational age. In addition, there was no significant association with cystatin C and maternal creatinine, while there was with infant creatinine and maternal creatinine.[12] Other novel biomarkers for detecting early AKI are G1 cell cycle arrest biomarkers. The combination of urinary tissue inhibitor of metalloproteinase 2 and insulin-like growth factor binding protein 7 has been shown to have a sensitivity of 89% and a specificity of 51% for predicting AKI in critically ill neonates.[13] Kidney injury molecule 1 is a transmembrane protein that is upregulated in kidney injury, and elevated levels have been shown to predict AKI as well.[14] More studies will be necessary to evaluate the use of additional biomarkers and their potential for implementation into clinical practice.

Preventative Measures

The first step in management of AKI before creating a medical intervention plan is to understand which patients may or may not be at risk and identifying them early on in their disease course. To better standardize this process and improve predictive abilities, the Renal Angina Index (RAI) was proposed by Basu et al. in 2012 and tested in 2014.[15] This is a scoring system that uses two variables, AKI risk levels and evidence of AKI injury. The two are then multiplied to obtain the final score. Risk-level point designations included 5 points for patients on a ventilator or who had cardiac surgery, 3 points for nephrotoxic drugs or burn injuries, 1 point for trauma or sepsis, and varying scores for high-risk clinical procedures based upon respective risk level. AKI injury points were allotted proportionally based upon set increases in SCr, oliguria, and hemodynamic instability. A score of ≥ 8 would indicate high probability of AKI. The efficacy of RAI has been extensively investigated, with many studies reporting improved accuracy in AKI prediction in comparison to SCr.[16,17] A study by Raina et al. suggests use of biomarkers in conjunction with RAI increases the predictive capabilities.[16]

The STARZ (Sethi, Tibrewal, Agrawal, Raina, waZir) scoring system has been developed specifically for rapidly predicting the risk of AKI in neonates. The STARZ study was a multicenter, national, prospective cohort study performed in 11 centers in India. A multivariable logistic regression technique with stepwise backward elimination method was used, and a "Risk Prediction Scoring" was devised. The STARZ score delineates AKI risk in the first 7 days postadmission and is calculated any time after 12 hours of admission in NICU. According to a validation cohort, The STARZ score predicts the risk of AKI in neonates with a sensitivity, specificity, positive predictive value, negative predictive value, and accuracy of 92.8%, 87.4%, 80.5%, 95.6%, and 89.4%, respectively.[18] Table 3.3 describes the 10 variables considered and the scoring system. Out of 0–100, a value of ≥31.5 indicates a high probability of AKI within 7 days post-NICU admission. Based on the findings from the validation cohort, the following cutoff scores were proposed: less than 31.5 predicts low probability of AKI; less than 59 predicts low probabil-

ity of severe AKI; less than 66 predicts low probability of severe AKI with the need for peritoneal dialysis (PD). The cutoff scores were found to increase with increased AKI severity. However, more studies are still required to validate the cutoff.[18,19]

The use of methylxanthines in pharmacologic management of AKI has proven to successfully aid in prevention of disease progression. Examples of these medications include theophylline and caffeine, which act as adenosine-receptor antagonists. Adenosine exerts its effects on the kidney by mediating preglomerular arteriolar vasoconstriction and postglomerular efferent arteriolar vasodilation. By inhibiting these actions, renal blood flow is effectively preserved.[17] Though theophylline is sparingly used as a first-line agent in the general clinical setting due to its narrow therapeutic index, multiple studies have confirmed its safety within neonates.[17] Prophylactic theophylline, given soon after birth, resulted in better kidney function, according to several independent randomized investigations in infants who had been asphyxiated.[20–23] Dopaminergic agonists such as dopamine and fenoldopam are additional medications that have been investigated for their ability to halt the onset of AKI and enhance renal blood flow.[24–26] Increases in perfusion by use of theophylline allow for increased protection of renal tubules, maintenance of GFR, and other essential kidney functions such as fluid balance and urine output. Additional studies have found that caffeine exposure within the first week of life is associated with lower odds of AKI in ELBW neonates and a lower incidence of AKI in those with necrotizing enterocolitis.[3]

Management

Following an AKI diagnosis, it's crucial to tightly monitor the fluid balance and drugs to decrease the likelihood of complications. Optimizing fluid balance requires meticulous documentation of all fluid input and output along with daily weights. Nephrotoxic medications should be monitored daily and, if possible, discontinued.[27] Infants with volume depletion need volume repletion in addition to maintenance fluids. To maintain urine output (UOP) in newborns with volume overload, diuretics can be utilized.[28] Due to a lack of studies in neonates, no standardized dose

TABLE 3.3 STARZ Scoring Model

Variables		Assigned Score
Age at entry in NICU (h)	<25.5	6
	≥25.5	0
PPV in the delivery room	Yes	7
	No	0
Gestational age (weeks)	<28	7
	≥28	0
Sepsis (during the NICU stay)	Yes	6
	No	0
Significant cardiac disease	Yes	10
	No	0
Urine output[a] (mL/kg per h)	<1.32	7
	≥1.32	0
Serum creatinine[a] (mg/dL)	≥0.98	20
	<0.98	0
Use of nephrotoxic drugs	Yes	11
	No	0
Use of furosemide	Yes	9
	No	0
Use of inotropes	Yes	17
	No	0

[a]First 12 hours postadmission in NICU.
Nephrotoxic drugs included vancomycin or colistin or amphotericin B. Significant cardiac disease included hemodynamically significant patent ductus arteriosus, persistent pulmonary hypertension of the newborn, cardiogenic shock and other congenital heart disease. Inotropes included dopamine or dobutamine or epinephrine or norepinephrine.
NICU, neonatal intensive care unit; *PPV*, positive pressure ventilation; *STARZ*, Sethi, Tibrewal, Agrawal, Raina, waZir.

or definition for diuretic use has been established. Although diuretics may be tried in oliguric neonates, the primary therapy for severe cases of neonatal AKI is currently kidney replacement therapy (KRT).[29]

Indications for KRT in neonates include refractory acidosis, uremia, electrolyte abnormalities, inability to provide adequate nutrition, and fluid overload.[10] The two modalities of KRT commonly utilized in neonates are PD and continuous KRT (CKRT). Since most existing equipment was designed for older children, KRT in neonates is challenging. PD is technically simple, as there is no need for vascular access or an extracorporeal blood circuit. PD is also cost-effective and often used in regions with poor infrastructure.[30–32] For short-term PD, a temporary catheter can be placed. Because solute and fluid elimination are gradual, PD has been demonstrated to have great cardiovascular tolerance.[33,34] Furthermore, the peritoneal surface area–to–body weight ratio is significantly higher in pediatric patients, providing sufficient surface area for dialysis to occur. This is a distinct advantage of PD that is not found in the adult population.[35] Several studies describe successful PD by several different techniques in critically ill neonates as small as 830 g.[36–39] PD is a safer choice for small infants when specialized CKRT equipment, which allows low extracorporeal volumes, is not available. If PD is contraindicated or difficult, CKRT can be performed. CKRT is performed with a hemodialysis catheter placed in a central location and either regional or systemic anticoagulation. In the neonatal population, the extracorporeal circuit volume is

especially important. Frequently, these neonates will need to have the CKRT machine primed with blood if the circuit volume surpasses 10% to 15% of the total blood volume.[40]

In the past few years, CKRT for critically ill neonates has undergone tremendous advancements. Prior to this, adult-designed equipment and filters were used to perform CKRT, and substantial hemodynamic instability limited its use. Smaller filters, like the Prismaflex HF20, have recently been created and can be used to deliver CKRT in neonates. The management of neonatal AKI has been enhanced by the invention of CKRT devices intended exclusively for use in neonates. The first report on the usage of the Cardio-Renal Pediatric Dialysis Emergency Machine (CARPEDIEM) device was published in 2014 by Ronco et al.[41] Since then, comparable devices like the Nidus and the Aquadex have been created with circuit volumes less than half that of other available CKRT circuits.[42,43] These were created especially for neonatal patients to reduce hemodynamic instability and improve the CKRT delivery and tolerance. The challenges and advancements in KRT have been summarized in Table 3.4.

Long-Term Complications

The role that AKI plays in the development of CKD in the neonatal population is unknown. Large longitudinal studies on the same are lacking. Mammen et al. conducted a prospective cohort study to better understand

TABLE 3.4	Challenges and Advancements in Neonatal Kidney Replacement Therapy	
Challenges	**Advancements**
PD	
• Decreased filtration rates and decreased clearance • Mechanical complications (leaks, catheter displacement, and catheter obstruction) • Large delivery systems in comparison with patients • Requires intact peritoneum • Complications: peritonitis, raised intraabdominal pressure	• Tenckhoff catheters allow for higher dialysate flow and reduced mechanical complications • Insertion via laparoscopy for efficient catheter placement (alternatively can be performed via Seldinger technique) • Elimination of catheter dead space can increase efficiency in patients requiring small fill volumes • Automated PD systems allow for precisely measured input and output (e.g., HomeChoice Pro and Fresenius Sleep Safe Harmony device) • Various dialysis regimens to increase efficiency of PD, including acute intermittent PD, continuous PD, tidal PD, and continuous flow PD

TABLE 3.4 Challenges and Advancements in Neonatal Kidney Replacement Therapy—cont'd	
Challenges	**Advancements**
CKRT	
• Immature body temperature control • Difficulties establishing vascular access • Large-caliber catheters for venous catheterization • Hemodynamic instability from large extracorporeal volumes of adult system • Inaccurate control of volumes; can lead to fluid and electrolyte imbalances • Requirement of blood priming (risk of bradykinin release if AN69 membranes are used)	Novel equipment with low circuit volumes that operate at slow blood flow rates with more precise ultrafiltration CARPEDIEM • Can be used for infants 2.5 to 10 kg in size • Can perform both dialysis and hemofiltration • Dialysis/hemofiltration rates ranges from 2.5 to 5.0 mL/min • Blood flow rates range from 5 to 50 mL/min (can reach optimal blood flow rate of 40 mL/min with error, 10%) • Contains filters of different surface areas that can be altered based on the size of the patient • Small solute clearance (25–35 mL/kg per h) • Gravimetric controls for controlled fluid balances • Has a reduced priming volume required (27 mL) and microhemolysis index of 0.7 g of plasma-free hemoglobin released per 100 L of blood • Has automatic feedback system that adjusts flow rates as per the prescribed and actual flow rates, keeping the difference between prescribed and actual flow rate lower than 20 g/day NIDUS • Can be used for infants 800 g to 8 kg in size • Greater control of fluid balances in comparison to conventional modalities • Circuit volume of 4.3 mL; does not require blood priming • Precise fluid removal owing to direct control of the ultrafiltration rate • A single-lumen central venous line can be used for CKRT for up to 24 h Aquadex Flex Flow Machine • Offers a low extracorporeal volume for KRT (33 mL when using the 500-filter set) • Contains a continuous hematocrit sensor, which can regulate fluid removal at prescribed hematocrit limit • Can run continuously for 72 h • Ultrafiltration rates can reach up to 500 mL/h Prismaflex HF20 filter set • Created with polyarylethersulfone membrane (not associated with bradykinin release syndrome) • Low circuit volume (60 mL); does not require blood priming in majority of patients

CARPEDIEM, Cardio-Renal Pediatric Dialysis Emergency Machine; *CKRT*, continuous kidney replacement therapy; *KRT*, kidney replacement therapy; *PD*, peritoneal dialysis.

the long-term renal outcomes of AKI in pediatrics. According to this study, 10% of tertiary-care pediatric intensive care unit patients develop CKD 1–3 years after AKI.[44] However, of the 30 patients with neonatal AKI, 16.6% developed CKD, suggesting that this population may be at higher risk of developing CKD after AKI. Morgan et al. studied 264 neonates undergoing complex cardiac repair to characterize the epidemiology of neonatal cardiac surgery-associated AKI and determine its impact on clinical outcomes. It was deduced that height

was reduced in those with AKI after a 2-year follow-up.[45] Menon et al. performed a retrospective cohort study of children exposed to an aminoglycoside for ≥3 days or ≥3 nephrotoxic medications simultaneously for the development of CKD at 6 months. Residual renal damage was detected in 70% of children medication at the 6-month follow-up visit after their illness. This residual damage was in the form of reduced GFR, hyperfiltration, proteinuria, or hypertension. The mean age of children in this study was 9.3 years.[46]

REFERENCES

1. Momtaz HE, Sabzehei MK, Rasuli B, Torabian S. The main etiologies of acute kidney injury in the newborns hospitalized in the neonatal intensive care unit. *J Clin Neonatol.* 2014;3(2):99.
2. Section 2: AKI definition. *Kidney Int Suppl.* 2012;2(1):19–36.
3. Coleman C, Tambay Perez A, Selewski DT, Steflik HJ. Neonatal acute kidney injury. *Front Pediatr.* 2022;10:389.
4. Jetton JG, Boohaker LJ, Sethi SK, et al. Incidence and outcomes of neonatal acute kidney injury (AWAKEN): a multicentre, multinational, observational cohort study. *Lancet Child Adolesc Health.* 2017;1(3):184–194.
5. Timovska SN, Cekovska S, Tosheska-Trajkovska K. Acute kidney injury in newborns. *PRILOZI.* 2016;36(3):83–89.
6. Branagan A, Costigan CS, Stack M, Slagle C, Molloy EJ. Management of acute kidney injury in extremely low birth weight infants. *Front Pediatr.* 2022;10:867715.
7. Mussap M, Degrandi R, Fravega M, Fanos V. Acute kidney injury in critically ill infants: the role of urine Neutrophil Gelatinase-Associated Lipocalin (NGAL). *J Matern Fetal Neonatal Med.* 2010;23(suppl 3):70–72.
8. Rhone ET, Carmody JB, Swanson JR, Charlton JR. Nephrotoxic medication exposure in very low birth weight infants. *J Matern Fetal Neonatal Med.* 2014;27(14):1485–1490.
9. Fanos V, Antonucci R, Zaffanello M. Ibuprofen and acute kidney injury in the newborn. *Turk J Pediatr.* 2010;52(3):231–238.
10. Selewski DT, Charlton JR, Jetton JG, et al. Neonatal acute kidney injury. *Pediatrics.* 2015;136(2):e463–e473.
11. Sweetman DU, Onwuneme C, Watson WR, et al. Renal function and novel urinary biomarkers in infants with neonatal encephalopathy. *Acta Paediatr.* 2016;105(11):e513–e519.
12. Kandasamy Y, Rudd D. Cystatin C: a more reliable biomarker of renal function in young infants? A longitudinal cohort study. *Acta Paediatr.* 2021;110(4):1341–1345.
13. Chen J, Sun Y, Wang S, et al. The effectiveness of urinary TIMP-2 and IGFBP-7 in predicting acute kidney injury in critically ill neonates. *Pediatr Res.* 2020;87(6):1052–1059.
14. Stojanović VD, Barišić NA, Vučković NM, et al. Urinary kidney injury molecule-1 rapid test predicts acute kidney injury in extremely-low-birth-weight neonates. *Pediatr Res.* 2015;78(4):430–435.
15. Basu RK, Zappitelli M, Brunner L, et al. Derivation and validation of the renal angina index to improve the prediction of acute kidney injury in critically ill children. *Kidney Int.* 2014;85(3):659–667.
16. Raina R, Sethi SK, Mawby I, et al. Re-evaluating renal angina index: an authentic, evidence-based instrument for acute kidney injury assessment: critical appraisal. *Front Pediatr.* 2021;9:682672.
17. Raina A, Pandita A, Harish R, Yachha M, Jamwal A. Treating perinatal asphyxia with theophylline at birth helps to reduce the severity of renal dysfunction in term neonates. *Acta Paediatr.* 2016;105(10):e448–e451.
18. Sethi SK, Raina R, Rana A, et al. Validation of the STARZ neonatal acute kidney injury risk stratification score. *Pediatr Nephrol.* 2022;37(8):1923–1932.
19. Sethi SK, Raina R, Wazir S, et al. STARZ neonatal AKI risk stratification cut-off scores for severe AKI and need for dialysis in neonates. *Kidney Int Rep.* 2022;7(9):2108–2111.
20. Bakr AF. Prophylactic theophylline to prevent renal dysfunction in newborns exposed to perinatal asphyxia—a study in a developing country. *Pediatr Nephrol.* 2005;20(9):1249–1252.
21. Eslami Z, Shajari A, Kheyr AM, et al. Theophylline for prevention of kidney dysfunction in neonates with severe asphyxia. *Iran J Kidney Dis.* 2009;3(4):222–226.
22. Cattarelli D, Spandrio M, Gasparoni A, et al. A randomised, double blind, placebo controlled trial of the effect of theophylline in prevention of vasomotor nephropathy in very preterm neonates with respiratory distress syndrome. *Arch Dis Child Fetal Neonatal Ed.* 2006;91(2):F80–F84.
23. Jenik AG, Cernadas JM, Gorenstein A, et al. A randomized, double-blind, placebo-controlled trial of the effects of prophylactic theophylline on renal function in term neonates with perinatal asphyxia. *Pediatrics.* 2000;105(4):e45.
24. Landoni G, Biondi-Zoccai GG, Tumlin JA, et al. Beneficial impact of fenoldopam in critically ill patients with or at risk for acute renal failure: a meta-analysis of randomized clinical trials. *Am J Kidney Dis.* 2007;49(1):56–68.
25. Kellum JA, M Decker J. Use of dopamine in acute renal failure: a meta-analysis. *Crit Care Med.* 2001;29(8):1526–1531.
26. Bellomo R, Chapman M, Finfer S, Hickling K, Myburgh J. Low-dose dopamine in patients with early renal dysfunction: a placebo-controlled randomised trial. Australian and New Zealand Intensive Care Society (ANZICS) Clinical Trials Group. *Lancet.* 2000;356(9248):2139–2143.
27. Stoops C, Stone S, Evans E, et al. Baby NINJA (Nephrotoxic Injury Negated by Just-in-Time Action): reduction of nephrotoxic medication-associated acute kidney injury in the neonatal intensive care unit. *J Pediatr.* 2019;215:223–228.
28. Mohamed TH, Klamer B, Mahan JD, Spencer JD, Slaughter JL. Diuretic therapy and acute kidney injury in preterm neonates and infants. *Pediatr Nephrol.* 2021;36(12):3981–3991.
29. Starr MC, Charlton JR, Guillet R, et al. Advances in neonatal acute kidney injury. *Pediatrics.* 2021;148(5):1–9.
30. Reznik VM, Randolph G, Collins CM, Peterson BM, Lemire JM, Mendoza SA. Cost analysis of dialysis modalities for pediatric acute renal failure. *Perit Dial Int.* 1993;13(4):311–312.
31. Flynn JT. Choice of dialysis modality for management of pediatric acute renal failure. *Pediatr Nephrol.* 2002;17(1):61–69.
32. George J, Varma S, Kumar S, et al. Comparing continuous venovenous hemodiafiltration and peritoneal dialysis in critically ill patients with acute kidney injury: a pilot study. *Perit Dial Int.* 2011;31(4):422–429.
33. Flynn JT, Kershaw DB, Smoyer WE, et al. Peritoneal dialysis for management of pediatric acute renal failure. *Perit Dial Int.* 2001;21(4):390–394.
34. Golej J, Kitzmueller E, Hermon M, et al. Low-volume peritoneal dialysis in 116 neonatal and paediatric critical care patients. *Eur J Pediatr.* 2002;161(7):385–389.
35. Esperanca MJ, Collins DL. Peritoneal dialysis efficiency in relation to body weight. *J Pediatr Surg.* 1966;1(2):162–169.
36. Harshman LA, Muff-Luett M, Neuberger ML, et al. Peritoneal dialysis in an extremely-low-birth-weight infant with acute kidney injury. *Clin Kidney J.* 2014;7(6):582–585.
37. Alparslan C, Yavascan O, Bal A, et al. The performance of acute peritoneal dialysis treatment in neonatal period. *Ren Fail.* 2012;34(8):1015–1020.
38. Unal S, Bilgin L, Gunduz M, et al. The implementation of neonatal peritoneal dialysis in a clinical setting. *J Matern Fetal Neonatal Med.* 2012;25(10):2111–2114.
39. Yu JE, Park MS, Pai KS. Acute peritoneal dialysis in very low birth weight neonates using a vascular catheter. *Pediatr Nephrol.* 2010;25(2):367–371.

40. Bridges BC, Askenazi DJ, Smith J, Goldstein SL. Pediatric renal replacement therapy in the intensive care unit. *Blood Purif.* 2012;34(2):138–148.

41. Ronco C, Garzotto F, Brendolan A, et al. Continuous renal replacement therapy in neonates and small infants: development and first-in-human use of a miniaturised machine (CARPEDIEM). *Lancet.* 2014;383(9931):1807–1813.

42. Menon S, Broderick J, Munshi R, et al. Kidney support in children using an ultrafiltration device: a multicenter, retrospective study. *Clin J Am Soc Nephrol.* 2019;14(10):1432–1440.

43. Coulthard MG, Crosier J, Griffiths C, et al. Haemodialysing babies weighing< 8 kg with the Newcastle infant dialysis and ultrafiltration system (Nidus): comparison with peritoneal and conventional haemodialysis. *Pediatr Nephrol.* 2014;29:1873–1881.

44. Mammen C, Al Abbas A, Skippen P, et al. Long-term risk of CKD in children surviving episodes of acute kidney injury in the intensive care unit: a prospective cohort study. *Am J Kidney Dis.* 2012;59(4):523–530.

45. Morgan CJ, Zappitelli M, Robertson CM, et al. Risk factors for and outcomes of acute kidney injury in neonates undergoing complex cardiac surgery. *J Pediatr.* 2013;162(1):120–127.

46. Menon S, Kirkendall ES, Nguyen H, Goldstein SL. Acute kidney injury associated with high nephrotoxic medication exposure leads to chronic kidney disease after 6 months. *J Pediatr.* 2014;165(3):522–527.

47. Cataldi L, Leone R, Moretti U, et al. Potential risk factors for the development of acute renal failure in preterm newborn infants: a case-control study. *Arch Dis Child Fetal Neonatal Ed.* 2005;90(6):F514–F519.

48. Cuzzolin L, Fanos V, Pinna B, et al. Postnatal renal function in preterm newborns: a role of diseases, drugs and therapeutic interventions. *Pediatr Nephrol.* 2006;21:931–938.

49. Mathur NB, Agarwal HS, Maria A. Acute renal failure in neonatal sepsis. *Indian J Pediatr.* 2006;73(6):499–502.

50. Koralkar R, Ambalavanan N, Levitan EB, et al. Acute kidney injury reduces survival in very low birth weight infants. *Pediatr Res.* 2011;69(4):354–358.

51. Gadepalli SK, Selewski DT, Drongowski RA, Mychaliska GB. Acute kidney injury in congenital diaphragmatic hernia requiring extracorporeal life support: an insidious problem. *J Pediatr Surg.* 2011;46(4):630–635.

52. Türker G, Özsoy G, Günlemez A, et al. Acute renal failure SNAPPE and mortality. *Pediatr Int.* 2011;53(4):483–488.

53. Viswanathan S, Manyam B, Azhibekov T, Mhanna MJ. Risk factors associated with acute kidney injury in extremely low birth weight (ELBW) infants. *Pediatr Nephrol.* 2012;27:303–311.

54. Selewski DT, Jordan BK, Askenazi DJ, et al. Acute kidney injury in asphyxiated newborns treated with therapeutic hypothermia. *J Pediatr.* 2013;162(4):725–729.

55. Bruel A, Rozé JC, Flamant C, et al. Critical serum creatinine values in very preterm newborns. *PLoS One.* 2013;8(12):e84892.

56. Bolat F, Comert S, Bolat G, et al. Acute kidney injury in a single neonatal intensive care unit in Turkey. *World J Pediatr.* 2013; 9:323–329.

57. Askenazi DJ, Koralkar R, Hundley HE, et al. Fluid overload and mortality are associated with acute kidney injury in sick near-term/term neonate. *Pediatr Nephrol.* 2013;28:661–666.

58. El-Badawy AA, Makar S, Abdel-Razek AR, Abd Elaziz D. Incidence and risk factors of acute kidney injury among the critically ill neonates. *Saudi J Kidney Dis Transpl.* 2015;26(3):549.

59. Zhang Y, XJ, Liu YQ, Zhao RX, Hu T, Zhao FH. Relevant factor analysis of pathogenesis and prognosis of neonatal acute kidney injury. *Prog Mod Biomed.* 2016(24):4698–4701.

60. Kriplani DS, Sethna CB, Leisman DE, Schneider JB. Acute kidney injury in neonates in the PICU. *Pediatr Crit Care Med.* 2016;17(4):e159-e164.

61. Bansal SC, Nimbalkar AS, Kungwani AR, et al. Clinical profile and outcome of newborns with acute kidney injury in a level 3 neonatal unit in Western India. *J Clin Diagn Res.* 2017;11(3):SC01.

62. Ghobrial EE, Elhouchi SZ, Eltatawy SS, Beshara LO. Risk factors associated with acute kidney injury in newborns. *Saudi J Kidney Dis Transpl.* 2018;29(1):81–87.

63. El-Sadek AE, El-Gamasy MA, Behiry EG, et al. Plasma cystatin C versus renal resistive index as early predictors of acute kidney injury in critically ill neonates. *J Pediatr Urol.* 2020;16(2): 206.e1–206.e8.

64. Mazaheri M, Rambod M. Risk factors analysis for acute kidney injury in the newborn infants: predictive strategies. *Iran J Kidney Dis.* 2019;13(5):310–315.

65. Askenazi DJ, Heagerty PJ, Schmicker RH, et al. Prevalence of acute kidney injury (AKI) in extremely low gestational age neonates (ELGAN). *Pediatr Nephrol.* 2020;35:1737–1748.

66. Mwamanenge NA, Assenga E, Furia FF. Acute kidney injury among critically ill neonates in a tertiary hospital in Tanzania; prevalence, risk factors and outcome. *PLoS One.* 2020;15(2): e0229074.

67. Nesargi SV, Prashantha YN, John MA, Iyengar A. Acute kidney injury in sick neonates: a comparative study of diagnostic criteria, assessment of risk factors and outcomes. *J Matern Fetal Neonatal Med.* 2020:1–7.

Chapter 4

Pulmonary Hypoplasia in the Fetus With Oligohydramnios: Causes, Treatment, and Prevention

Khalid Taha, MD, and Douglas G. Matsell, MDCM

Chapter Outline

Introduction

Normal amniotic fluid production and volume are essential for normal fetal development. Oligohydramnios, or low amniotic fluid volume, when severe can impact normal lung development. As the fetal kidneys are the major source of amniotic fluid in the second half of pregnancy, anomalies associated with poor fetal kidney function lead to oligohydramnios, particularly in the second and third trimesters of pregnancy in humans.[1] Congenital anomalies of the kidney and urinary tract represent 20%–30% of all abnormalities identified on prenatal ultrasound imaging.[2,3] They include a wide spectrum of severity from mild, asymptomatic, self-resolving pelvicaliectasis to lethal bilateral renal agenesis. Postnatally congenital anomalies of the kidney and urinary tract are responsible for up to 50% of causes of kidney injury and chronic kidney disease in children and adolescents.[4–6] The more severe forms of kidney anomalies can impair fetal urine output, which often leads to oligohydramnios. Oligohydramnios is associated with pulmonary hypoplasia,[7,8] which is a major cause of morbidity and mortality for neonates and infants with renal anomalies.[9,10] The severity and timing of oligohydramnios contribute to the degree of pulmonary hypoplasia.

Intrauterine mechanical thoracic compression and decreased lung fluid volume due to oligohydramnios are the major mechanisms of developing pulmonary hypoplasia.[9] Cellular and genetic pathways connecting pulmonary hypoplasia and oligohydramnios due to fetal kidney anomalies, although intriguing, are yet to be clarified. In this chapter, the link between congenital kidney anomalies, oligohydramnios, and pulmonary hypoplasia will be explored. First, the normal fetal development of the kidneys and lungs will be discussed. In addition, the causes and consequences of kidney anomalies, oligohydramnios, and pulmonary hypoplasia will be defined. Finally, the current available preventative interventions and treatments of pulmonary hypoplasia will be reviewed. Although this chapter will focus on the cause, treatment, and prevention of pulmonary hypoplasia, it will lend the perspective of a pediatric nephrologist.

The Link Between Kidney and Lung Development

To understand the pathogenesis of oligohydramnios and subsequent pulmonary hypoplasia, it is helpful to review the normal development of the kidneys and lungs. These will be compared with reference to the embryologic timelines, similarities in branching morphogenesis, and potentially shared genetic pathways.

KIDNEY DEVELOPMENT

Human fetal kidneys arise sequentially from the embryonic mesoderm and nephrogenic cord over three distinct stages of overlapping rostral-to-caudal systems: the pronephros, mesonephros, and metanephros. The earliest pronephric ducts are nonfunctional vestigial ducts that form at the cervical region of the nephrogenic cord, appearing at the beginning of the fourth week of gestation then regressing by the end of the same week. In the next stage, the mesonephros emerges in the fourth week of gestation, arising from the upper thoracic to upper lumbar segments of the nephrogenic cord. The mesonephros and mesonephric ducts differentiate in a rostral-to-caudal fashion, developing early renal corpuscles that include a glomerulus, tubules, and collecting ducts. These early nephrons excrete small amounts of "urine" into the amnion during the second month of gestation. However, by the end of the second month of gestation, the majority of the mesonephros degenerates. In males, select structures persist and develop into parts of the reproductive system.[11,12] The final stage, the metanephros, becomes the definitive mammalian kidney. It appears in the fifth week of gestation and is derived from the sacral region of the nephrogenic duct (Fig. 4.1A). The undifferentiated and pluripotent cells or blastema of the metanephros develop into nephrons in a similar fashion as in the mesonephros, leading to the formation of glomeruli, Bowman's capsules, and the proximal and distal tubules. The collecting ducts of the metanephros, on the other hand, develop from the ureteric bud, which is an extension of the mesonephric duct proximal to the cloaca. Through reciprocal induction with the metanephric blastema, the extending ureteric bud begins branching in the sixth week of gestation and gives rise to the collecting tubules, renal calyces, renal pelvis, and ureters.[11,13,14] The metanephros is functional around the 12th week of gestation.[12] Urine passing into the amnion and eventually comprises approximately 90% of the composition of the amniotic fluid in the third trimester. However, the placenta, not the kidney, serves as the main source of fetal blood filtration and the elimination of fetal waste products until birth.[15]

A detailed description of the regulation of normal nephrogenesis is beyond the scope of this chapter, and excellent reviews can be found elsewhere.[16–20] However, shared biological pathways in both kidney and lung development may offer a link between congenital kidney anomalies and pulmonary hypoplasia and the potential for therapeutic intervention. The ureteric bud and the surrounding metanephric blastema or cap mesenchyme differentiate though reciprocal signaling. The ligands glial cell–derived neurotropic factor and hepatocyte growth factor from the cap mesenchyme and Rearranged during transfection (RET), the glial cell–derived neurotropic factor receptor in the ureteric bud tip, are fundamental for the growth and branching of the ureteric ducts. Several hierarchical transcription factors, such as Six2, Wnt4, and WT1, guide the differentiation of the blastema into nephrons through regulation of mesenchymal to epithelial differentiation. Later, Notch proteins regulate tubule segment-specific differentiation. Similarly, the ureteric bud secretes signaling factors including fibroblast growth factor (FGF) 2 and bone morphogenetic protein 7, which are involved in normal glomerular, tubule, and collecting duct development.[13,18,21–25] Renal branching morphogenesis therefore is a crucial process in the formation of fetal kidneys and in the determination of the final number of nephrons, of effective glomerular filtration rate (GFR), and of postnatal renal function. Interestingly, many of the proteins encoded by these genes, such as transforming growth factor-β, FGF, and members of the retinoid signaling pathways, are soluble growth factors that can be recovered in the urine and amniotic fluid.[26,27] In humans, kidney branching morphogenesis and the acquisition of new nephrons

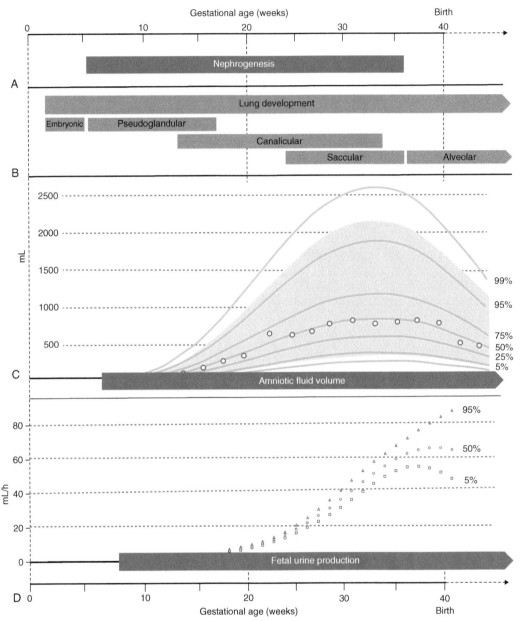

Fig. 4.1 Overlay and temporal relationship of fetal kidney and lung development. (A) Nephrogenesis. Metanephric kidney development starts at approximately 6–8 weeks' gestation and is complete by 36 weeks. (B) Lung development. Lung development begins at approximately 3.5 weeks' gestation, and the final stage of alveolar development continues into the postnatal period. (Modified from Wu C-S, Chen C-M, Chou H-C. Pulmonary hypoplasia induced by oligohydramnios: findings from animal models and a population-based study. *Pediatr Neonatol.* 2017;58(1):3–7.) (C) Amniotic fluid volume. Appreciable increase in total amniotic fluid volume from about 20 mL at 10 weeks' gestation to a maximum mean of 800 mL at term gestation. Postterm amniotic fluid volume decreases. (Modified from Beall MH, van den Wijngaard JP, van Gemert MJ, Ross MG. Amniotic fluid water dynamics. *Placenta.* 2007;28(8–9):816–823.) (D) Fetal urine production. Fetal urine production begins upon induction of the metanephric kidney, increasing from approximately 2 mL/h at 20 weeks' gestation to a mean of approximately 67 mL/h at 36 weeks' gestation. The rapid increase in fetal urine production is reflected by the parallel increase in amniotic fluid volume, the onset of which occurs at the critical stage of pseudoglandular lung development. (Modified from Peixoto-Filho FM, de Sa RA, Velarde LG, Lopes LM, Ville Y. Normal range for fetal urine production rate by 3-D ultrasound in Brazilian population. *Arch Gynecol Obstet.* 2011;283(3):497–500.)

are complete by 36 weeks' gestation.[18] The average number of nephrons in a human kidney is approximately 1 million, with a wide range between 200,000 up to 2.7 million nephrons. Consequently, a number of factors that disrupt normal kidney development (including genetic mutations, alterations of the normal fetal environment, and preterm birth) have been associated with reduced nephron number.[28]

LUNG DEVELOPMENT

The organogenesis of the human lungs shares some similarities with the kidney, yet with some key differences. Both organs rely on branching morphogenesis to establish the number of functional units (i.e., alveoli in the lung and nephrons in the kidney). Unlike the kidney, the lung continues to develop and mature postnatally; humans acquire their final number of alveoli in the first decade of life. The human lung also develops in multiple stages, namely the embryonic, pseudoglandular, canalicular, saccular, and alveolar stages (Fig. 4.1B). These stages occur in chronological sequence and are determined morphologically. The first embryonic stage starts with the appearance of the respiratory diverticulum (lung bud) as an outgrowth from the ventral foregut endoderm at 4 weeks' gestation. Two bronchial buds emerge and enlarge during the fifth week, determining the right and left main bronchi.[8,12,29,30] During the fifth week of gestation, the pseudoglandular stage occurs and is characterized by continued lung growth through dichotomous branching morphogenesis with simultaneous blood vessel branching. At the end of this stage, and by the 16th week of gestation, the airway tree, cartilage, smooth muscle, and mucous glands have branched and differentiated into terminal bronchioles. In the canalicular stage, terminal bronchioles branch into respiratory bronchioles, leading to future alveoli. This canicular stage starts in the 16th week and ends by the 26th week of gestation. By the end of this stage, the most distal epithelial branches start to widen and thin with proximity to the capillary network, leading to the first sign of alveolar epithelial cell differentiation.[8,29–31] Between the 24th week and term gestation, the saccular stage occurs during which branching morphogenesis continues. This stage is also characterized by further differentiation of the terminal airspaces into clusters of thin-walled saccules to become alveoli. The alveolar epithelium differentiates into type I and type II alveolar cells, which is surrounded by capillaries and fibroblasts. Surfactant production and recycling starts in this stage. By the end of the saccular stage, the lung is composed of numerous saccules, suitable for gas exchange. The fifth and final alveolar stage occurs postnatally and ends in childhood; however, recent imaging studies suggest that it continues into early adulthood. In the alveolar stage, the saccular walls septate and divide into mature alveoli. The vascular capillary systems also mature around the alveoli, leading to increase surface area for gas exchange.[29,32–34]

Similar to the kidneys, the lungs rely on branching morphogenesis for normal development. Lung development also depends on reciprocal signaling between the airway epithelium and the supporting mesenchymal cells. The initial budding of the respiratory diverticulum is induced by increased retinoic acid levels in the surrounding embryonic mesoderm. Retinoic acid upregulates transcription factor TBX4 in the adjacent area of the foregut, leading to the formation of the lung bud. After that, branching is dependent on multiple secretory signals from the mesenchymal cells including FGF10, Sonic Hedgehog (Shh), bone morphogenic protein 4, Wingless-related integration site (WNT), retinoic acid, Notch, transforming growth factor-β, and others.[33,35–39] As an example of reciprocal signaling, FGF10 expressed by distal mesenchymal cells drives the expression of Shh in the epithelial cells at the tip of the branch. In turn, Shh signals the smooth muscle at the tip, which splits and bifurcates the growing bud into two branches.[32] Notably there is an overlap of signaling pathways responsible for branching morphogenesis in the lungs and in the kidneys. An alteration in these common branching signaling pathways, either in response to an abnormal intrauterine environment (as seen in lower urinary tract obstruction and associated oligohydramnios) or through genetic mutation, could help explain the association of and relationship between renal dysplasia and lung hypoplasia, particularly in genetic syndromes such as the ciliopathies and nephronophthises.

In addition to signaling pathways, two main mechanical forces, episodic fetal breathing movement and distending pressure of the luminal airway, are unique in and critical to normal fetal lung development. Fetal breathing movements are first noted during the pseudoglandular stage of lung development corresponding to the 10th to 11th week of gestation. Fetal breathing movements lead to repetitive changes in the distal lung surface area and thus lead to mechanical stretching. This stretching promotes epithelial cell differentiation via mechanosensitive channels, the maturation of type II epithelial cells, and the secretion of surfactant.[9] Distending intraluminal fluid is the second mechanical force critical for normal lung development. Lung fluid is secreted into the lumen and creates distending pressure. Peristaltic waves of intraluminal fluid with rhythmic contraction of the airway smooth muscles are thought to promote branching morphogenesis.[7] The amniotic fluid therefore represents a link between kidney and lung development.

Amniotic Fluid

Amniotic fluid is essential for normal fetal development, providing a protected and buffered environment for the rapidly growing fetus. In the early fetal period, most of the amniotic fluid is produced by the epithelium of the amnion, the underlying placental fetal maternal circulation, and the umbilical cord. Amniotic fluid volume increases from approximately 20 mL at 10 weeks' gestation to approximately 630 mL at 22 weeks' gestation when fetal kidneys become the main source, although the total volume of amniotic fluid can vary substantially (Fig. 4.1C).[15] By 28 weeks' gestation, amniotic fluid volume reaches a plateau of approximately 800 mL until term, with a slight decline postterm.[40] Any impairment of fetal kidney function, including urinary tract obstruction, can manifest as oligohydramnios from midtrimester onward. However, amniotic fluid volume is a coarse estimation of absolute fetal GFR with poor correlation with actual GFR. Establishment of the amniotic fluid environment is more complex than fetal urine production alone.[40] The balance, mechanics, and exchange of fetal water flow to and from the amniotic cavity involves the amniotic membrane, the lung epithelium, the fetal kidney, and the fetal gut through amniotic fluid swallowing.

Fetal kidney urine flow and its contribution to amniotic fluid volume increases from a mean of approximately 2 mL/h at 20 weeks' gestation up to a mean as high as of 67 mL/h at 36 weeks' gestation.[41–43] Fetal urinary flow rates and amniotic fluid volume have also been used as indirect measures of fetal GFR during the second half of pregnancy and can be calculated from

changes in fetal bladder volumes on repeat ultrasound examinations over time (Fig 4.1D).[44,45] The composition of fetal urine also changes with increasing gestational age, the acquisition of nephrons, and maturation of kidney tubule epithelial transporters.[46] The kidneys increase their capacity to reabsorb electrolytes such as sodium, potassium, and calcium, and the fetal urine consequently becomes more dilute. This becomes complicated by the opposite effect of the fetal kidney's increasing responsiveness to antidiuretic hormone, which increases its capacity to concentrate the urine. Urinary sodium concentration has been used as an index of fetal renal tubular function, with values less than 90 mmol/L being normal at 20–30 weeks of gestation. Fetal urinary sodium or chloride values in excess of 100 mmol/L have also been shown to be highly predictive of fetal or perinatal death from terminal renal or pulmonary failure.[47,48]

The developing fetal lung epithelium also contributes to the production and maintenance of amniotic fluid volume. In the second and third trimesters, with lung maturation, fetal lung fluid is estimated to contribute approximately one-sixth of the total amniotic fluid volume. In fetal sheep, total lung fluid production in the third trimester has been estimated to be as high as 100 mL/kg per day.[15] During fetal life the respiratory epithelium is largely secretory, through the function of apical chloride channels. This lung fluid production is essential for normal lung development and for ongoing lung branching morphogenesis. In fetal sheep experiments, removal of fetal lung fluid starting at approximately 120 days' gestation in the sheep (equivalent to approximately 30–32 weeks' gestation in humans) results in significant lung developmental abnormalities, including pulmonary hypoplasia.[49]

Early in gestation, before the initiation of kidney function and production of fetal urine, the fetal membranes effect water exchange and thus amniotic fluid production between the amniotic cavity and the fetal-maternal circulation. In particular, the interposed amnion epithelium is permeable to water and solute flow, through intercellular channels and the action of intracellular aquaporin proteins.[40,50] Transmembrane flow is likely regulated and responsive to changes in maternal and fetal hydration status as reflected by serum osmolality. This is supported by the experimental observation that the instillation of hypotonic fluid into the amniotic cavity results in a corresponding decrease in fetal serum osmolality.[51] This suggests that, in part, fluid is exchanged across the amnion and then into the fetal maternal circulation of the placenta. Furthermore, pregnant women who are dehydrated with an increase in serum osmolality have been shown to have lower amniotic fluid production and total amniotic fluid volumes, suggesting movement of fluid from the maternal circulation across the amnion into the amniotic fluid cavity.[52]

The movement of fluid across the fetal skin barrier is an underrecognized contribution to total amniotic fluid production, particularly in the first trimester. Normally fetal skin becomes keratinized at approximately 19–25 weeks' gestation and thereafter its permeability to the free movement of water is reduced significantly.[40] Prior to this keratinization, fluid movement from the fetus though the skin and into the amniotic cavity is bidirectional and contributes to the total volume of amniotic fluid, which increases from 25 mL at 10 weeks' gestation to 400 mL by 20 weeks' gestation. In fact, this significant fluid movement is an important consideration in the neonatal intensive care of extreme preterm infants when skin losses must be adjusted and accounted for in daily fluid intake requirements.

When the total volume of amniotic fluid is calculated from the contributions from fetal urine output, lung fluid production, and movement of water across the amniotic and fetal skin membranes, the total exceeds the actual gestational age-specific measured amount of amniotic fluid. This is accounted for by amniotic fluid that is swallowed by the fetus and absorbed through the gut epithelium. In fetal sheep, fluid absorbed by the gut is estimated to be approximately 130 mL/kg day in late gestation and as high as 400 mL/kg day near term.[53] Experimental models of esophageal ligation result in significant increases of amniotic fluid accumulation, or polyhydramnios, accounted for by the inability to swallow and absorb the amniotic fluid.[54] Human conditions, such as variants of tracheoesophageal fistula with a blind end esophagus and duodenal atresia are also associated with excessive amniotic fluid accumulation. In fact, polyhydramnios is a red flag on antenatal screening for these conditions. Although amniotic fluid contains protein, amino acids, carbohydrates, and lipids, their roles are

not well described. However, they likely also serve as important trophic factors for gut development and maturation.[40]

OLIGOHYDRAMNIOS

Estimates of amniotic fluid volume and amniotic fluid composition factor frequently into decisions about fetal health, in utero interventions, and pregnancy management. Oligohydramnios is defined as a decrease in the total amount of amniotic fluid expected at a specific gestational age. Both oligohydramnios and polyhydramnios (an increase in normal amniotic fluid volume) may be important indicators of significant fetal abnormalities, which can affect intrauterine and postnatal health. In addition, low amniotic volume can impact on further fetal development, as previously described. Oligohydramnios is most commonly an acute process, resulting from spontaneous premature rupture of the amniotic membrane.[55] However, chronic forms of oligohydramnios can result from the pregnancy extending postterm, from fetal growth restriction, and from severe congenital kidney anomalies of the kidney and urinary tract. In these instances, kidney anomalies can be either genetic or acquired. If normal kidney development is interrupted (developmental kidney injury[56]), normal nephron number is reduced, resulting in a decrease in glomerular filtration. To affect normal urine output, total urine volume, and amniotic fluid volume, the insult or developmental injury must be extreme, with a significant decrease in nephron number.[28] In children born with certain kidney anomalies, glomerular filtration can be reduced to as low as 10%–15% of normal without an appreciable change in urine output. In other words, oligohydramnios due to a congenital kidney anomaly is often associated with a poor postnatal outcome in the newborn and infant.

Any defect in fetal kidney development when severe enough can result in oligohydramnios. Most commonly these conditions include bladder outlet obstruction in male fetuses, renal agenesis, renal hypodysplasia (isolated or associated with specific genetic mutations affecting normal kidney development), and various forms and combinations of ureteric obstruction, which affects both kidneys or in the case of unilateral obstruction, associated with anomalies in the contralateral kidney.[57,58] Congenital urinary tract obstruction (CUTO), when severe and occurring early in gestation, is often associated with oligohydramnios. In fact, oligohydramnios is a well-described risk factor for poor postnatal kidney outcome in these children.[59,60] Bladder outlet obstruction due to posterior urethral valves in the fetus not only affects amniotic fluid volume by impeding urine flow but also interrupts normal kidney function. In experimental animals CUTO is associated with severe kidney injury including the development of kidney dysplasia, disruption of normal kidney architecture, and a decrease in kidney size and in glomerular number.[61–64] The effect on amniotic fluid volume therefore is not due simply to mechanical obstruction but also due to irreversible fetal kidney injury. These considerations are underlined by the body of experience with in utero surgical urinary diversion in fetuses with CUTO. In recent systematic reviews and metanalyses of the published experience, in utero intervention with vesicoamniotic shunting does not ultimately change the postnatal and long-term kidney outcome of these fetuses.[65–67] The PLUTO study, a multicenter, international, nonrandomized cohort of pregnancies, demonstrated a slight survival benefit of in utero intervention in fetuses with bladder outlet obstruction,[68] but without differences in postnatal kidney outcome. All deaths in this trial were caused by respiratory failure due to pulmonary hypoplasia. Since vesicoamniotic shunting can potentially restore amniotic fluid volume, it can attenuate the deleterious effects of oligohydramnios on lung development if successful.

The antenatal assessment of amniotic fluid volume therefore becomes an important clinical tool in helping to identify fetuses with congenital anomalies, in determining antenatal management of these fetuses, in pregnancy planning, and in prognostication of postnatal outcomes. There is, however, a surprising lack of consensus on how best to routinely determine amniotic fluid volume in pregnant women at the bedside. Several methods are subjective and can be affected by variability in operator skill and technique. In the clinic, amniotic fluid is measured using ultrasound almost exclusively. It is relatively inexpensive and noninvasive. In extraordinary circumstances, other modalities such as MRI or CT scanning can be used. Not surprisingly, subjective evaluation of amniotic fluid volume adequacy, which includes assessments such as paucity of amniotic fluid, crowding of fetal parts, and the fluid to fetal interspace,[69,70] has low sensitivity as a test of

postnatal outcomes of conditions such as intrauterine growth restriction. Subjective assessment by itself probably should not be used in higher-risk pregnancies. Other objective quantitative measurements signifying low amniotic fluid volume include a largest fluid pocket less than 1 cm in largest diameter,[71] a fluid pocket diameter less than 2 cm in two perpendicular planes,[72] and a total 5-cm pocket diameter using a four-quadrant technique of amniotic fluid assessment.[73] The latter has been termed the amniotic fluid index (AFI) and has been used extensively and routinely since 1987. Since then, it has been revised to improve its performance as a diagnostic test. The AFI is obtained by performing a four-quadrant ultrasound assessment for amniotic fluid; the transducer is held perpendicular to the plane of the floor and the largest diameter of the fluid pocket is obtained (values are combined for a final score). Although an absolute value of less than 5 cm was associated with adverse fetal outcomes, a standardized value corrected for gestational age of less than the 2.5 percentile has been developed as a prognosticator for adverse fetal outcomes. The optimal amniotic fluid volume assessment has yet to be determined. When the strengths of the various methods were assessed as tests of perinatal outcomes, there was no difference between AFI and the depth of the largest vertical pocket assessments.[74]

Pulmonary Hypoplasia

Fetuses with severe congenital anomalies of the kidney and urinary tract, as seen in cases of early and complete bladder outlet obstruction, bilateral renal agenesis, or bilateral severe renal hypodysplasia, among others, have a high perinatal mortality rate and increased morbidity.[58,75] Disruption of normal fetal kidney development results in a decrease in kidney function and urine production, manifesting as severe oligohydramnios. This oligohydramnios or decrease in amniotic fluid in turn is associated with pulmonary hypoplasia. In fact, the most common cause of neonatal death in these infants is due to respiratory failure due to pulmonary hypoplasia.

The diagnosis of pulmonary hypoplasia in the fetus and neonate, however, is not straightforward. Pulmonary hypoplasia is defined as a reduction in normal functioning lung tissue.[76,77] Pulmonary hypoplasia is the result of abnormal fetal and postnatal lung development. In theory, interruption of the normal sequence of development results in correspondingly different forms of lung anomalies. For example, a disruption early in gestation, before and during the pseudoglandular phase of development, has profound effects on fetal lung branching morphogenesis, with a reduction in the formation of the bronchial tree elements, including terminal bronchioles acini, saccules, alveoli, and their corresponding vascular supply. Disruption in lung development at later stages, on the other hand, affects the maturation of the formed elements such as alveolar sacs, acini, and radial alveolar counts (a marker of branching morphogenesis).[7,77,78]

There are primary and secondary causes of pulmonary hypoplasia. Secondary causes are more common and include conditions that affect fetal breathing movements such as congenital diaphragmatic hernia, skeletal dysplasias, fetal hydrops, brain malformations, and neuromuscular malformations.[79] Many of these result from monogenic mutations, are hereditary, and are associated with malformations in other organ systems. Illustrative examples include mutations in the retinoic acid receptor (RARB, STRA6),[80,81] T-box (TBX4),[82] and Wnt (WNT3)[83] gene families, which have multiple organ congenital anomalies including pulmonary hypoplasia. Pulmonary hypoplasia associated with oligohydramnios can be due to premature rupture of membranes (PROM).[84] Congenital kidney anomalies are a more common association, with up to 20% of these due to monogenic mutations in *HNF1B, PAX2, SIX1, EYA1* genes among others.[4] Notably, there is a paucity of reports of isolated primary pulmonary hypoplasia, and familial occurrence is rare.[79,85] Surprisingly there have been few reports of mutations that affect both lung and kidney branching morphogenesis.[86] The lung effects in these cases with genetic mutations are almost exclusively a consequence of oligohydramnios secondary to kidney developmental abnormalities.

The exact mechanism by which oligohydramnios causes pulmonary hypoplasia is unknown. Normal lung development is directly influenced by the physical forces of fetal breathing movements and transluminal lung pressures.[7] The production of luminal fluid by the lung epithelium is essential for the maintenance of normal airway distension and subsequent airway development. There also seems to be an interplay between lung fluid and fetal breathing movements, with the latter allowing for distribution of lung fluid throughout the proximal and distal airways. Through a variety of proposed cellular pathways, including the upregulation of Platelet-derived growth factor (PDGF), Connective tissue growth factor (CTGF), Vascular endothelial growth factor (VEGF),[9,87] airway stretching is then responsible for epithelial proliferation, maturation, and differentiation, and ultimately the production of surfactant.[88] Oligohydramnios leads to compression of the fetal thorax, thereby restricting fetal breathing movements and affecting the normal dynamics of fetal lung fluid distribution and mechanical stretching of the fetal lung. This paradigm is supported by experiments in which the removal of fluid lung fluid in fetal sheep by fetal tracheostomy at 117–122 days' gestation resulted in decreased lung weight and volume and altered lung DNA concentration and structural development of the acinus.[89] As well, oligohydramnios produced in fetal sheep by drainage of amniotic fluid during the last third of gestation led to a reduction in lung liquid volume and caused a significant reduction in fetal lung expansion.[49]

The precise diagnosis of pulmonary hypoplasia or reduction in lung tissue is best accomplished on postmortem examination and has been found in up to 20% of neonatal autopsies.[90] Measurements of pulmonary hypoplasia include gestational age-specific total lung DNA content and lung weight–to–body weight ratio of less than 0.012 for fetuses 28 weeks or older and less than 0.015 for fetuses less than 28 weeks' gestation[91]; however, a measure of lung volume to body weight may be more appropriate as it mitigates the effects of changes in lung water content and lung edema. Radial alveolar counts, obtained by microscopic evaluation of sectioned lung tissue, reflects the extent of branching morphogenesis in the lung and is an assessment of total number of alveoli (and alveolar septa) formed. A value of less than 75% normal is deemed diagnostic of hypoplasia.[92]

Prenatal diagnosis of pulmonary hypoplasia and defining its severity is essential in guiding decisions around fetal intervention, pregnancy termination, and discussions around postnatal prognosis and outcome. The most common and available technique for antenatal assessment of lung hypoplasia is two-dimensional ultrasonography. The most commonly measured parameters include thoracic circumference, thoracic circumference–to–abdominal circumference ratio, lung area, and lung circumference–to–head circumference ratio.[93] When their performance as tests for pulmonary hypoplasia (postmortem lung weight) is measured, there is significant and wide variability, related in part to technical limitations and to the underlying reason for the hypoplasia. In general, two-dimensional ultrasound is not a reliable tool for predicting postnatal pulmonary hypoplasia. Volumetric sonography has also been used, in which the three-dimensional structure of the lung is reconstructed, and the lung volume is calculated. This improves the predictive value of two-dimensional ultrasounds, but again is limited by technical reasons and artifact.[94] Total lung volume has also been calculated using MRI.[95] In fetuses with congenital diaphragmatic hernia, it has been shown to be a "significant" predictor of postnatal fetal outcome; however, its clinical usefulness is also limited given the area under the receiver operator curve of 0.79. Taken together, ultrasound and MRI imaging are limited in their ability to antenatally diagnose pulmonary hypoplasia in the affected fetus. As emphasized by Triebwasser and colleagues, these limitations should be included in discussions at the time of family counseling.[93]

The perinatal mortality rate of infants born with pulmonary hypoplasia is high, and variable, with rates quoted from 55% to 100%.[77] This variability is notable and is also an important issue when having discussions with families about in utero intervention and postnatal prognosis. There are a few variables that influence outcome. The first is the era from which the data are being selected. Overall, outcomes have improved over the years, in part because of more aggressive interventions both in the fetal and postnatal period. The second issue is that the outcome data are influenced by unaccounted fetal losses, including in utero deaths and pregnancy terminations. Finally, and maybe most importantly, is that the postnatal outcome is influenced by the underlying cause of the pulmonary hypoplasia. For example, with the advent of in utero intervention and postnatal intensive care support including extracorporeal membrane oxygenation, recent mortality rates in infants born with congenital diaphragmatic hernia are as low as 29%,[96] which is increased

to 45% when fetal losses or "hidden mortality" is included.[97] In pregnancies complicated by PROM, the mortality rate is also variable, dependent on the timing of membrane rupture and the duration of oligohydramnios.[98] In a Brazilian cohort, perinatal mortality following PROM at gestational age between 18 to 26 weeks was as high as 54%,[99] with lower mortality rates in other centers. In fetuses with congenital anomalies of the kidney, the neonatal mortality has been determined to be as high as 24%, with variation depending on underlying diagnosis.[100] In fetuses with lower urinary tract obstruction, including male fetuses with posterior urethral valves, the mortality is as high as 90% in those with oligohydramnios and pulmonary hypoplasia.[101]

The relationship of severe oligohydramnios at various stages of gestation to underlying diagnosis and outcome has also been studied.[75] The diagnosis of severe oligohydramnios was made by subjective evaluation using ultrasound assessment in 250 singleton pregnancies between 13 and 42 weeks' gestation. Of pregnancies in the second trimester (13–24 weeks' gestation) with associated severe oligohydramnios, 51% (65/128) had fetal anomalies, most of which were considered lethal anomalies and ending in pregnancy termination. Of these, 74% (48/65) were congenital anomalies of the kidney including kidney hypoplasia, dysplasia, agenesis, and posterior urethral valves. There was a 10% overall survival. Of pregnancies in the third trimester (25–42 weeks' gestation) with associated severe oligohydramnios, 22% (27/122) had fetal anomalies, the majority of which were genitourinary anomalies. Thirty percent of these (8/27) had Potter's syndrome, 19% (5/27) had polycystic kidney disease, and 11% (3/27) had posterior urethral valves. There was an overall survival of 85%, which was higher than in the second trimester.

Not surprisingly, fetuses with early pregnancy renal anhydramnios (EPRA) have the worst prognosis. EPRA, defined as a fetus that is anuric before 22 weeks' gestation, is considered universally fatal due to the associated anhydramnios and pulmonary hypoplasia.[57,102] In postmortem analyses the severity of pulmonary hypoplasia is proportional to the length of the anhydramnios.[103] The causes of EPRA include congenital bilateral renal agenesis, forms of cystic kidney disease including autosomal recessive and dominant polycystic kidney disease, bilateral multi-cystic kidney disease, and severe lower urinary tract obstruction.[58] There are no reports of survivors in singleton pregnancies with bilateral renal agenesis.[104]

The postnatal diagnosis of pulmonary hypoplasia is based on the clinical picture and postnatal imaging. The immediate postnatal clinical presentation can vary from transient tachypnea to early death due to respiratory failure, depending on the severity of the pulmonary hypoplasia. Newborns with severe pulmonary hypoplasia have immediate onset of respiratory difficulty, are difficult to ventilate by mechanical ventilation, and usually require escalating ventilatory pressure and oxygen support. Their course is often complicated by air leak that is either spontaneous or iatrogenic, with the development of pneumothorax and pneumomediastinum, requiring escalation of invasive support.[77] In addition to pneumothorax and pneumomediastinum, radiologic findings usually include small lung fields with elevated diaphragmatic domes and a bell-shaped thorax. However, these clinical features have limited diagnostic value for pulmonary hypoplasia.[105]

Treatment and Prevention of Pulmonary Hypoplasia Due to Oligohydramnios

As discussed, the morbidity and mortality of cases with fetal kidney anomalies are variable. Outcomes depend on the severity of kidney impairment and the severity and gestational age at onset of oligohydramnios, which ultimately affect the degree of pulmonary hypoplasia and respiratory compromise at birth.[9,10] In cases of severe kidney impairment, pregnancy termination or palliative care are options historically offered to families. Multiple fetal interventions for urinary tract obstruction or oligohydramnios, including vesicocentesis, vesicoamniotic shunting, fetal cystoscopy, and amnioinfusions, have been described.[106] In the following section these major fetal interventions and neonatal outcomes will be reviewed with a focus on their effects on pulmonary hypoplasia.

VESICOCENTESIS

Vesicocentesis is the procedure of percutaneous aspiration of urine from the bladder usually in cases of fetal bladder outlet obstruction. There has been conflicting evidence regarding its efficacy in relieving urethral obstruction in these cases.[107–109] It is mostly used as a diagnostic tool to analyze fetal urine and to indirectly estimate renal function accordingly.[106] Vesicocentesis is only offered when there is suspected lower urinary tract obstruction and normally would not be considered in cases of anuria with severe renal impairment or bilateral renal agenesis. Vesicocentesis by itself does not affect the severity of oligohydramnios and its usefulness in preventing pulmonary hypoplasia and improving postnatal outcome is limited.

VESICOAMNIOTIC SHUNTING

Vesicoamniotic shunting is another procedure used in fetuses with bladder outlet obstruction to decompress the upper urinary tracts and mitigate in utero kidney injury. It is performed by the percutaneous placement of a catheter connecting the fetal bladder and the amniotic cavity. Like vesicocentesis, shunting is offered in cases of obstruction and would not be indicated in the cases of fetal anuria with an empty fetal bladder or in bilateral renal agenesis. In a recent updated meta-analysis of cohort studies of vesicoamniotic shunting for fetal lower urinary tract obstruction, a total of nine studies were included with 112 fetuses treated with shunting and 134 managed conservatively.[47,68,111–117] Although 57.1% of fetuses survived pregnancy after vesicoamniotic shunting (compared with 38.8% in the conservative arm), patient survival and renal function were not significantly different at 6-month to 2-year follow-up.[118] The PLUTO trial is notable, as it was the first multicenter prospective study performed to evaluate the role of fetal vesicoamniotic shunting; however, it was stopped early due to poor recruitment. In this study, as expected, the cause of mortality in early neonatal period was due to pulmonary hypoplasia. Vesicoamniotic shunting showed a marginal improvement in fetal survival but failed to show benefit in long-term survival or renal function.[68] Further prospective trials stratifying severity of obstruction and studying long-term renal and pulmonary outcomes are still required.

FETAL CYSTOSCOPY

Fetal cystoscopy using in utero antegrade insertion of a flexible fetoscope into the fetal bladder through the urethra has been proposed as a diagnostic and possible therapeutic tool in fetal lower urinary tract obstruction, particularly cases with posterior urethral valve.[119] Multiple therapeutic techniques are available for ablation of the valves, including guide-wire perforation, hydroablation, and laser fulguration.[106] Fetal cystoscopy is technically challenging and, like the other fetal interventions, carries the risk of PROM, placental abruption, preterm labor, and chorioamnionitis.[120] Risks specific to fetal cystoscopy include urinary ascites[121] and vesicocutaneous or vesicoenteral fistulas.[122] A retrospective cohort study of 30 cases of fetal cystoscopies for posterior urethral valve showed a 57% and 56% survival rate and 77% and 73% with normal kidney function at 1 and 2 years of age, respectively. However, 58% of cases required postnatal ablation of the posterior urethral valve.[123] A systematic review showed no significant improvement in fetal survival when comparing fetal cystoscopy and vesicoamniotic shunting.[124] In conclusion, fetal cystoscopy can offer a therapeutic treatment for lower urinary tract obstruction, but, like vesicocentesis and vesicoamniotic shunting, future prospective trials are required to determine its effect on the development of pulmonary hypoplasia and survival when cases are stratified according to severity of kidney involvement at enrollment.[106,119,121–129]

SERIAL AMNIOINFUSIONS

Amnioinfusions involve instillation of fluid, usually normal saline, into the amniotic cavity in cases of fetal oligohydramnios or anhydramnios related to underlying fetal kidney anomalies. This process is usually repeated multiple times during the pregnancy. Although amnioinfusions do not address the cause of kidney dysfunction and do not offer a means to relieve obstruction in cases of lower urinary tract obstruction, they do offer the possibility of pulmonary palliation and theoretically decrease the risk of pulmonary hypoplasia due to oligohydramnios. In cases of congenital bilateral renal agenesis, amnioinfusions have been proposed as therapy to improve chances of fetal survival in a condition that is otherwise universally lethal because of the anhydramnios and resultant pulmonary hypoplasia.[106,120,130]

A recent systematic review evaluating outcomes of fetuses with severe renal anomalies showed that serial amnioinfusion therapy improved survival and decreased risk of respiratory compromise at birth.[130] A total of eight reports were included in the analysis

with 17 cases receiving serial amnioinfusions.[120,130–139] There was considerable study-to-study heterogeneity in the review, with large variability in the fetal kidney diagnosis, and remarkably in only one case report was there a comment about oligohydramnios, with most reports lacking sufficient detail. The analysis included nine cases with severe lower urinary tract obstruction (of which one was partial obstruction), three with bilateral renal agenesis, three with bilateral renal hypodysplasia, one with a solitary hypodysplastic kidney, and one with autosomal recessive polycystic kidney disease. The cohort received a range of 2–22 amnioinfusions, with the first infusion at 16–27 weeks' gestation. The gestational age at delivery varied from 28 to 41 weeks' gestation. Of the cases with lower urinary tract obstruction, 3/9 (33%) died in the neonatal period; the remaining cases (6/6; 100%) were all started on dialysis, and 3 (50%) of these went on to receive a successful kidney transplant. Of the remaining cases, 5/8 (63%) died in the neonatal period, 2/8 were started on dialysis after birth but died before 6 months of age, and only 1 case was alive after 6 months of age.[130] Unfortunately, given the small numbers, the heterogeneity of cases, and the lack of detail in the case reports, the value of serial amnioinfusion is uncertain and based on anecdotal evidence.

Successful case reports of the use of serial amnioinfusions have led to development of the National Institutes of Health–sponsored Renal Anhydramnios Fetal Therapy (RAFT) Trial.[102] The primary aims of the RAFT trial are to determine the safety, feasibility, and efficacy of serial amnioinfusions in fetuses with EPRA. In the trial, cases will not be randomized, nor is there a control group. Concurrently a national ethics symposium concluded that serial amnioinfusions should not be offered as a treatment modality outside of an ethics-board approved research study.[141]

Summary

Pulmonary hypoplasia is a congenital reduction in normal functioning lung tissue that results from abnormal lung development. In most cases it is associated with low amniotic fluid volume. The pathogenesis of pulmonary hypoplasia is multifactorial, including an alteration in normal fetal breathing movements and chest excursion, an interruption in normal growth factor signaling pathways, and genetic mutations in select cases. Pregnancies complicated by severe congenital anomalies of the kidney and urinary tract are important examples. They are often associated with oligohydramnios, pulmonary hypoplasia, increased morbidity, and a high perinatal mortality rate. Although postnatal outcomes are directly related to the severity of pulmonary hypoplasia, the assessment and treatment of both oligohydramnios and pulmonary hypoplasia are challenging. These pregnancies require multidisciplinary assessments with the input and expertise of pediatric nephrologists, maternal fetal medicine specialists, geneticists and counsellors, ethicists, and neonatologists, among others. Pediatric nephrologists can lend expertise in helping to determine the initial and differential diagnoses, providing an understanding and explanation of the impact of in utero injury and its timing on normal in utero kidney development, assessing the severity of kidney injury and its effect on fetal kidney function. This information can help predict the postnatal kidney outcome, with and without in utero intervention. Most importantly, however, is the nephrologists' role in discussions with affected families. Frank and informed discussions are often required when discussing postnatal outcome, particularly when the situation might require palliation or escalation of care. In situations that predict an outcome needing renal replacement therapy, either immediately in the neonatal period or later in infancy, the nephrologist can provide objective, balanced, practical, and relevant information for the family.

REFERENCES

1. Lindower JB. Water balance in the fetus and neonate. *Semin Fetal Neonatal Med.* 2017;22(2):71–75. doi:10.1016/j.siny.2017.01.002
2. Queißer-Luft A, Stolz G, Wiesel A, Schlaefer K, Spranger J. Malformations in newborn: results based on 30940 infants and fetuses from the Mainz congenital birth defect monitoring system (1990-1998). *Arch Gynecol Obstet.* 2002;266(3): 163–167. doi:10.1007/s00404-001-0265-4
3. Rosenblum S, Pal A, Reidy K. Renal development in the fetus and premature infant. *Semin Fetal Neonatal Med.* 2017;22(2): 58–66. doi:10.1016/j.siny.2017.01.001
4. Murugapoopathy V, Gupta IR. A primer on congenital anomalies of the kidneys and urinary tracts (CAKUT). *Clin J Am Soc Nephrol.* 2020;15(5):723–731. doi:10.2215/CJN.12581019
5. Ardissino G, Dacco V, Testa S, et al. Epidemiology of chronic renal failure in children: data from the ItalKid project. *Pediatrics.* 2003;111(4 Pt 1):e382–e387.
6. Furth SL, Pierce C, Hui WF, et al. Estimating time to ESRD in children with CKD. *Am J Kidney Dis.* 2018;71(6):783–792. doi:10.1053/j.ajkd.2017.12.011
7. Cotten CM. Pulmonary hypoplasia. *Semin Fetal Neonatal Med.* 2017;22(4):250–255. doi:10.1016/j.siny.2017.06.004
8. Mullassery D, Smith NP. Lung development. *Semin Pediatr Surg.* 2015;24(4):152–155. doi:10.1053/j.sempedsurg.2015.01.011
9. Wu C-S, Chen C-M, Chou H-C. Pulmonary hypoplasia induced by oligohydramnios: findings from animal models and a population-based study. *Pediatr Neonatol.* 2017;58(1):3–7. doi:10.1016/j.pedneo.2016.04.001
10. Ibirogba ER, Haeri S, Ruano R. Fetal lower urinary tract obstruction: what should we tell the prospective parents? *Prenat Diagn.* 2020;40(6):661–668. doi:10.1002/pd.5669
11. Rehman S, Ahmed D. Embryology, kidney, bladder, and ureter. In: *StatPearls.* StatPearls Publishing; 2021. https://www.ncbi.nlm.nih.gov/books/NBK547747/
12. Sadler TW, Langman J. *Langman's Medical Embryology.* 12th ed. Wolters Kluwer Health/Lippincott Williams & Wilkins; 2012:xiii.
13. Upadhyay KK, Silverstein DM. Renal development: a complex process dependent on inductive interaction. *Curr Pediatr Rev.* 2014;10(2):107–114. doi:10.2174/15733963100214051310 1950
14. Ludwig KS, Landmann L. Early development of the human mesonephros. *Anat Embryol (Berl).* 2005;209(6):439–447. doi:10.1007/s00429-005-0460-3
15. Beall MH, van den Wijngaard JP, van Gemert MJ, Ross MG. Amniotic fluid water dynamics. *Placenta.* 2007;28(8-9): 816–823. doi:10.1016/j.placenta.2006.11.009
16. Oxburgh L. Kidney nephron determination. *Annu Rev Cell Dev Biol.* 2018;34:427–450. doi:10.1146/annurev-cellbio-100616-060647
17. Little MH. Returning to kidney development to deliver synthetic kidneys. *Dev Biol.* 2021;474:22–36. doi:10.1016/j.ydbio.2020.12.009
18. Short KM, Smyth IM. Branching morphogenesis as a driver of renal development. *Anat Rec (Hoboken).* 2020;303(10): 2578–2587. doi:10.1002/ar.24486
19. Nagata M. Glomerulogenesis and the role of endothelium. *Curr Opin Nephrol Hypertens.* 2018;27(3):159–164. doi: 10.1097/MNH.0000000000000402
20. Glassberg KI. Normal and abnormal development of the kidney: a clinician's interpretation of current knowledge. *J Urol.* 2002;167(6):2339–2350; discussion 2350-2351.
21. Kurtzeborn K, Kwon HN, Kuure S. MAPK/ERK signaling in regulation of renal differentiation. *Int J Mol Sci.* 2019;20(7): 1779. doi:10.3390/ijms20071779
22. Ivanova L, Butt MJ, Matsell DG. Mesenchymal transition in kidney collecting duct epithelial cells. *Am J Physiol Renal Physiol.* 2008;294(5):F1238–F1248. doi:10.1152/ajprenal.00326.2007
23. Dressler GR. The cellular basis of kidney development. *Annu Rev Cell Dev Biol.* 2006;22:509–529. doi:10.1146/annurev.cellbio.22.010305.104340
24. Michael EL, Richard NS. Molecular genetics of renal development. *Curr Urol Rep.* 2003;4(2):171–176. doi:10.1007/s11934-003-0046-7
25. Kim CM, Glassberg KI. Molecular mechanisms of renal development. *Curr Urol Rep.* 2003;4(2):164–170. doi:10.1007/s11934-003-0045-8
26. Ichiba H, Saito M, Yamano T. Amniotic fluid transforming growth factor-β1 and the risk for the development of neonatal

bronchopulmonary dysplasia. *Neonatology.* 2009;96(3):156–161. doi:10.1159/000210088

27. Tong X. Amniotic fluid may act as a transporting pathway for signaling molecules and stem cells during the embryonic development of amniotes. *J Chin Med Assoc.* 2013;76(11): 606–610. doi:10.1016/j.jcma.2013.07.006

28. Charlton JR, Springsteen CH, Carmody JB. Nephron number and its determinants in early life: a primer. *Pediatr Nephrol.* 2014;29(12):2299–2308. doi:10.1007/s00467-014-2758-y

29. Schittny JC. Development of the lung. *Cell Tissue Res.* 2017;367(3):427–444. doi:10.1007/s00441-016-2545-0

30. Warburton D, El-Hashash A, Carraro G, et al. *Lung Organogenesis.* Elsevier; 2010:73–158.

31. Nikolić MZ, Sun D, Rawlins EL. Human lung development: recent progress and new challenges. *Development.* 2018; 145(16):dev163485. doi:10.1242/dev.163485

32. Goodwin K, Nelson CM. Branching morphogenesis. *Development.* 2020;147(10):dev184499. doi:10.1242/dev.184499

33. Miura T. Models of lung branching morphogenesis. *J Biochem.* 2015;157(3):121–127. doi:10.1093/jb/mvu087

34. Miura T. *Modeling Lung Branching Morphogenesis.* Elsevier; 2008:291–310.

35. Fernandes-Silva H, Araújo-Silva H, Correia-Pinto J, Moura RS. Retinoic acid: a key regulator of lung development. *Biomolecules.* 2020;10(1):152. doi:10.3390/biom10010152

36. Herriges M, Morrisey EE. Lung development: orchestrating the generation and regeneration of a complex organ. *Development.* 2014;141(3):502–513. doi:10.1242/dev.098186

37. Warburton D, Bellusci S, De Langhe S, et al. Molecular mechanisms of early lung specification and branching morphogenesis. *Pediatr Res.* 2005;57(5 Part 2):26R–37R. doi:10.1203/01.pdr.0000159570.01327.ed

38. Roth-Kleiner M, Post M. Similarities and dissimilarities of branching and septation during lung development. *Pediatr Pulmonol.* 2005;40(2):113–134. doi:10.1002/ppul.20252

39. Chuang P-T, McMahon AP. Branching morphogenesis of the lung: new molecular insights into an old problem. *Trends Cell Biol.* 2003;13(2):86–91. doi:10.1016/s0962-8924(02)00031-4

40. Underwood MA, Gilbert WM, Sherman MP. Amniotic fluid: not just fetal urine anymore. *J Perinatol.* 2005;25(5):341–348. doi:10.1038/sj.jp.7211290

41. Touboul C, Boulvain M, Picone O, Levaillant JM, Frydman R, Senat MV. Normal fetal urine production rate estimated with 3-dimensional ultrasonography using the rotational technique (virtual organ computer-aided analysis). *Am J Obstet Gynecol.* 2008;199(1):57.e1–5. doi:10.1016/j.ajog.2007.12.012

42. Magann EF, Sanderson M, Martin JN, Chauhan S. The amniotic fluid index, single deepest pocket, and two-diameter pocket in normal human pregnancy. *Am J Obstet Gynecol.* 2000;182(6):1581–1588. doi:10.1067/mob.2000.107325

43. Peixoto-Filho FM, de Sa RA, Velarde LG, Lopes LM, Ville Y. Normal range for fetal urine production rate by 3-D ultrasound in Brazilian population. *Arch Gynecol Obstet.* 2011;283(3):497–500. doi:10.1007/s00404-010-1397-1

44. Rabinowitz R, Peters MT, Vyas S, Campbell S, Nicolaides KH. Measurement of fetal urine production in normal pregnancy by real-time ultrasonography. *Am J Obstet Gynecol.* 1989;161(5): 1264–1266.

45. Hedriana HL. Ultrasound measurement of fetal urine flow. *Clin Obstet Gynecol.* 1997;40(2):337–351.

46. Nicolini U, Spelzini F. Invasive assessment of fetal renal abnormalities: urinalysis, fetal blood sampling and biopsy. *Prenat Diagn.* 2001;21(11):964–969. doi:10.1002/pd.212

47. Glick PL, Harrison MR, Golbus MS, et al. Management of the fetus with congenital hydronephrosis II: prognostic criteria and selection for treatment. *J Pediatr Surg.* 1985;20(4):376–387.

48. Crombleholme TM, Harrison MR, Golbus MS, et al. Fetal intervention in obstructive uropathy: prognostic indicators and efficacy of intervention. *Am J Obstet Gynecol.* 1990;162(5): 1239–1244. doi:10.1016/0002-9378(90)90026-4

40. Harding R, Hooper SB, Dickson KA. A mechanism leading to reduced lung expansion and lung hypoplasia in fetal sheep during oligohydramnios. *Am J Obstet Gynecol.* 1990;163(6 Pt 1): 1904–1913. doi:10.1016/0002-9378(90)90772-y

50. Prat C, Blanchon L, Borel V, et al. Ontogeny of aquaporins in human fetal membranes. *Biol Reprod.* 2012;86(2):48. doi:10.1095/biolreprod.111.095448

51. Gilbert WM, Brace RA. The missing link in amniotic fluid volume regulation: intramembranous absorption. *Obstet Gynecol.* 1989;74(5):748–754.

52. Hanson RS, Powrie RO, Larson L. Diabetes insipidus in pregnancy: a treatable cause of oligohydramnios. *Obstet Gynecol.* 1997;89(5 Pt 2):816–817. doi:10.1016/s0029-7844(97)00029-x

53. Nijland MJ, Day L, Ross MG. Ovine fetal swallowing: expression of preterm neurobehavioral rhythms. *J Matern Fetal Med.* 2001;10(4):251–257. doi:10.1080/714904334

54. Fujino Y, Agnew CL, Schreyer P, Ervin MG, Sherman DJ, Ross MG. Amniotic fluid volume response to esophageal occlusion in fetal sheep. *Am J Obstet Gynecol.* 1991;165(6 Pt 1):1620–1626. doi:10.1016/0002-9378(91)90005-c

55. Mercer BM. Preterm premature rupture of the membranes: diagnosis and management. *Clin Perinatol.* 2004;31(4): 765–782, vi. doi:10.1016/j.clp.2004.06.004

56. Trnka P, Hiatt MJ, Tarantal AF, Matsell DG. Congenital urinary tract obstruction: defining markers of developmental kidney injury. *Pediatr Res.* 2012;72(5):446–454. doi:10.1038/pr.2012.113

57. Grijseels EW, van-Hornstra PT, Govaerts LC, et al. Outcome of pregnancies complicated by oligohydramnios or anhydramnios of renal origin. *Prenat Diagn.* 2011;31(11):1039–1045. doi:10.1002/pd.2827

58. Jelin AC, Sagaser KG, Forster KR, Ibekwe T, Norton ME, Jelin EB. Etiology and management of early pregnancy renal anhydramnios: is there a place for serial amnioinfusions? *Prenat Diagn.* 2020;40(5):528–537. doi:10.1002/pd.5658

59. Matsell DG, Yu S, Morrison SJ. Antenatal determinants of long-term kidney outcome in boys with posterior urethral valves. *Fetal Diagn Ther.* 2016;39(3):214–221. doi:10.1159/000439302

60. Morris RK, Kilby MD. An overview of the literature on congenital lower urinary tract obstruction and introduction to the PLUTO trial: percutaneous shunting in lower urinary tract obstruction. *Aust N Z J Obstet Gynaecol.* 2009;49(1):6–10. doi:10.1111/j.1479-828X.2008.00940.x

61. Peters CA, Carr MC, Lais A, Retik AB, Mandell J. The response of the fetal kidney to obstruction. *J Urol.* 1992;148(2 Pt 2): 503–509.

62. Matsell DG, Mok A, Tarantal AF. Altered primate glomerular development due to in utero urinary tract obstruction. *Kidney Int.* 2002;61(4):1263–1269. doi:10.1046/j.1523-1755.2002.00274.x

63. Chevalier RL, Thornhill BA, Forbes MS, Kiley SC. Mechanisms of renal injury and progression of renal disease in congenital obstructive nephropathy. *Pediatr Nephrol.* 2010;25(4): 687–697. doi:10.1007/s00467-009-1316-5

64. Singh S, Robinson M, Nahi F, et al. Identification of a unique transgenic mouse line that develops megabladder, obstructive uropathy, and renal dysfunction. *J Am Soc Nephrol.* 2007; 18(2):461–471. doi:10.1681/ASN.2006040405

65. Clark TJ, Martin WL, Divakaran TG, Whittle MJ, Kilby MD, Khan KS. Prenatal bladder drainage in the management of fetal lower urinary tract obstruction: a systematic review and meta-analysis. *Obstet Gynecol.* 2003;102(2):367–382. doi:10.1016/s0029-7844(03)00577-5

66. Holmes N, Harrison MR, Baskin LS. Fetal surgery for posterior urethral valves: long-term postnatal outcomes. *Pediatrics.* 2001;108(1):E7.

67. Biard JM, Johnson MP, Carr MC, et al. Long-term outcomes in children treated by prenatal vesicoamniotic shunting for lower urinary tract obstruction. *Obstet Gynecol.* 2005;106(3): 503–508. doi:10.1097/01.AOG.0000171117.38929.eb

68. Morris RK, Malin GL, Quinlan-Jones E, et al. Percutaneous vesicoamniotic shunting versus conservative management for fetal lower urinary tract obstruction (PLUTO): a randomised trial. *Lancet.* 2013;382(9903):1496–1506. doi:10.1016/S0140-6736(13)60992-7

69. Philipson EH, Sokol RJ, Williams T. Oligohydramnios: clinical associations and predictive value for intrauterine growth retardation. *Am J Obstet Gynecol.* 1983;146(3):271–278. doi:10.1016/0002-9378(83)90748-2

70. Crowley P. Non quantitative estimation of amniotic fluid volume in suspected prolonged pregnancy. *J Perinat Med.* 1980;8(5):249–251. doi:10.1515/jpme.1980.8.5.249

71. Bottoms SF, Welch RA, Zador IE, Sokol RJ. Limitations of using maximum vertical pocket and other sonographic evaluations of amniotic fluid volume to predict fetal growth: technical or physiologic? *Am J Obstet Gynecol.* 1986;155(1):154–158. doi:10.1016/0002-9378(86)90101-8

72. Chamberlain PF, Manning FA, Morrison I, Harman CR, Lange IR. Ultrasound evaluation of amniotic fluid volume. I. The relationship of marginal and decreased amniotic fluid volumes to perinatal outcome. *Am J Obstet Gynecol.* 1984;150(3): 245–249. doi:10.1016/s0002-9378(84)90359-4

73. Rutherford SE, Phelan JP, Smith CV, Jacobs N. The four-quadrant assessment of amniotic fluid volume: an adjunct to antepartum fetal heart rate testing. *Obstet Gynecol.* 1987;70(3 Pt 1):353–356.

74. Moses J, Doherty DA, Magann EF, Chauhan SP, Morrison JC. A randomized clinical trial of the intrapartum assessment of amniotic fluid volume: amniotic fluid index versus the single deepest pocket technique. *Am J Obstet Gynecol.* 2004;190(6):1564–1569; discussion 1569–1570. doi:10.1016/j.ajog.2004.03.046

75. Shipp TD, Bromley B, Pauker S, Frigoletto FD Jr, Benacerraf BR. Outcome of singleton pregnancies with severe oligohydramnios in the second and third trimesters. *Ultrasound Obstet Gynecol.* 1996;7(2):108–113. doi:10.1046/j.1469-0705.1996.07020108.x

76. Matsell DG, Cojocaru D, Matsell EW, Eddy AA. The impact of small kidneys. *Pediatr Nephrol.* 2015;30(9):1501–1509. doi:10.1007/s00467-015-3079-5

77. Laudy JA, Wladimiroff JW. The fetal lung. 2: pulmonary hypoplasia. *Ultrasound Obstet Gynecol.* 2000;16(5):482–494. doi:10.1046/j.1469-0705.2000.00252.x

78. Mullassery D, Smith NP. Lung development. *Semin Pediatr Surg.* 2015;24(4):152–155. doi:10.1053/j.sempedsurg.2015.01.011

79. Frey B, Fleischhauer A, Gersbach M. Familial isolated pulmonary hypoplasia: a case report, suggesting autosomal recessive inheritance. *Eur J Pediatr.* 1994;153(6):460–463. doi:10.1007/BF01983413

80. Srour M, Chitayat D, Caron V, et al. Recessive and dominant mutations in retinoic acid receptor beta in cases with microphthalmia and diaphragmatic hernia. *Am J Hum Genet.* 2013;93(4):765–772. doi:10.1016/j.ajhg.2013.08.014

81. Marcadier JL, Mears AJ, Woods EA, et al. A novel mutation in two Hmong families broadens the range of STRA6-related malformations to include contractures and camptodactyly. *Am J Med Genet A.* 2016;170A(1):11–18. doi:10.1002/ajmg.a.37389

82. Kariminejad A, Szenker-Ravi E, Lekszas C, et al. Homozygous null TBX4 mutations lead to posterior amelia with pelvic and pulmonary hypoplasia. *Am J Hum Genet.* 2019;105(6): 1294–1301. doi:10.1016/j.ajhg.2019.10.013

83. Kosaki K, Jones MC, Stayboldt C. Zimmer phocomelia: delineation by principal coordinate analysis. *Am J Med Genet.* 1996;66(1):55–59. doi:10.1002/(SICI)1096-8628(19961202)66:1<55::AID-AJMG12>3.0.CO;2-P

84. Rubin LP. Pulmonary hypoplasia resulting from prolonged rupture of membranes: a distinct clinical entity with instructive experimental models. *Pediatr Pulmonol.* 2017;52(11): 1378–1380. doi:10.1002/ppul.23764

85. Boylan P, Howe A, Gearty J, O'Brien NG. Familial pulmonary hypoplasia. *Ir J Med Sci.* 1977;146(6):179–180. doi:10.1007/BF03030956

86. Smith NP, Losty PD, Connell MG, Mayer U, Jesudason EC. Abnormal lung development precedes oligohydramnios in a transgenic murine model of renal dysgenesis. *J Urol.* 2006; 175(2):783–786. doi:10.1016/S0022-5347(05)00169-2

87. Williams O, Hutchings G, Hubinont C, Debauche C, Greenough A. Pulmonary effects of prolonged oligohydramnios following mid-trimester rupture of the membranes—antenatal and postnatal management. *Neonatology.* 2012;101(2): 83–90. doi:10.1159/000329445

88. Koos BJ, Rajaee A. Fetal breathing movements and changes at birth. *Adv Exp Med Biol.* 2014;814:89–101. doi:10.1007/978-1-4939-1031-1_8

89. Fewell JE, Hislop AA, Kitterman JA, Johnson P. Effect of tracheostomy on lung development in fetal lambs. *J Appl Physiol Respir Environ Exerc Physiol.* 1983;55(4):1103–1108. doi:10.1152/jappl.1983.55.4.1103

90. Wigglesworth JS, Desai R. Is fetal respiratory function a major determinant of perinatal survival? *Lancet.* 1982;1(8266): 264–267. doi:10.1016/s0140-6736(82)90986-2

91. Wigglesworth JS, Desai R. Use of DNA estimation for growth assessment in normal and hypoplastic fetal lungs. *Arch Dis Child.* 1981;56(8):601–605. doi:10.1136/adc.56.8.601

92. Askenazi SS, Perlman M. Pulmonary hypoplasia: lung weight and radial alveolar count as criteria of diagnosis. *Arch Dis Child.* 1979;54(8):614–618. doi:10.1136/adc.54.8.614

93. Triebwasser JE, Treadwell MC. Prenatal prediction of pulmonary hypoplasia. *Semin Fetal Neonatal Med.* 2017;22(4): 245–249. doi:10.1016/j.siny.2017.03.001

94. Peralta CF, Kazan-Tannus JF, Bunduki V, et al. Evaluation of the agreement between 3-dimensional ultrasonography and magnetic resonance imaging for fetal lung volume measurement. *J Ultrasound Med.* 2006;25(4):461–467. doi:10.7863/jum.2006.25.4.461

95. Jani J, Cannie M, Sonigo P, et al. Value of prenatal magnetic resonance imaging in the prediction of postnatal outcome in fetuses with diaphragmatic hernia. *Ultrasound Obstet Gynecol.* 2008;32(6):793–799. doi:10.1002/uog.6234

96. Putnam LR, Harting MT, Tsao K, et al. Congenital diaphragmatic hernia defect size and infant morbidity at discharge. *Pediatrics.* 2016;138(5):e20162043. doi:10.1542/peds.2016-2043

97. Burgos CM, Frenckner B. Addressing the hidden mortality in CDH: a population-based study. *J Pediatr Surg.* 2017;52(4): 522–525. doi:10.1016/j.jpedsurg.2016.09.061

98. Baser E, Aydogan Kirmizi D, Ulubas Isik D, et al. The effects of latency period in PPROM cases managed expectantly. *J Matern Fetal Neonatal Med.* 2020;33(13):2274–2283. doi:10.1080/14767058.2020.1731465

99. Esteves JS, de Sa RA, de Carvalho PR, Coca Velarde LG. Neonatal outcome in women with preterm premature rupture of membranes (PPROM) between 18 and 26 weeks. *J Matern Fetal Neonatal Med.* 2016;29(7):1108–1112. doi:10.3109/14767058.2015.1035643

100. Melo BF, Aguiar MB, Bouzada MC, et al. Early risk factors for neonatal mortality in CAKUT: analysis of 524 affected newborns. *Pediatr Nephrol.* 2012;27(6):965–972. doi:10.1007/s00467-012-2107-y

101. Irfan A, O'Hare E, Jelin E. Fetal interventions for congenital renal anomalies. *Transl Pediatr.* 2021;10(5):1506–1517. doi:10.21037/tp-2020-fs-05

102. O'Hare EM, Jelin AC, Miller JL, et al. Amnioinfusions to treat early onset anhydramnios caused by renal anomalies: background and rationale for the renal anhydramnios fetal therapy trial. *Fetal Diagn Ther.* 2019;45(6):365–372. doi:10.1159/000497472

103. Jelin EB, Hooper JE, Duregon E, et al. Pulmonary hypoplasia correlates with the length of anhydramnios in patients with early pregnancy renal anhydramnios (EPRA). *J Perinatol.* 2021;41(8):1924–1929. doi:10.1038/s41372-021-01128-0

104. Huber C, Shazly SA, Blumenfeld YJ, Jelin E, Ruano R. Update on the prenatal diagnosis and outcomes of fetal bilateral renal agenesis. *Obstet Gynecol Surv.* 2019;74(5):298–302. doi:10.1097/OGX.0000000000000670

105. Leonidas JC, Bhan I, Beatty EC. Radiographic chest contour and pulmonary air leaks in oligohydramnios-related pulmonary hypoplasia (Potter's syndrome). *Invest Radiol.* 1982;17(1):6–10. doi:10.1097/00004424-198201000-00002

106. Irfan A, O'Hare E, Jelin E. Fetal interventions for congenital renal anomalies. *Transl Pediatr.* 2021;10(5):1506–1517. doi:10.21037/tp-2020-fs-05

107. Carroll SG, Soothill PW, Tizard J, Kyle PM. Vesicocentesis at 10-14 weeks of gestation for treatment of fetal megacystis. *Ultrasound Obstet Gynecol.* 2001;18(4):366–370. doi:10.1046/j.0960-7692.2001.00531.x

108. Jouannic JM, Hyett JA, Pandya PP, Gulbis B, Rodeck CH, Jauniaux E. Perinatal outcome in fetuses with megacystis in the first half of pregnancy. *Prenat Diagn.* 2003;23(4):340–344. doi:10.1002/pd.593

109. Evans MI, Sacks AJ, Johnson MP, Robichaux AG III, May M, Moghissi KS. Sequential invasive assessment of fetal renal function and the intrauterine treatment of fetal obstructive uropathies. *Obstet Gynecol.* 1991;77(4):545–550.

110. Favre R, Kohler M, Gasser B, Muller F, Nisand I. Early fetal megacystis between 11 and 15 weeks of gestation. *Ultrasound Obstet Gynecol.* 1999;14(6):402–406. doi:10.1046/j.1469-0705.1999.14060402.x

111. Morris RK, Middleton LJ, Malin GL, et al. Outcome in fetal lower urinary tract obstruction: a prospective registry study. *Ultrasound Obstet Gynecol.* 2015;46(4):424–431. doi:10.1002/uog.14808

112. Ruano R, Sananes N, Sangi-Haghpeykar H, et al. Fetal intervention for severe lower urinary tract obstruction: a multicenter case-control study comparing fetal cystoscopy with vesicoamniotic shunting. *Ultrasound Obstet Gynecol.* 2015;45(4):452–458. doi:10.1002/uog.14652

113. McLorie G, Farhat W, Khoury A, Geary D, Ryan G. Outcome analysis of vesicoamniotic shunting in a comprehensive population. *J Urol.* 2001;166(3):1036–1040.

114. Freedman AL, Bukowski TP, Smith CA, Evans MI, Johnson MP, Gonzalez R. Fetal therapy for obstructive uropathy: diagnosis specific outcomes [corrected]. *J Urol.* 1996;156(2 Pt 2):720–723; discussion 723–724.

115. Johnson MP, Bukowski TP, Reitleman C, Isada NB, Pryde PG, Evans MI. In utero surgical treatment of fetal obstructive uropathy: a new comprehensive approach to identify appropriate candidates for vesicoamniotic shunt therapy. *Am J Obstet Gynecol.* 1994;170(6):1770–1776; discussion 1776–1779. doi:10.1016/s0002-9378(94)70353-1

116. Lipitz S, Ryan G, Samuell C, et al. Fetal urine analysis for the assessment of renal function in obstructive uropathy. *Am J Obstet Gynecol.* 1993;168(1 Pt 1):174–179. doi:10.1016/s0002-9378(12)90909-6

117. Nicolini U, Tannirandorn Y, Vaughan J, Fisk NM, Nicolaidis P, Rodeck CH. Further predictors of renal dysplasia in fetal obstructive uropathy: bladder pressure and biochemistry of "fresh" urine. *Prenat Diagn.* 1991;11(3):159–166. doi:10.1002/pd.1970110305

118. Nassr AA, Shazly SAM, Abdelmagied AM, et al. Effectiveness of vesicoamniotic shunt in fetuses with congenital lower urinary tract obstruction: an updated systematic review and meta-analysis. *Ultrasound Obstet Gynecol.* 2017;49(6):696–703. doi:10.1002/uog.15988

119. Farrugia M-K. Fetal bladder outflow obstruction: interventions, outcomes and management uncertainties. *Early Hum Dev.* 2020;150:105189. doi:10.1016/j.earlhumdev.2020.105189

120. O'Hare EM, Jelin AC, Miller JL, et al. Amnioinfusions to treat early onset anhydramnios caused by renal anomalies: background and rationale for the renal anhydramnios fetal therapy trial. *Fetal Diagn Ther.* 2019;45(6):365–372. doi:10.1159/000497472

121. Welsh A, Agarwal S, Kumar S, Smith RP, Fisk NM. Fetal cystoscopy in the management of fetal obstructive uropathy: experience in a single European centre. *Prenat Diagn.* 2003;23(13):1033–1041. doi:10.1002/pd.717

122. Ruano R, Duarte S, Bunduki V, Giron AM, Srougi M, Zugaib M. Fetal cystoscopy for severe lower urinary tract obstruction-initial experience of a single center. *Prenat Diagn.* 2010;30(1):30–39. doi:10.1002/pd.2418

123. Sananes N, Cruz-Martinez R, Favre R, et al. Two-year outcomes after diagnostic and therapeutic fetal cystoscopy for lower urinary tract obstruction. *Prenat Diagn.* 2016;36(4):297–303. doi:10.1002/pd.4771

124. Morris RK, Ruano R, Kilby MD. Effectiveness of fetal cystoscopy as a diagnostic and therapeutic intervention for lower urinary tract obstruction: a systematic review. *Ultrasound Obstet Gynecol.* 2011;37(6):629–637. doi:10.1002/uog.8981

125. Ruano R, Sananes N, Wilson C, et al. Fetal lower urinary tract obstruction: proposal for standardized multidisciplinary prenatal management based on disease severity. *Ultrasound Obstet Gynecol.* 2016;48(4):476–482. doi:10.1002/uog.15844

126. Ruano R, Sananes N, Sangi-Haghpeykar H, et al. Fetal intervention for severe lower urinary tract obstruction: a multicenter case-control study comparing fetal cystoscopy with vesicoamniotic shunting. *Ultrasound Obstet Gynecol.* 2015;45(4):452–458. doi:10.1002/uog.14652

127. Ruano R, Yoshizaki CT, Giron AM, Srougi M, Zugaib M. Cystoscopic placement of transurethral stent in a fetus with urethral stenosis. *Ultrasound Obstet Gynecol.* 2014;44(2):238–240. doi:10.1002/uog.13293

128. Ruano R, Yoshisaki CT, Salustiano EMA, Giron AM, Srougi M, Zugaib M. Early fetal cystoscopy for first-trimester severe megacystis. *Ultrasound Obstet Gynecol.* 2011;37(6):696–701. doi:10.1002/uog.8963

129. Morris RK, Malin GL, Khan KS, Kilby MD. Systematic review of the effectiveness of antenatal intervention for the treatment of congenital lower urinary tract obstruction. *BJOG.* 2010; 117(4):382–390. doi:10.1111/j.1471-0528.2010.02500.x

130. Warring SK, Novoa V, Shazly S, et al. Serial amnioinfusion as regenerative therapy for pulmonary hypoplasia in fetuses with intrauterine renal failure or severe renal anomalies: systematic review and future perspectives. *Mayo Clin Proc Innov Qual Outcomes.* 2020;4(4):391–409. doi:10.1016/j.mayocpiqo.2020.04.008

131. Riddle S, Habli M, Tabbah S, et al. Contemporary outcomes of patients with isolated bilateral renal agenesis with and without fetal intervention. *Fetal Diagn Ther.* 2020;47(9): 675–681. doi:10.1159/000507700

132. Jelin AC, Sagaser KG, Forster KR, Ibekwe T, Norton ME, Jelin EB. Etiology and management of early pregnancy renal anhydramnios: is there a place for serial amnioinfusions? *Prenat Diagn.* 2020;40(5):528–537. doi:10.1002/pd.5658

133. Polzin WJ, Lim FY, Habli M, et al. Use of an amnioport to maintain amniotic fluid volume in fetuses with oligohydramnios secondary to lower urinary tract obstruction or fetal renal anomalies. *Fetal Diagn Ther.* 2017;41(1):51–57. doi:10.1159/000445946

134. Whittaker N, Leonardi M. Five-month survival of neonate after serial amnioinfusions for fetal bilateral renal agenesis [18D]. *Obstet Gynecol.* 2016;127:39S. doi:10.1097/01.AOG.0000483396.15861.e1

135. Haeri S. Fetal Lower Urinary Tract Obstruction (LUTO): a practical review for providers. *Matern Health Neonatol Perinatol.* 2015;1:26. doi:10.1186/s40748-015-0026-1

136. Bienstock JL, Birsner ML, Coleman F, Hueppchen NA. Successful in utero intervention for bilateral renal agenesis. *Obstet Gynecol.* 2014;124(2 Pt 2 suppl 1):413–415. doi:10.1097/AOG.0000000000000339

137. Hsu TL, Hsu TY, Tsai CC, Ou CY. The experience of amnioinfusion for oligohydramnios during the early second trimester. *Taiwan J Obstet Gynecol.* 2007;46(4):395–398. doi:10.1016/S1028-4559(08)60009-1

138. Cameron D, Lupton BA, Farquharson D, Hiruki T. Amnioinfusions in renal agenesis. *Obstet Gynecol.* 1994;83(5 Pt 2): 872–876.

139. Hansmann M, Chatterjee MS, Schuh S, Gembruch U, Bald R. Multiple antepartum amnioinfusions in selected cases of oligohydramnios. *J Reprod Med.* 1991;36(12):847–851.

140. Fisk NM, Ronderos-Dumit D, Soliani A, Nicolini U, Vaughan J, Rodeck CH. Diagnostic and therapeutic transabdominal amnioinfusion in oligohydramnios. *Obstet Gynecol.* 1991; 78(2):270–278.

141. Sugarman J, Anderson J, Baschat AA, et al. Ethical considerations concerning amnioinfusions for treating fetal bilateral renal agenesis. *Obstet Gynecol.* 2018;131(1):130–134. doi:10.1097/AOG.0000000000002416

Chapter 5

Pathophysiology and Management of Hyperkalemia in the Neonate

Xamayta Negroni, MD, MS and Melvin Bonilla-Felix, MD, FAAP

Chapter Outline

Potassium (K), the major intracellular (IC) cation (98% of [K] is located inside the cells), is responsible for protein synthesis, cell growth, and regulation of cell volume. Sodium-potassium ATPase (Na-K-ATPase) in cell membranes is responsible for maintaining this gradient, which is critical for excitable cells.

Compared with children and adults, neonates have a higher serum potassium concentration ([K]), with very preterm and very low birth weight neonates showing even higher levels. This is why it is important to use reference values for age to make therapeutic decisions. Serum [K] usually peaks between 9 and 72 hours, followed by a decreasing trend after the second or third day of life with the onset on postnatal diuresis/natriuresis.[1] Prior to the more prevalent use of antenatal steroids for threatened preterm delivery,[2] a third of these neonates had a peak [K] above 6.7 mEq/L in one study.[1]

In adults, [K] balance requires [K] excretion to equal dietary [K] intake. The kidneys are responsible for excreting 90% of [K] intake, with remaining excreted by the gastrointestinal tract. Changes in [K] intake trigger changes in [K] excretion, but the immediate shifting of [K] into or out of the IC compartment maintains normal serum concentrations while renal compensation occurs to blunt changes in serum [K].[3]

Intestinal Potassium Handling

Dietary [K] is 90% absorbed in the gastrointestinal tract, primarily in the small intestine. When renal excretion of [K] is limited, the colon (which under normal conditions plays a minimal role in absorption and secretion of K) acquires a more prominent role. The messenger RNA encoding the colonic alpha isoform of the H-K-ATPase[4,5] upregulates in conditions that favor [K] absorption.[5]

The kidney is the major regulator of extracellular (EC) [K]. A chronic oral [K] load is needed to cause a significant rise in EC potassium. This increases [K] secretion in the distal nephron mediated by aldosterone.[6] Conversely, limited [K] intake inhibits aldosterone.

Minor changes in dietary [K] can induce kaliuresis without hyperkalemia or changes in aldosterone. Increase in [K] in the splenic circulation stimulates local sensors that can directly induce a kaliuretic response through a phenomenon known as the feedforward mechanism.[7] This effect is blunted by loop diuretics such as bumetanide, suggesting that an Na-K-Cl cotransporter in the hepatoportal system signals the kidneys and consequently causes kaliuresis.[8,9] With low potassium intake the inverse occurs, possibly due to sensors in the gastric or hepatoportal circulation inactivating renal outer medullary [K] channels (ROMK).[10]

A positive [K] balance is necessary in neonates for somatic growth. This is achieved via maximal intestinal absorption of [K] and decreased renal excretion. There are experimental data demonstrating that the immature intestine absorbs [K] more avidly because of lower activity of the basolateral Na-K-ATPase and increased activity of apical [K] absorptive pumps (H-K-ATPase and Na-independent K-ATPase). As a consequence, a lower IC [K] promotes intestinal absorption in the neonate vs. secretion in the adult colon. This results in total body [K] retention with higher EC [K] in the neonate.[11,12]

Extrarenal Potassium Regulation

The [K] that is absorbed is rapidly shifted into the IC compartment preventing a dangerous rise in plasma [K]. This is due to coordination between active uptake by cells via Na-K-ATPase pump (principally in skeletal muscle) and passive back leak of [K] from the cells through [K] channels.[3] This mechanism is not fully developed in preterm neonates. Premature infants with hyperkalemia exhibit lower Na-K-ATPase activity associated with lower IC K–to–serum [K] ratios when compared to normokalemic premature infants.[13] These immature mechanisms are the most likely cause of nonoliguric hyperkalemia of premature infants, defined as a plasma [K$^+$] higher than 6.5 mEq/L within the first 72 hours of life in very low birth weight (birth weight lower than 1500 g) or very preterm (less than 32 weeks' postmenstrual age) infants in the presence of normal renal function for age.[14]

ß2 agonist and insulin regulate [K] by increasing IC uptake via stimulation of Na-K-ATPase pump, primarily in the skeletal muscle.[15] Metabolic acidosis reduces the activity of Na-K-ATPase decreasing [K] entry to the cell.

Renal Potassium Regulation

Potassium is freely filtered in the glomerulus. In the mature kidney 60%–70% is absorbed in the proximal tubule with sodium, chlorine, and fluid. At the thick ascending limb of the loop of Henle another 25% is reabsorbed primarily via Na-K-2Cl cotransporter. Immature kidneys preserve K.[3] Studies in humans have shown the ability of children to excrete a [K] load is decreased until 10–11 years of age.[11] This is important to ensure somatic growth.

GLOMERULAR FILTRATION

This is the initial step of renal [K] excretion and might play a role in premature infants. In adults and older children with advanced chronic kidney disease, once estimated glomerular filtration rate (GFR) is below 25 mL/min per 1.73 m^2, this low glomerular filtration of [K] may lead to clinical hyperkalemia. Almost all premature infants will have estimated GFR less than 25 during the first week of life and up to a month in those with very low birth weight (1.5 kg). Therefore, low GFR in neonates is a limiting factor for renal [K] excretion. However, even after correction for low GFR, clearances of [K] in this population are low, suggesting immature tubular handling.[16]

PROXIMAL TUBULE

Mature kidneys reabsorb about 60%–70% of filtered [K] primarily via paracellular pathways. This process is the result of solvent drag from sodium absorption via Na-K-ATPase.[17,18] The mean activity of Na-K-ATPase during the first week of life is one-third of the adult level until 7 weeks of age.[19] This lower activity results in a diminished solvent drag effect.

LOOP OF HENLE

Twenty-five percent of filtered [K] is absorbed through transcellular and paracellular pathways in the mature loop of Henle.[20] Na-K-ATPase at the basolateral membrane maintains a low IC [Na] driving this way the luminal Na-K-2Cl transporter (NKCC2).[21] High IC [K] promotes recycling into the lumen via the ROMK secretory [K] channel.[22] Consequently, this provides [K] for NKCC2 pump and keeps a positive intraluminal voltage that drives [K] absorption through paracellular pathways with magnesium and calcium jointly. IC [K] moves to the basolateral membrane cotransporter with Cl or via a [K] channel (see Fig. 5.1).

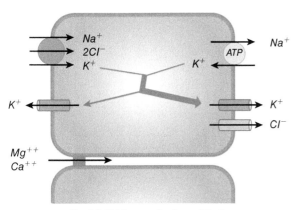

Fig. 5.1 Thick ascending loop of Henle.

ALDOSTERONE-SENSITIVE DISTAL NEPHRON

In this segment, Na-K-ATPase, apical [K] secretory channels and the epithelial sodium channel (ENaC) are responsible for net [K] secretion. ENaC absorbs sodium, creating a negative luminal charge favoring potassium efflux, which is further enhanced by high flow rates, probably a result of big conductance channel activation.[23–25]

Newborn infants exhibit high levels of aldosterone and renin; therefore, hyperkalemia and urinary sodium losses are the result of resistance to mineralocorticoids at the distal nephron.[26] Low renal expression of mineralocorticoid receptors in high aldosterone states was shown in human and mouse kidney at birth, which could explain in part this resistance.[27] As previously noted, activity of the Na-K-ATPase is as well very low during early development, resulting in high IC [Na] sodium and lowering apical sodium absorption and potassium secretion.[28] The ROMK (small conductance, calcium activated potassium (SK) channel) is responsible for basal [K] secretion from the thick ascending loop (TAL) through the CD. The large conductance calcium activated potassium channel (Maxi-K), or big conductance, channel is responsible for flow-dependent [K] secretion in the distal nephron mostly at the apical membrane of intercalated cells.[29–33]

The thiazide-sensitive NaCl cotransporter (NCC) located in the distal convoluted tubule (DCT) is very sensitive to EC [K] and has an important role in [K] excretion.[34] Although the DCT does not secrete [K] itself, it plays a major role regulating Na delivery to the CD, thereby regulating voltage-dependent [K] secretion

in that segment. This involves the with-no-lysine kinases (WNK) WNK1 and WNK 4, which activate NCC. Increased Na absorption in DCT decreases Na delivery and absorption in the CD, consequently decreasing [K] secretion. Conversely, high [K] intake inhibits NCC, causing decreased sodium absorption in the DCT and increased sodium delivery to the connecting tubule and CD. This causes activation of ENaC, which increases [K] secretion in the CD.[35] Maturation of the with-no-lysine kinases WNK1 and WNK 4 was characterized in a study using in situ hybridization in mouse tissue and showed more prominent renal expression of WNK1 in the postnatal period compared with embryos.[36–38]

Premature infants, especially those less than 30 weeks, have decreased transtubular [K] gradient (TTKG).[39] Data from rabbits showed absent [K] secretion at birth and initial appearance by 4 weeks, reaching maturity by 6 weeks.[40] Other studies have shown an increase in ROMK channel activity between 2 and 5 weeks of age.[41] In human fetuses ENaC expression is limited until 32 weeks, when expression increases. The abilities to absorb sodium seem to precede [K] secretion maturation.[42]

H-K-ATPASE

The H-K-ATPase pump absorbs [K] in exchange for protons in the CCD. Potassium depletion induces upregulation of alpha-2c subunit of H-K-ATPase pump (HKα2) for [K] preservation. In neonatal rats, messenger RNA and protein expression of one of the splice variants of HKα2 (HKα2c) is upregulated, but in adults it is undetectable. This suggests a mechanism favoring [K] absorption in the neonate.[43]

Hyperkalemia in the Neonate

Hyperkalemia in the neonatal period could be defined as a serum [K] higher than 6 mEq/L in full-term and higher than 6.5 mEq/L in premature infants. Very premature infants (less than 32 weeks of postmenstrual age) can have serum [K] > 6.5 mEq/L during the first week of life.[2,44] Hyperkalemia is life-threatening as it causes cardiac arrhythmias. Therefore, identification of its cause and treatment are essential to prevent complications.

The first step to identify the etiology of hyperkalemia is ruling out pseudohyperkalemia from in vitro hemolysis due to technical difficulties in obtaining an adequate blood sample. This is the most common source of an elevated [K$^+$] in the neonate, as K$^+$ is released from the red blood cells with hemolysis during or after blood sampling. In most instances, assessment of the degree of hemolysis in a blood sample is subjective, based on visual inspection of the color of the plasma. Therefore, all samples obtained by a heel stick, from fingertip, or after prolonged use of tourniquet should be considered a hemolyzed sample and should not be used to make therapeutic decisions. Other rare causes of pseudohyperkalemia are pathologically elevated platelet, leukocyte, or red blood cell counts in the blood sample.[45]

Nonoliguric hyperkalemia is common in the first 48–72 hours of life in the very preterm infant who has not been exposed to antenatal steroids, and its possibility should be anticipated in these infants.[1] It is thought to be the result of immaturity of the mechanisms that regulate internal distribution of potassium as previously described.[12] It is speculated that antenatal steroid upregulates Na-K-ATPase in cell membranes in the fetus. Because hyperkalemia can cause serious complications, it is important to monitor serum [K] during the first 72 hours of life in all very premature and very low birth weight infants.[46,47] During this period, [K] intake should be withheld until serum [K] is normal and is not rising.

Metabolic acidosis promotes shift of [K] from the cell to the EC space. Several medications can also promote cellular shifts of potassium. Succinylcholine, by depolarizing the muscle membrane, induces efflux of K$^+$ from the cell. Digoxin overdose and β_2 adrenergic blockers cause hyperkalemia by inhibiting Na-K-ATPase.[48] Other medications induce hyperkalemia by affecting angiotensin-aldosterone. Spironolactone is a mineralocorticoid antagonist. Indomethacin produces hyporeninemic hypoaldosteronism and decreases GFR. Angiotensin-converting enzyme inhibitors can block angiotensin II synthesis and the subsequent generation of aldosterone. Amiloride and trimethoprim inhibit ENaC, which reduces sodium reabsorption and [K] excretion.[49] Neonates are more susceptible to the effects of these medications as they have an already compromised Na-K-ATPase activity, ability to shift [K] into the cell, and the tubular response to mineralocorticoids.

Urinary potassium excretion is impaired with acute kidney injury and chronic kidney disease, primarily as a result of decreased glomerular filtration and resistance to aldosterone due to tubular injury.

Decreased aldosterone activity results from deficiency of or resistance to mineralocorticoids. Both result in variable degrees of metabolic acidosis, renal salt wasting, and hyperkalemia. Hypoaldosteronism occurs with congenital adrenal hyperplasia secondary to C-21-hydroxilase deficiency or 3 β-OL-dehydrogenate deficiency. These are relatively rare causes of hyperkalemia. Although detected in newborn screening programs, the results of the latter are not available before the onset of symptoms. Presenting signs include vomiting, salt wasting (which can lead to life-threatening dehydration), hyperkalemia, and virilization of females (with C-21-hydroxylase deficiency or hypospadias/ambiguous genitalia in males with 3 β-OL-dehydrogenate deficiency. Aldosterone synthase deficiency, a rare autosomal recessive disease, causes hypoaldosteronism due to defective biosynthesis of aldosterone. Patients present with salt wasting, recurrent dehydration, hyperkalemia, and failure to thrive. Neonatal screening fails to detect aldosterone synthase deficiency, for which patients are diagnosed when presenting with salt-wasting crisis.[50,51] Pseudohypoaldosteronism is another rare disorder that results from end-organ resistance to aldosterone, consequently causing high plasma aldosterone and renin. Type 1 is caused by a defect in the mineralocorticoid receptor and presents in the neonatal period with hypovolemia, hyponatremia, hyperkalemia, vomiting, failure to thrive, metabolic acidosis, and dehydration or shock.[52] Type 2 pseudohypoaldosteronism, also known as Gordon syndrome, is a rare form of familial hypertension caused by mutations in WNK kinases.[53] Patients typically present during adolescence with hypertension and hyperkalemic acidosis. Gordon syndrome responds to treatment with salt restriction and thiazide diuretics. Hypertension develops in late childhood, but the electrolyte disturbances (hyperkalemic acidosis) can be present from the neonatal period.[54]

Renal tubular acidosis type 4, which is characterized by hyperkalemia and metabolic acidosis, is a common finding in infants with urinary tract obstruction. Therefore, a renal ultrasound, looking for hydronephrosis, should be done in a every infant with hyperkalemia.[55,56]

Caution must be exercised with excessive oral or intravenous [K] supplementation/nutrition, medications with [K] salts, or blood transfusions in clinical circumstances in which renal [K] secretion is limited.

On the other hand, an endogenous [K] load results from tissue breakdown, as in hemolysis, gastrointestinal bleeding, and tissue necrosis. An example of an endogenous [K] load is a cephalohematoma, although hyperkalemia is a rare complication of cephalohematomas. The neonate usually has high urine [K] excretion, adequate intake of K, and onset/recession of hyperkalemia during the presence and resection of cephalohematoma.[57]

EVALUATION OF NEONATAL HYPERKALEMIA

As noted previously, pseudohyperkalemia should always be considered and the blood collection technique identified.

The evaluation of hyperkalemia starts with an ECG to check for life-threatening signs. Initial ECG changes are prolonged PR interval and peaked T waves, followed by absence of P wave and widened QRS with S-T depression and persistent peaked T waves. The QRS continues to widen as serum [K] increases until ventricular fibrillation develops.

In true hyperkalemia, plasma concentrations of sodium, chloride, bicarbonate, and creatinine should be measured as well as a complete blood count. If the GFR is normal and no other etiology is identified (e.g., nonoliguric hyperkalemia), hypoaldosteronism should be ruled out. In these patients, hyperkalemia will be accompanied by hyponatremia and metabolic acidosis. Despite its limitations, the TTKG could assist to discriminate between renal and extrarenal causes in term infants. The TTKG provides an indirect measure of the mineralocorticoid activity in the distal nephron and is calculated using the equation:

$$TTKG = \frac{(Urine\,[K])\,/\,(Plasma\,[K])}{(Urine\,Osmolality)\,/\,(Plasma\,Osmolality)}$$

The TTKG in preterm infants is low and does not correlate with plasma aldosterone. In children with hyperkalemia due to a nonrenal cause, the urinary [K] excretion is very high and, therefore, the TTKG is high (>11). In newborns with hypoaldosteronism and pseudohypoaldosteronism, the TTKG is very low (1.4–4.1).[58] When adrenal etiology is suspected, serum levels of aldosterone, renin, and cortisol should be measured. It is important to note that in states where urea excretion is high, urine sodium is low (<25 mEq/L) or the urine is not hypertonic compared with plasma TTKG should not be used.[59]

MANAGEMENT OF NEONATAL HYPERKALEMIA

Therapy targets for hyperkalemia are to prevent arrhythmias and to decrease the serum [K]. This can be achieved by stimulating IC shift of [K] or by body depletion. If the ECG shows changes consistent with hyperkalemia, the first step should be administration of calcium gluconate 10% at a dose of 0.5 mL/kg over 5–15 minutes for cardiac membrane stabilization (Fig. 5.2). The effect should be seen in 1–3 minutes and lasts for 30–60 minutes. An additional dose can be given after 5 minutes if ECG changes persist.[60] Insulin/glucose administration and albuterol nebulization shift [K] into the cell. Insulin can be administered at a dose of 0.1–0.6 units/kg per hour with glucose infusion of 0.5–1 g/kg per hour (5–10 mL/kg per hour of glucose 10%).[61] Onset of action is approximately 15 minutes and lasts a few hours. β agonists have a rapid onset of action. Albuterol can be administered by nebulizer at a dose of 400 μg to 2.5 mg diluted in 2 mL of normal saline.[62] This decreases plasma [K] by 0.5–1 mEq/L and is a great alternative for neonates as albuterol nebulizer is readily available in most neonatal intensive care units. Intravenous albuterol at a dose of 4 μg/kg, given slowly over 5 minutes, decreases plasma [K] by 0.9–1.5 mEq/L.[63,64] If metabolic acidosis is present, sodium bicarbonate infusion can also promote [K] shifting into the cell. It should be given judiciously due to it being hyperosmolar and the potential association with intraventricular hemorrhages in premature infants.[65–67] A dose of 1 mEq/kg diluted 1:4 in sterile water, administered over 30–60 minutes to decrease the adverse hemodynamic effects, is recommended. To remove body [K] stores, if the patient is making urine, one could use loop or thiazide diuretics. For severe, unremitting hyperkalemia, dialysis is required. The use of resins (sodium polystyrene 1 g/kg orally or as enema) is of questionable efficacy in neonates.[68] Moreover, because of its risk of intestinal perforation and obstruction, it is contraindicated in infants with necrotizing enterocolitis or premature infants.[69,70] None of the newer [K] binders (patiromer sorbitex calcium and sodium zirconium cyclosilicate) are approved for use in neonates.

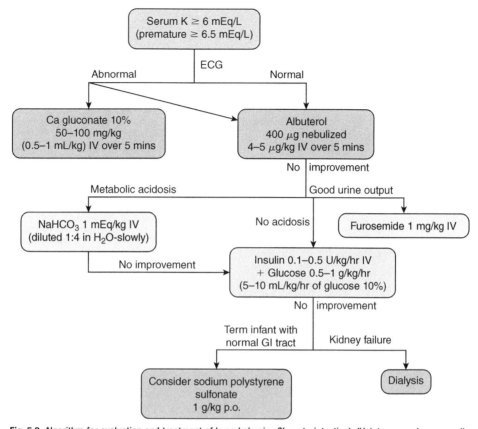

Fig. 5.2 Algorithm for evaluation and treatment of hyperkalemia. *GI,* gastrointestinal; *IV.,* intravenously; *p.o.,* orally.

REFERENCES

1. Lorenz JM, Kleinman LI, Markarian K. Potassium metabolism in extremely low birth weight infants in the first week of life. *J Pediatr.* 1997;131:81–86.
2. Omar SA, DeCristofaro JD, Agarwal BI, LaGamma EF. Effect of prenatal steroids on potassium balance in extremely low birth weight neonates. *Pediatrics.* 2000;106:561–567.
3. Bonilla-Félix M. Potassium regulation in the neonate. *Pediatr Nephrol.* 2017;32:2037–2049. doi:10.1007/s00467-017-3635-2
4. Agarwal R, Afzalpurkar R, Fordtran JS. Pathophysiology of potassium absorption and secretion by the human intestine. *Gastroenterology.* 1994;107:548–571.
5. Codina J, Pressley TA, DuBose TD Jr. Effect of chronic hypokalemia on H-K-ATPase expression in rat colon. *Am J Physiol.* 1997;272:F22–F30.
6. Giebisch G, Krapf R, Wagner C. Renal and extrarenal regulation of potassium. *Kidney Int.* 2007;72:397–410.
7. Rabinowitz L. Aldosterone and potassium homeostasis. *Kidney Int.* 1996;49:1738–1742.
8. Morita H, Fujiki N, Miyahara T, Lee K, Tanaka K. Hepatoportal bumetanide-sensitive K-sensor mechanism controls urinary K excretion. *Am J Physiol.* 2000;278:R1134–R1139.
9. Tsuchiya Y, Nakashima S, Banno Y, Suzuki Y, Morita H. Effect of high-NaCl or high-KCl diet on hepatic Na+- and K+-receptor

sensitivity and NKCC1 expression in rats. *Am J Physiol.* 2004; 286:R591–R596.
10. Chen P, Guzman JP, Leong PK, et al. Modest dietary K+ restriction provokes insulin resistance of cellular K+ uptake and phosphorylation of renal outer medulla K+ channel without fall in plasma K+ concentration. *Am J Physiol.* 2006;290:C1355–C1363.
11. Aizman R, Grahnquist L, Celsi G. Potassium homeostasis: ontogenic aspects. *Acta Pædiatr.* 1998;87:609–617.
12. Aizman R, Celsi G, Grahnquist L, Wang Z, Finkel Y, Aperia A. Ontogeny of K+ transport in rat distal colon. *Am J Physiol.* 1996;271:G268–G274.
13. Stefano JL, Norman ME, Morales MC, Goplerud JM, Mishra OP, Delivoria-Papadopoulos M. Decreased erythrocyte Na+,K+-ATPase activity associated with cellular potassium loss in extremely low birth weight infants with nonoliguric hyperkalemia. *J Pediatr.* 1993;122:276–284.
14. Sato K, Kondo T, Iwao H, Honda S, Ueda K. Internal potassium shift in premature infants: cause of nonoliguric hyperkalemia. *J Pediatr.* 1995;126:109–113.
15. Palmer BF. Regulation of potassium homeostasis. *Clin J Am Soc Nephrol.* 2015;10:1050–1060.
16. Vieux R, Hascoet JM, Merdariu D, Fresson J, Guillemin F. Glomerular filtration rate reference values in very preterm infants. *Pediatrics.* 2010;125:e1186–e1192.

17. Wareing M, Wilson RW, Kibble JD, Green R. Estimated potassium reflection coefficient in perfused proximal convoluted tubules of the anaesthetized rat in vivo. *J Physiol*. 1995;488:153–161.
18. Kibble JD, Wareing M, Wilson RW, Green R. Effect of barium on potassium diffusion across the proximal convoluted tubule of the anaesthetized rat. *Am J Physiol*. 1995;268:F778–F783.
19. Schwartz GJ, Evan AP. Development of solute transport in rabbit proximal tubule. III. Na-K-ATPase activity. *Am J Physiol*. 1984;246:F845–F852.
20. Palmer LG, Schnermann J. Integrated control of Na transport along the nephron. *Clin J Am Soc Nephrol*. 2015;10:676–687.
21. Mount DB. Thick ascending limb of the loop of Henle. *Clin J Am Soc Nephrol*. 2014;9:1974–1986.
22. Welling PA, Ho K. A comprehensive guide to the ROMK potassium channel: form and function in health and disease. *Am J Physiol*. 2009;29:F849–F863.
23. Kunau RT Jr, Webb HL, Borman SC. Characteristics of the relationship between the flow rate of tubular fluid and potassium transport in the distal tubule of the rat. *J Clin Invest*. 1974;54:1488–1495.
24. Engbretson BG, Stoner LC. Flow-dependent potassium secretion by rabbit cortical collecting tubule in vitro. *Am J Physiol*. 1987;253:F896–F903.
25. Carrisoza-Gaytan R, Carattino MD, Kleyman TR, Satlin LM. An unexpected journey: conceptual evolution of mechanoregulated potassium transport in the distal nephron. *Am J Physiol*. 2016;310:C243–C259.
26. Martinerie L, Pussard E, Foix-L'hélias L, et al. Physiological partial aldosterone resistance in human newborns. *Pediatr Res*. 2009;66:323–328.
27. Martinerie L, Viengchareun S, Delezoide AL, et al. Low renal mineralocorticoid receptor expression at birth contributes to partial aldosterone resistance in neonates. *Endocrinology*. 2009;150:4414–4424.
28. Schmidt U, Horster M. Na-K-activated ATPase: activity maturation in rabbit nephron segments dissected in vitro. *Am J Physiol*. 1977;233:F55–F60.
29. Wang WH, Woda CB, Bragin A, Kleyman TR, Satlin LM. Flow-dependent K+ secretion in the cortical collecting duct is mediated by a maxi-K channel. *Am J Physiol*. 2001;280:F786–F793.
30. Woda CB, Bragin A, Kleyman TR, Satlin LM. Flow-dependent K+ secretion in the cortical collecting duct is mediated by a maxi-K channel. *Am J Physiol*. 2001;280:F786–F793.
31. Satlin LM. Developmental regulation of expression of renal potassium secretory channels. *Curr Opin Nephrol Hypertens*. 2004;13:445–450.
32. Pácha J, Frindt G, Sackin H, Palmer LG. Apical maxi K channels in intercalated cells of CCT. *Am J Physiol*. 1991;261:F696–F705.
33. Nüsing RM, Pantalone F, Gröne HJ, Seyberth HW, Wegmann M. Expression of the potassium channel ROMK in adult and fetal human kidney. *Histochem Cell Biol*. 2005;123:553–559.
34. Velázquez H, Ellison DH, Wright FS. Chloride dependent potassium secretion in early and late renal distal tubules. *Am J Physiol*. 1987;253:F555–F562.
35. Ellison DH, Terker AS, Gamba G. Potassium and its discontents: new insight, new treatments. *J Am Soc Nephrol*. 2016;27:981–989.
36. Kahle KT, Wilson FH, Leng Q, et al. WNK4 regulates the balance between renal NaCl reabsorption and K+ secretion. *Nat Genet*. 2003;35:372–376.
37. O'Shaughnessy KM. Gordon syndrome: a continuing story. *Pediatr Nephrol*. 2015;30:1903–1908.
38. Shekarabi M, Lafrenière RG, Gaudet R, et al. Comparative analysis of the expression profile of Wnk1 and Wnk1/Hsn2 splice variants in developing and adult mouse tissues. *PLoS One*. 2013;8:e57807.
39. Nako Y, Ohki Y, Harigaya A, Tomomasa T, Morikawa A. Transtubular potassium concentration gradient in preterm neonates. *Pediatr Nephrol*. 1999;13:880–885.
40. Satlin LM. Postnatal maturation of potassium transport in rabbit cortical collecting duct. *Am J Physiol*. 1994;266:F57–F65.
41. Satlin LM, Palmer LG. Apical K+ conductance in maturing rabbit principal cell. *Am J Physiol*. 1997;272:F397–F404.
42. Delgado MM, Rohatgi R, Khan S, Holzman IR, Satlin LM. Sodium and potassium clearances by the maturing kidney: clinical-molecular correlates. *Pediatr Nephrol*. 2003;18:759–767.
43. Codina J, DuBose TD Jr. Molecular regulation and physiology of the H+, K+-ATPases in kidney. *Semin Nephrol*. 2006;26:345–351.
44. Chevalier RL. What are normal potassium concentrations in the neonate? What is a reasonable approach to hyperkalemia in the newborn with normal renal function? *Sem Nephrol*. 1998;18:360–361.
45. Ong YL, Deore R, El-Agnaf M. Pseudohyperkalaemia is a common finding in myeloproliferative disorders that may lead to inappropriate management of patients. *Int J Lab Hematol*. 2010;32:151–157.
46. Lehnhardt A, Markus J. Kemper MJ. Pathogenesis, diagnosis and management of hyperkalemia. *Pediatr Nephrol*. 2011;26:377–384.
47. Perazella MA. Trimethoprim-induced hyperkalaemia: clinical data, mechanism, prevention and management. *Drug Saf*. 2000;22:227–236.
48. White PC. Abnormalities of aldosterone synthesis and action in children. *Curr Opin Pediatr*. 1997;9:424–430.
49. White PC. Aldosterone synthase deficiency and related disorders. *Mol Cell Endocrinol*. 2004;217:81–87.
50. Sudeep K, Rajpoot SK, Maggi C, Bhangoo A. Pseudohypoaldosteronism in a neonate presenting as life-threatening arrhythmia. *Endocrinol Diabetes Metab Case Rep*. 2014;2014:130077.
51. O'Shaughnessy KM. Gordon syndrome: a continuing story. *Pediatr Nephrol*. 2015;30:1903–1908.
52. Gereda JE, Bonilla-Felix M, Kalil B, Dewitt SJ. Neonatal presentation of Gordon syndrome. *J Pediatr*. 1996;129:615–617.
53. Chung-Hsiang Y, Ming-Chou C, Jhao-Jhuang D, Shih-Hua L, Min-Hua T. Incidental hyperkalemia in the infant: answers. *Ped Nephrol*. 2021;36:1139–1141.
54. Shortland D, Trounce JQ, Levene MI. Hyperkalaemia, cardiac arrhythmias, and cerebral lesions in high risk neonates. *Arch Dis Child*. 1987;62:1139–1143.
55. Yaseen H. Nonoliguric hyperkalemia in neonates: a case-controlled study. *Am J Perinatol*. 2009;26:185–189.
56. Batlle DC, Arruda JA, Kurtzman NA. Hyperkalemic distal renal tubular acidosis associated with obstructive uropathy. *N Engl J Med*. 1981;304:373–380.
57. Rodríguez-Soriano J, Vallo A, Oliveros R, Castillo G. Transient pseudohypoaldosteronism secondary to obstructive uropathy in infancy. *J Pediatr*. 1983;103:375–380.
58. Rodriguez-Soriano J, Ubetagoyena M, Vallo A. Transtubular potassium concentration gradient: a useful test to estimate renal aldosterone bio-activity in infants and children. *Pediatr Nephrol*. 1990;4:105–110.

59. Kamel KS, Halperin ML. Intrarenal urea recycling leads to a higher rate of renal excretion of potassium: an hypothesis with clinical implications. *Curr Opin Nephrol Hypertens.* 2011;20: 547–554.
60. Masilamani K, van der Voort J. The management of acute hyperkalaemia in neonates and children. *Arch Dis Child.* 2012; 97:376–380.
61. Ditzenberger GR, Collins SD, Binder N. Continuous insulin intravenous infusion therapy for VLBW infants. *J Perinat Neonatal Nurs.* 1999;13:70–82.
62. Singh BS, Sadiq HF, Noguchi A, Keenan WJ. Efficacy of albuterol inhalation in treatment of hyperkalemia in premature neonates. *J Pediatr.* 2002;141:16–20.
63. Helfrich E, de Vries TW, van Roon EN. Salbutamol for hyperkalaemia in children. *Acta Paediatr.* 2001;90:1213–1216.
64. Yaseen H, Khalaf M, Dana A, Yaseen N, Darwich M. Salbutamol versus cation-exchange resin (kayexalate) for the treatment of nonoliguric hyperkalemia in preterm infants. *Am J Perinatol.* 2008;25:193–197.
65. Wigglesworth JS, Keith IH, Girling DJ, Slade SA. Hyaline membrane disease, alkali, and intraventricular haemorrhage. *Arch Dis Child.* 1976;51:755–762.
66. Papile LA, Burstein J, Burstein R, Koffler H, Koops B. Relationship of intravenous sodium bicarbonate infusions and cerebral intraventricular hemorrhage. *J Pediatr.* 1978;93:834–836.
67. Szpecht D, Szymankiewicz M, Nowak I, Gadzinowski J. Intraventricular hemorrhage in neonates born before 32 weeks of gestation-retrospective analysis of risk factors. *Childs Nerv Syst.* 2016;32:1399–1404.
68. Vemgal P, Ohlsson A. Interventions for non-oliguric hyperkalaemia in preterm neonates. *Cochrane Database Syst Rev.* 2012; 5:CD005257.
69. Ohlsson A, Hosking M. Complications following oral administration of exchange resins in extremely low-birth-weight infants. *Eur J Pediatr.* 1987;146:571–574.
70. Bennett LN, Myers TF, Lambert GH. Cecal perforation associated with sodium polystyrene sulfonate-sorbitol enemas in a 650 grams infant with hyperkalemia. *Am J Perinatol.* 1996;13:167–170.

Chapter 6

Physiological Management of Fluid and Electrolyte Therapy in Newborns

Steven Ringer, MD, PhD

Chapter Outline

Introduction

Water is critical to the support of all life, and ensuring appropriate balance of fluid and electrolytes is a central aspect of the clinical management of patients. It has been extremely difficult to study and define optimal fluid and electrolyte management in premature infants, despite the fact that this is a population that is essentially completely dependent on what is administered. Study in this area is difficult because each individual patient is different, the impact of maturation changes with each day of gestational age (GA) or postnatal age, and environmental factors and clinical conditions are quite variable.

Management should be based on understanding the basic physiological processes and particular environmental factors in each case and then making judgments about the impact of these factors on an individual patient. It is equally important to then monitor each patient, to assess the infant's individual fluid and electrolyte status, and then to empirically adjust therapy and reassess at a later time point. This pattern of repeated refinements as needed is continued until clinical stability is assured, and the frequency of these assessments is determined by individual factors including GA birth weight and environment. These and other variables make it almost impossible to make perfect calculations of fluid and electrolyte needs at one point in time. At the same time, it is encouraging to understand that the system is dynamic, and most often even the most immature kidneys will function well enough to aid in achieving homeostasis.

Water and electrolyte homeostasis in newborn infants is variable because each patient's status is affected by numerous factors, including GA, postnatal physiological changes in renal function, altered response to hormones, redistribution of total body water (TBW), and water loss secondary to environmental factors including the use of radiant warmers or humidified environments. The water content of the newborn is higher than that of the adult, ranging from 73% to 80% in term and premature infant, to as high as 90% in infants of 23 weeks' gestation.[1] As a result, management of neonatal fluid and electrolyte therapy is challenging, as these factors and the clinical setting need to be accounted for while caring for neonates, especially preterm infants.

Examples that demonstrate how the understanding of physiology can be translated into clinical practice are interspersed within the following discussion. A few caveats and principles are worth noting:

1. Not every situation can be illustrated.
2. The best fluid management depends on calculations based on physiology and to some extent, reasonable approximations. It is essential to follow up any therapy or changes with repeat laboratory determinations and to then adjust that therapy based on the individual patient.
3. It is unnecessary to attempt to put too fine a point on calculations. The system is dynamic and even the immature kidney has mechanisms that are aimed at achieving homeostasis (see following discussion). Maturation is ongoing as each day passes and, in most instances, renal function changes progressively.

Neonatal Management Is Uniquely Difficult

Water and electrolyte physiology are primarily dependent on renal function and the balance between fluid intake and fluid losses. In the newborn period, there is an increased risk of derangements in water and electrolyte homeostasis, in large part because the intake and environment are completely controlled by caregivers, and there are progressive changes in body water components, functional immaturity of the neonatal kidney, and skin that are rapidly evolving. Newborns have increased insensible water losses and a greater dependence on environment compared with older patients, and they lack the ability to independently access water. The magnitude of postnatal diuresis, immaturity of renal function, and insensible fluid loss all increase as GA decreases. Water and electrolyte balance are of course integrally linked, but to better understand the basic physiologic mechanisms that regulate them, it is worth considering them separately at first.

PROGRESSIVE CHANGES IN TOTAL BODY WATER

TBW is composed of extracellular fluid (ECF), which includes intravascular and interstitial fluid and intracellular fluid. The amount of TBW as a percentage of body weight and its distribution in various fluid compartments vary with GA. In a newborn term infant, the TBW is 75% of the body weight as compared with 80% in an infant born at 27 weeks' gestation and may be as high as 90% in the most immature infants at 22–23 weeks' gestation. ECF volumes are 45% and 70%, respectively.[1]

Water in the newborn is the balance between intake (which also includes the tiny amount of water derived from metabolism) and losses including insensible water loss and urine losses (including the tiny amounts for stool and negligible water for growth in the days immediately following birth). Functionally this means that the fluid balance can be considered as the difference between intake and the sum of insensible and urine losses. This difference is reflected in weight loss or gain.

After birth, there is a physiologic, isotonic diuresis of ECF resulting in an expected weight loss during the first week of life,[2,3] and this weight loss is essentially the difference in water balance. The mechanism for this necessary diuresis and the relative loss of weight is as yet not identified, but the percent of weight loss decreases with increasing GA. Preterm infants normally lose 10% to 15% of birth weight, and term[4] breastfed infants average about a 5% loss of birth weight in the first day.[5] The postnatal diuresis is approximately 1 to 3 mL/kg per hour in term infants and is greater in preterm infants.[6] Since fluid administration in these infants is entirely regulated by caregivers, recognition of this normal physiologic fluid loss is a major determinant for fluid management. In addition, other concomitant fluid losses vary depending on the clinical setting. As a result, monitoring of intake and output is important to ensure adequate fluid intake. For the term infant, prior to discharge, parents are counseled on assessing intake and urinary output, and a follow-up appointment is scheduled within 48 to 72 hours after discharge to monitor weight loss and fluid intake.

FLUID AND ELECTROLYTES IN THE PREMATURE INFANT

Prospective studies involving very low birth weight infants (birth weight ≤ 1500 g) and extremely low birth weight infants (birth weight ≤ 1000 g) have demonstrated a consistent pattern of fluid and sodium homeostasis despite varying intakes of sodium and water over the first 5 to 7 days of life.[7] In this study infants were randomized to different fluid regimens intended to produce different degrees of negative water balance. When infants with birth weights of 750–1000 g were allowed a weight loss of 1%–2% per day (up to 10% during the first 5 days of life), their mean weight loss was only marginally smaller than that in the group allowed a 3%–5% weight loss per day (up to 15% during the first 5 days of life), despite a much higher fluid intake. This demonstrates that negative water balance in the first few days of life is physiologic and that even immature kidneys that are capable of compensating for varying fluid intakes at least to some degree. There was no difference in rates of major morbidities including patent ductus arteriosus, bronchopulmonary dysplasia, intraventricular hemorrhage, and necrotizing enterocolitis, and the mortality rates were similar.

In another study,[8] premature infants (23–33 weeks) were randomized to receive either 60–70 mL/kg per day on day 1, increasing to 150 mL/kg per day by day 7, or to an intake restricted to 80% of these volumes. Weight loss and both short- and long-term morbidities were similar between the groups. These results demonstrate that as long as regimens allow for contraction of the ECF and a goal weight loss of 6%–12% without hypernatremia, it is not possible to define a single optimal approach. When the postnatal weight loss is prevented[9,10] by high rates of fluid administration, the risks of bronchopulmonary dysplasia or death may be increased.

Shaffer and Meade[11] randomized infants to 1 or 3 mEq/kg per day of sodium intake over the first 10 days of life and found no difference between the groups in weight loss, decrease in extracellular volume, or sodium balance. This demonstrates that, as with water intake, negative sodium balance is physiologic in the first week of life and that even immature kidneys are capable of compensating for varying sodium intakes at least to some degree.

The underlying physiology of the early water, sodium, and weight loss in premature infants occurs in three sequential phases of water and sodium changes[12]:
- Prediuretic phase—The first day after birth is characterized by oliguria (<1 mL/kg per hour) with low glomerular filtration rate (GFR) and low fractional excretion of sodium (FENa). There is a normal rise in sympathetic nervous system activity that results from the processes of birth, including the changes in temperature and cardiac output. This leads to increased renal vascular resistance and the suppression of renal blood flow and decreased GFR. Fluid requirements are much lower on this day, and there is little need for supplemental sodium administration.
- Diuretic and natriuretic phase—On days 2 to 3 after birth, urine output and sodium losses normally increase abruptly along with sodium losses. The reabsorption of lung fluid leads to an increase in the ECF volume, which results in an inhibition of renal sympathetic activity. Renal vascular resistance decreases, causing an increase in GFR, FENa, and urine output and resulting in negative water and sodium balance. Weight loss during this phase is both normal and expected, and urine output may exceed the level of 2 mL/kg per hour (45 mL/kg per day) that is expected with later equilibration. Caregivers should be vigilant to neither interfere with this nor to ignore possible causes should it fail to occur.
- Postdiuretic phase—On days 4 to 5 urine output is more directly dependent on fluid intake, and the ongoing equilibration of the ECF volume results in a reduction of GFR and FENa compared with the prior phase. Weight loss due to fluid shifts becomes smaller during this phase.
- These phases unfold in the patient with otherwise normal renal function and blood pressure.
- Illnesses, including but not limited to hypoxic ischemic injury, hypotension, and infection, may significantly disrupt these stages. Fluid management must be appropriately adjusted as necessary.

WATER LOSSES

As noted previously, water loss occurs primarily through insensible losses (via the skin and respiratory tract) and renal output. Sensible water loss from the skin (sweating) is negligible in newborn infants.[13] The absolute and relative amounts of water loss through these routes change with GA and postnatal age. Other sources of fluid losses may include stool (usually negligible in the first several days) and those losses that are unique to individual patients, such as gastric or ileostomy drainage or thoracostomy output.

Skin

Evaporation through the skin is a major component of insensible water losses in newborns. Rates of loss are highest in extremely low birth weight (<1000 g) infants with very thin skin (increased skin permeability). In addition, the surface area–to–body volume (related to body weight) ratio increases with decreasing GA and size, resulting in increased rates of fluid loss per kilogram body weight.

As the skin matures with increasing GA and postnatal age, these evaporative losses diminish, and with growth the surface area–to–volume ratio ultimately decreases as well. The impact of skin maturity is less significant for infants born after 28 weeks' GA and even less for more mature infants. Progressive changes in the skin contribute to a marked diminution in these losses by about 1 week after birth. As an example, insensible water loss in an infant born at 24 weeks' gestation may be as high as 200 mL/kg per day in the first 24–48 hours compared with a loss of 20 mL/kg per day for a term infant, but will be only a fraction of that amount by 7–10 days.[14] There are less common conditions in which skin integrity is compromised (e.g., epidermolysis bullosa, abdominal wall defect)[15–17] and insensible skin losses will be very high.

Environmental factors can contribute to increased insensible losses, although many are less commonly used than previously. Radiant warmers for care may increase evaporative water loss by approximately 50%,[18] although this can be mitigated by introducing humidification and covering the bed with plastic wrap.[19] With the introduction of hybrid incubators, these warmers are rarely used in care.[20] These modern incubators include systems for humidification, which reduces the water losses significantly, but not entirely.[21]

Older heat-emitting phototherapy devices also increase transepidermal water loss,[22,23] but these too are much less commonly employed in care today. The newer devices employ high-intensity gallium nitride light-emitting diode phototherapy, which have no effect on transepidermal water loss.[24]

Most neonatal units aim to provide higher levels of ambient humidity, which reduces the insensible losses

from the respiratory system. In ambient humidity, about half of insensible losses are from the respiratory system in spontaneously breathing term infants.[25,26] Respiratory insensible water loss is independent of GA,[27] although the portion of insensible water loss that is respiratory is less because transepidermal water loss is less. Insensible water loss via the respiratory tract increases as respiratory rate rises. Respiratory losses are decreased for infants who are cared for in humidified air and are especially low in those who are intubated and mechanically ventilated using humidified gases. This is also true for continuous positive airway pressure and high-flow systems that include humidification, but in all cases the amount of respiratory water loss increases at lower gestational age. In comparison, however, the major losses in these immature infants are transepidermal.[26]

Changes in care practices themselves may also impact water losses. The antenatal administration of glucocorticoids to women with threatened premature deliveries affects organ maturation that extends to the skin and kidneys. In one report, infants who were exposed to antenatal glucocorticoids had lower insensible water loss, less hypernatremia, and an earlier diuresis and natriuresis over the first several days after birth than a similar group of infants who were unexposed, presumably due to accelerated maturation of the skin.[28] In vitro studies have demonstrated that glucocorticoid exposure results in maturation of ion channels in the proximal renal tubular epithelium,[29,30] and other reports have noted that accelerated renal maturation and upregulation of sodium-potassium ATPase (Na-K-ATPase) activity may be the mechanism by which glucocorticoid exposure prevents nonoliguric hyperkalemia.[31]

RENAL FUNCTION

Neonatal renal function varies between patients and changes over time for each individual patient. Especially in the premature infant, the kidneys are developmentally immature and function improves with increasing GA. In addition, the postnatal hemodynamic changes that follow birth affect function, and these are impacted by GA and illness severity.

Developmental immaturity has greater impact in the more immature preterm infant, and it can result in water and electrolyte imbalance by impacting the GFR and the ability to concentrate urine. The balance between the reabsorption of sodium and bicarbonate and the secretion of potassium and hydrogen is also affected by the shorter length of renal tubules, and thus there is a greater risk of derangement in the levels of these critical electrolytes.

The newborn kidney is limited in the ability to create a medullary osmotic gradient needed for the concentration of urine, in part because of the anatomically shortened loop of Henle. This limits the countercurrent multiplication needed to form the osmotic gradient from the corticomedullary junction to the inner medulla. As a result, the maximum level of urine concentration is only 400 mOsmol/kg in the first few days after birth (and only about 300 mOsmol/kg in the premature infant), with maturation to 1200 mOsmol/kg at 1 year of age.[32] The relatively low levels of sodium and protein in human milk and premature formula and the typically anabolic metabolic state result in lower concentration of osmolar molecules (e.g., urea) to be excreted, and the obligate urine volume is at least 50 mL/kg per day per risk for hypovolemia and hypernatremia. Fluid intake must be adequate to account for these renal losses as well as insensible losses noted previously.

The immature kidney also has a diminished response to antidiuretic hormone (ADH) because of immaturity and reduced surface area in the tubules and a lack of activation of ADH receptors. Water permeability in the collecting tubules is diminished, and as a result urine concentration is limited. Maturation of ADH response is, like most aspects, inversely related to GA.[33]

In all infants the maturation of concentrating ability increases after birth, but the pace of this maturation is lower in infants of lower GA. Understanding these processes allows caregivers to assess the status of each individual patient and adjust the intake of water and electrolytes as needed.

ELECTROLYTE BALANCE

Sodium reabsorption is limited in the neonatal kidney, primarily due to tubular immaturity and tubuloglomerular imbalance, both of which improve as GA increases. It is further affected by reduced responsiveness to aldosterone.[34-36] Sodium, bicarbonate, and potassium are all dependent on the Na-K-ATPase pump located on the basolateral membrane of various sections of the tubule and membrane transporters, and the expression and function of this pump are immature in the newborn, especially in premature infants born before 32 weeks. As a result, sodium resorption is decreased[37] and the FENa is as high as 5% in infants less than 30 weeks' gestation. It does mature as GA increases, dropping to about 2% in term infants.

The reduced activity and expression of the Na-K-ATPase pump also results in a lower resorptive threshold for bicarbonate of 19–21 mmol/L in term infants and as low as 16–20 mmol/L in premature infants. This, along with reduced activity of carbonic anhydrase and the sodium-hydrogen antiporter, results in lower serum bicarbonate levels in the newborn.[38,39]

The diminished activity of the Na-K-ATPase pump also results in decreased potassium excretion in the newborn, exacerbated by the decreased responsiveness to aldosterone and the lower Glomerular Filtration Rate (GFRA). As a result, newborns, including especially premature newborns, normally have higher levels of serum potassium than those in older infants, especially in the first several days after birth, putting them at higher risk of clinically significant hyperkalemia.[40]

Renal function in the newborn is also significantly impacted by the reduction in GFR. The embryogenesis of the kidney is complete at about 35 weeks' gestation when between 0.6 and 1.2 million nephrons are present. At lower GAs there are proportionately fewer nephrons, and as a result the GFR is proportionately reduced. A full-term infant has a GFR of about 26 mL/min per 1.73 m^2, and the reduced nephron number in an infant of 27 weeks' gestation results in a GFR that is about one half that value. GFR does rise after birth as renal vascular resistance decreases. In the term infant, the GFR will double over the first 2 weeks, and the increase in the very premature infant is only about 25%, increasing from 13.0 to 16.2 mL/min/m^2 in the first 2 weeks of life.[41]

The use of serum creatinine (SCr) to assess renal function and GFR is hampered by variations resulting from maturity and postnatal age. The SCr concentration at birth is essentially the same as the maternal value, and in term infants it falls rapidly to low values (SCr 0.2–0.4 mg/dL [18–35 μmol/L]) by 7–14 days. In preterm newborns, SCr may actually increase shortly after birth, then decline (Bateman DA, Thomas W, Parravicini E, Polesana E, Locatelli C, Lorenz JM. Patterns of change in SCr concentration in very low birth weight infants with uncomplicated clinical courses during the first 2 months of life. *Pediatr Res.* 2015;77:696–702). It may take up to 2 months to reach normal baseline. Abnormal change in SCr for GA and postnatal age over time may be helpful in the diagnosis of renal injury. In preterm infants, blood urea nitrogen is not a reliable marker for renal function or protein intolerance, especially for infants who receive parenteral amino acid.[42–44]

Monitoring and Management

FLUID MANAGEMENT

Fluid and electrolyte management in the newborn is guided by several physiologic changes that occur at birth and the impact of ongoing maturation determined by GA and postnatal age. Both the clinical setting and environmental factors must be taken into consideration as well. To adequately assess the patient and adjust fluid and electrolyte management effectively, several aspects of monitoring are important.

Determination of fluid need depends on an assessment of likely fluid losses. Key information includes GA and an assessment of skin maturity, as well as the environmental factors such as use of humidified gases or incubators or the rare use of a radiant warmer.

Especially in the first several days, body weight should be measured at least daily to aid in the assessment of fluid balance. As stressed previously, fluid administration should be done in a manner that allows for the expected physiologic weight loss in the first several days of life of 5% to 10% in term infants (roughly 1% per day)[1] and as high as 15% in preterm infants (2% per day).[45] The absence of this normal weight loss, or a weight gain over the first few days, usually suggests excess fluid intake that must be adjusted.

A reasonable goal in fluid management is to calculate intake to allow weight to reach a nadir at approximately 3 to 4 days after birth, mirroring the physiology. With fluids and nutrition the weight should then rebound to near birth weight by 7 days, although a significant percentage of otherwise normal infants may not regain birth weight for 14 days or longer. Serum sodium provides a guide to hydration status if sodium intake is balanced against losses. Because fluid intake is normalized to body weight and as weight normally decreases after birth, there is a risk of inadvertently providing less and less intake as weight decreases. Most neonatal units employ the convention of using birth weight for calculations for the first 7 days or until it is regained.

Monitoring will permit caregivers to appropriately readjust fluid and electrolyte intake as required. Weight gain and a low serum sodium concentration in the first few days suggests excess body water (i.e., volume overload). In infants with diminished renal function, volume overload may also manifest with an increase in blood pressure and peripheral edema. Weight loss in excess of expected suggests inadequate fluid intake, often accompanied by an elevated sodium concentration, tachycardia, and poor capillary refill. Blood pressure is initially preserved even in the early stages of shock.

In certain illnesses, such as sepsis or ileus, third spacing of fluid may occur. Typical signs may include an increase in weight, without evidence of peripheral edema, and a decrease in serum sodium concentration.

INTAKE AND OUTPUT

A general approach to fluid management is illustrated by the following example. An infant is born at 27 weeks' gestation weighing 1000 g and is breathing spontaneously in a humidified incubator. The caregivers estimate that a 3% weight loss per day should be expected over the first few days after birth. The input is calculated to exceed the renal output plus estimated insensible fluid needs of the infant (based on the GA and environmental setting) minus the expected or anticipated weight loss. Administered fluids include initial parenteral nutrition to provide 2 g/kg of protein per day and minimal sodium intake of 2 mEq/kg per day with no added potassium. Obligate urine volume is a function of renal solute load and maximum renal concentration capacity. The NaCl provides a solute load of 4 mOsm/kg per day and the protein will be metabolized to about 12 mOsm/kg of urea. To excrete this solute load in a urine that can be maximally concentrated to 300 mOsm/L, the urine volume will need to be 16 (12 mOsm/kg per day)/300 mOsm/L = 0.053 L /kg or 53 mL of urine per day for this 1-kg infant. If the insensible water losses are estimated at 50 mL/kg per day, the caregivers should administer (53 mL/kg per day + 50 mL/kg per day) − 30 mL/kg per day (desired weight loss) = 73 mL/kg per day. Given that many estimates are included in this calculation, the rate could be rounded to 70 mL/kg per day for ease in administration.

The key to optimal management is to make reasonable estimates and then adjust by frequent assessment of output and electrolyte levels. In our example of this extremely premature infant, it may be that the skin permeability is greater than estimated, such that the insensible losses are really 70 mL/kg per day. The infant's weight will decrease by 5% (too rapidly) in 1 day and the measured serum sodium level may increase. The intake for the subsequent day should be adjusted to replete the fluid loss and avoid further excess losses.

Serial serum sodium determinations should be done to monitor fluid and electrolyte balance, especially in ill and or extremely premature neonates. Along with body weight measurements, caregivers can then determine the etiology of serum sodium derangements. Because sodium losses and requirements are low in the first days after birth, most alterations in serum sodium concentrations reflect water imbalance rather than abnormal sodium losses or intake. Thus, hyponatremia suggests excess free water (hypervolemia) and hypernatremia suggests depletion of free water or dehydration (hypovolemia). Measurement of urine sodium losses can confirm this suggestion but will be misleading if these losses are measure after the onset of diuresis/natriuresis. In any case, elucidation of the cause of perturbations in serum sodium concentration must always take into account estimation of *both* sodium and water balance.

The frequency at which serum sodium should be measured should be based on the estimated risk of abnormalities, GA, and postnatal age, as well as the infant's clinical condition. Extremely premature infants with diminished skin integrity may require monitoring as frequently as every 6 to 8 hours over the first 2 to 3 days after birth, although daily determinations are adequate as GA increases.[46] As soon as clinical stability is established, the frequency of monitoring should be reduced.

ADJUSTMENTS IN FLUID ADMINISTRATION

Repeated or daily calculation of fluid and electrolyte requirements must account for correction of identified fluid abnormalities (deficit of water or excess water) and ongoing maintenance requirements. Maintenance fluid requirements are those needed for neutral water balance after accounting for obligatory losses (e.g., urine and stool) and insensible losses (e.g., skin and lungs). Requirements will be influenced by factors that include GA and postnatal age, environmental temperature and humidity, renal function, and ventilator dependence (which affects respiratory water losses). In specific cases, excessive or additional losses of other fluids, such as ileostomy or gastric drainage and thoracostomy output, must also be measured and replaced.

Management should be adjusted at appropriate frequency to permit corrections and avoid allowing derangements to reach critical levels. Changes in clinical condition (for example, septic shock) may manifest with acute changes in cardiovascular status such as tachycardia and poor perfusion. When severe, extracellular water deficits may require prompt partial correction with boluses of normal saline. Renal dysfunction or acute kidney injury may be associated with decreased urine output and weight gain. Fluid administration should be restricted until the condition improves. Abnormally high urine output with normal intake suggests a defect in renal concentrating ability (that may be GA associated) or an inherent renal tubular disorder. In these cases, fluid administration rates must be increased until balance is achieved.

ELECTROLYTE MAINTENANCE

Maintenance requirements for sodium, potassium, and chloride are approximately 2–3 mEq/kg per day. There is no need for these electrolytes, and they generally are not given intravenously during the first 48 hours after birth because of the low initial urinary excretion expected during this period and the risk of nonoliguric hypernatremia in extremely preterm infants. Sodium is added with the onset of diuresis/natriuresis if serum sodium concentration is not rising as body weight decreases; potassium is added when urine output is adequate and serum potassium intake is not increasing. In individual patients, additional deficits of electrolytes are replaced based on estimates or measurements of the actual losses. Gastric fluid typically contains 20–80 mEq/L sodium, 5–20 mEq/L potassium, and 100–150 mEq/L chloride, and fluid from the small bowel contains 100–140 mEq/L sodium, 5–15 mEq/L potassium, 90–130 mEq/L chloride, and 40–75 mEq/L bicarbonate. Thoracostomy drainage has an electrolyte composition that is similar to serum. These are reasonable initial estimates; monitoring of serum levels will allow for refined calculations.

EXAMPLE FLUID ORDERS

Some examples of standard fluid orders may illustrate how the physiologic principles are applied in fluid management. Newborns are typically given 10% glucose concentration to provide normal glucose requirements (4–7 mg/kg per minute) while limiting overall fluid volume, but extremely premature infants are often intolerant of these rates of glucose administration and will require 5% glucose concentration as the base fluid. Infants born at GA less than 30–32 weeks will receive fluids as parenteral nutrition, the details of which are beyond the scope of this discussion. IV pumps usually dispense fluid in increments as small as 0.1 mL/h, so fluid rates should be rounded to one decimal place.

A. For a 28-week-gestation infant, 1.1 kg, similar to the example given previously:
   a. Day of birth, fluids are begun IV 10 percent dextrose in water (D10W) at 80/mL/kg per day. For this infant, this is 80 × 1.1 = 88 mL per day, or 3.7 mL/h. The estimate is based on an expected weight loss of 2%–3% or 25–30 g, which is fluid loss. The estimated insensible loss in a humidified environment is 60 mL/kg per day. Assuming maximum urine concentration of 300 mOsm/L and a solute load of 16 mOsm from urea and small amounts of sodium in flushes and so on, the urine volume will be about 53 mL/kg per day, so total losses are about 110 mL/kg. Administering 80 mL/kg per day should allow about a 30-g weight loss.
   b. Day 1–2 has good urine output as infant enters the diuretic phase. Fluids are increased to 100 mL/kg per day and electrolytes added to give infant ~ 3 mEq/kg per day of sodium per kilogram and 2 mEq/kg per day of potassium. For this infant, that is 3.3 of sodium and 2.2 mEq of potassium.

Since fluid total is 110 mL/d, the required sodium concentration is 3.3 mEq/110 mL or 3 mEq/100 mL. Similarly, for potassium, a concentration of 2 mEq/100 mL will supply the planned 2.2 mEq. If the pharmacy convention is to provide fluids in 250-mL bags, the order should read:
   D10W plus 7.5 mEq Na (as chloride) and 5 mEq K (as chloride) per 250 mL. Please run at 110 mL/d, or 4.6 mL/h.

B. For a term infant, 3.4 kg:
   a. Day of birth, fluids IV D10W at 80 mL/kg per day. For this infant, this is 3.4 × 80 = 272 mL/d, so order should be D10W at 11.3 mL/h.
   b. Day 1–2, urine output has been good, and fluids are increased to 100 mL/kg per day. Measured electrolytes are normal, but excretion will continue so electrolytes are added to provide 3 mEq/kg per day of sodium and 2 mEq/kg per day of potassium. For this infant that is 10.2 mEq/d of sodium and 6.8 mEq/d of potassium. Fluid volume per day is 340 mL (3.4 × 100), so sodium concentration is 10.2 mEq Na/340 mL= 3 mEq Na per 100 mL and potassium concentration is 6.8 mEq/340 mL = 2 mEq K/100 mL. As previously, this is given in D10W, so the order for a 250 mL bag will be: D10W plus 7.5 mEq Na (as chloride) and 5 mEq K (as chloride) per 250 mL. Please run at 100 mL/kg per day = 14.2 mL/h.

Sodium Balance Disorders

HYPONATREMIA

It can be difficult to maintain the balance between sodium and water in extremely premature infants with birth weights < 1000 g.[47] The most common causes of aberrant levels are discussed here.

Hyponatremia (serum sodium concentration of 128 mEq/L or less) in the first several days after birth is almost always the result of excessive free water intake with a normal total body sodium, because sodium losses are minimal at this time. Correction usually occurs if fluid volume is reduced and the normal physiologic diuresis occurs. Water retention may rarely result from the syndrome of inappropriate ADH related to severe illnesses such as pneumonia, meningitis, pneumothorax, or severe intraventricular hemorrhage.[48] This aberration is initially treated by markedly restricting water intake and making serial readjustments based on measured sodium levels.

If adequate sodium content is not added to fluids beyond the first few days after birth, hyponatremia may result when renal sodium losses are proportionately greater than total water loss during the postnatal diuresis/natriuresis. After diuresis/natriuresis, hyponatremia in the absence of fluid retention is due to inadequate sodium intake. Measurement of urine sodium levels is often helpful to confirm this condition and estimate the magnitude of the losses during the postdiuretic phase, aiding in the calculation of how much additional sodium should be administered to replete the deficit. One can calculate the existing deficit from the product of the TBW volume times the sodium deficit per liter (140 minus the serum sodium concentration). The TBW volume is approximately the volume of distribution of sodium because of the rapid osmotic equilibration between the extracellular and intracellular fluid. Although the TBW is usually about 75% or higher in the newborn, the conventional approach is to use an estimated volume of distribution of 60% to ensure that the correction occurs in a slow controlled manner. It is important to include normal maintenance requirements in addition to the calculated deficit.

For example, a 2-week-old 0.9-kg infant has a serum sodium level of 127 after receiving furosemide therapy. Urinary sodium losses during that therapy were greater than the amount the infant is receiving in her intravenous fluids, which is her sole source of fluids at this time. Now that diuretic therapy has completed, her TBW is not in excess and her ongoing urinary sodium losses are 2.5 mEq/kg per day or (2.5 × 0.9 kg) = 2.25 mEq per day. Her fluids are being administered at 130 mL/kg per day. To correct her sodium deficit, you calculate her total sodium deficit using a "desired" level of 140 as the goal. Since her volume of distribution for sodium is estimated as 0.6, you calculate her total body sodium deficit as follows: (goal Na – actual Na) × weight × volume of distribution or (140 − 127) × 0.9 × 0.6 = 7.02 mEq Na.

You want to correct this slowly and choose to do this over 36 hours to avoid rapid fluid shifts. Thus, you will add an additional 7 mEq to 36 hours' worth of fluids or an additional 4.7 mEq per day. She is receiving 130 mL/kg per day or (130 × 0.9 kg) = 117 mL per day. So, in each 117 mL of fluid you would add 4.7 mEq of sodium plus her maintenance sodium (2.25 mEq), for a total of 6.95 (rounded to 7 mEq). Thus each 250 mL of IV fluid should contain (7/117) × 250 = 15 mEq of sodium. Your order would be: add 15 mEq sodium as chloride to every 250 mL of IV fluids, to run at 130 mL/kg per day. This would be 117 mL per day or 4.9 mL/h. Recheck sodium after 12 and 24 hours on the new fluids. You have calculated a rise in the sodium level of 0.36 mEq/L per hour (total of 13 over 36 hours) so you expect a rise of (0.36 × 12) = 4.33 (or 4–5) at 12 hours, to a serum sodium of 131–132 mEq/L. If the level approximates this, stay the course. If the level does not change as expected, you must explore the reasons why not.

Factitious Hyponatremia

Markedly high serum glucose levels may result in factitious hyponatremia being reported by the laboratory. Hyperglycemia results in a shift of water from the intracellular to extracellular space, which results in a decrease in the extracellular sodium concentration (with no change in extracellular sodium content by about 1.6 mEq/L for every 100 mg/dL increase in glucose level). Erroneously low sodium level may also be caused by sample collection errors from access lines from which fluid with a low sodium concentration is not fully cleared from the line before sampling.

HYPERNATREMIA

Neonatal hypernatremia is serum sodium concentration ≥ 150 mEq/L that usually results from either excessive fluid loss but can result from excessive sodium intake.

Neonatal hypernatremia is most commonly due to excessive water deficit with associated high weight loss. Incorrect estimates of insensible losses or measurement of urine volumes alter the calculations of the necessary administered volume of fluid. In full-term infants, this is most frequently caused by an overestimate of the fluid volume obtained by breastfeeding in the first days after birth,[49] resulting in a weight loss in excess of that normally expected.

When the hypernatremia is due to excessive fluid loss from any cause, it is corrected by judiciously increasing the administered volume of free water administration and frequently reassessing sodium levels to avoid correcting the hypernatremia more quickly than 0.5 mEq/L per hour (see Chapter 7). This slow approach allows time for tissue equilibration and helps avoid cerebral edema and seizures.[50]

For example, analogous to the example for hyponatremia above: You are caring for a 2.8-kg, late preterm infant who has excessively high urine output, signs of volume contraction, and a weight loss of 0.3 kg. His serum sodium is 150 mEq/L. You endeavor to reduce this to a goal of 140 mEq/L, at a rate of no more than 0.5 mEq/L per hour.

For simplicity you calculate a plan to reduce it to a normal level of 140 mEq/L over a period of 36 hours, or a rate of (150 − 140)/36 hours = ~0.28 mEq/h. You plan to replace the deficit of 300 mL of fluid over this period, or an additional 12.5 mL/h added to the ongoing fluid administration. You expect that the serum sodium will decrease by ~ 3.4 mEq/L (approximately 3–4) over 12 hours. You remeasure the sodium level after 12 hours on the new fluids and anticipate that the level will have decreased to about 146–147 mEq/L. Again, if the measured level is very different from this, you must explore to identify what factor you have not considered.

Hypernatremia without significant weight loss should prompt a search for inadvertent high sodium administration from errors in parenteral fluid preparation or sodium sources for which you have not accounted, such as medications or blood products.[51] In these cases, removal of the exogenous source should lead to improvement.

See Chapter 7 for discussion of other pathologic causes of hypernatremia.

Potassium Disorders

HYPOKALEMIA

Hypokalemia (<3 mEq/L serum level) can occur due to kaliuresis associated with postnatal diuresis/natriuresis if potassium administration is not initiated in a timely manner during this phase. It also may occur with diuretic use (see Chapter 9), renal tubular defects, or unaccounted losses from gastric or intestinal fluids. Most hypokalemia is asymptomatic, but it can cause weakness and paralysis, ileus, urinary retention, or cardiac conduction defects. It is usually readily correctable by

supplementing intake by 1 to 2 mEq/kg. Rarely, it is necessary to intravenously administer a dose of 0.5–1 mEq/kg with appropriate cardiac monitoring.

HYPERKALEMIA

Hyperkalemia when using the definition of serum concentration >6 mEq/L for older children and adults often occurs normally in neonates in the first days after birth, because of reduced urinary potassium excretion caused by aldosterone insensitivity and decreased GFR, factors that are more prominent in preterm infants.[52]

In the absence of pathologic conditions, clinically significant hyperkalemia is most likely to occur in extremely preterm infants in the prediuretic phase as a result of a shift of potassium from the intracellular to the ECF compartment.[53-55] It is best prevented by withholding potassium intake until urine output is confirmed to be >1 mL/kg per hour and serum potassium concentration is not increasing. Antenatal glucocorticoid administration appears to prevent this.[21] Pathologic hyperkalemia can occur as a result of decreased potassium clearance (e.g., renal failure, certain forms of congenital adrenal hyperplasia), increased potassium release from tissue destruction, internal bleeding, or accidental excess administration.

Severe or acute elevations in potassium levels can result in life-threatening brady- or tachyarrhythmias and cardiovascular instability, manifested on the electrocardiogram as peaked T waves, flattened P waves, increased PR interval, and widening of the QRS complex. Bradycardia, supraventricular or ventricular tachycardia, and ventricular fibrillation may occur. Vigorous treatment (see Chapter X) should include the cessation of all potassium administration, stabilization of cardiac cells with calcium chloride or gluconate infusion, and rapid promotion of potassium flux into cells by administering insulin and glucose. Second-line therapies include the correction of metabolic acidosis, the use of beta agonists, and kaliuretic diuretics.

REFERENCES

1. Friis-Hansen B. Body water compartments in children: changes during growth and related changes in body composition. *Pediatrics*. 1961;28:169–181.
2. Shaffer SG, Weismann DN. Fluid requirements in the preterm infant. *Clin Perinatol*. 1992;19(1):233–250.
3. Bauer K, Versmold H. Postnatal weight loss in preterm neonates less than 1,500 g is due to isotonic dehydration of the

extracellular volume. *Acta Paediatr Scand Suppl.* 1989;360: 37–42. doi:10.1111/j.1651-2227.1989.tb11280.x

4. Shaffer SG, Quimiro CL, Anderson JV, Hall RT. Postnatal weight changes in low birth weight infants. *Pediatrics.* 1987;79(5): 702–705.

5. Flaherman VJ, Schaefer EW, Kuzniewicz MW, et al. Early weight loss nomograms for exclusively breastfed newborns. *Pediatrics.* 2015;135(1):e16–e23. doi:10.1542/peds.2014-1532

6. Modi N, Bétrémieux P, Midgely J, et al. Postnatal weight loss and contraction of the extracellular compartment is triggered by atrial naturetic peptide. *Early Hum Dev.* 2000;59:201–208.

7. Lorenz JM, Kleinman LI, Kotagal UR, Reller MD. Water balance in very low-birth-weight infants: relationship to water and sodium intake and effect on outcome. *J Pediatr.* 1982;101: 423–432.

8. Kavvadia V, Greenough A, Dimitrou G, Hooper R. Randomized trial of fluid restriction in ventilated very low birthweight infants. *Arch Dis Child Fetal Neonatal Ed.* 2000;83(2):F91–F96. doi:10.1136/fn.83.2.f91

9. Oh W, Poindexer BB, Perritt R, et al. Association between fluid intake and weight loss during the first ten days of life and risk of bronchopulmonary dysplasia in extremely low birthweight infants. *J Pediar.* 2005;147:786–790.

10. Palta M, Gabbert D, Weinstein MR, Peters ME. Multivariate assessment of traditional risk factors for chronic lung disease in very low birthweight neonates. The Newborn Lung Project. *J Pediatr.* 1991;119:285–292.

11. Shaffer SG, Meade VM. Sodium balance and extracellular volume regulation in very low birth weight infants. *J Pediatr.* 1989;115(2):285–290. doi:10.1016/s0022-3476(89)80087-3

12. Lorenz JM, Kleinman LI, Ahmed G, Markarian K. Phases of fluid and electrolyte homeostasis in the extremely low birth weight infant. *Pediatrics.* 1995;96(3 Pt 1):484–489.

13. Hammarlund K, Sedin G, Strömberg B. Transepidermal water loss in newborn infants. VIII. Relation to gestational age and post-natal age in appropriate and small for gestational age infants. *Acta Paediatr Scand.* 1983;72(5):721–728. doi:10.1111/j.1651-2227.1983.tb09801.x

14. Agren J, Sjörs G, Sedin G. Transepidermal water loss in infants born at 24 and 25 weeks of gestation. *Acta Paediatr.* 1998;87(11):1185–1190. doi:10.1080/080352598750031194

15. Kjartansson S, Arsan S, Hammarlund K, et al. Water loss from the skin of term and preterm infants nursed under a radiant heater. *Pediatr Res.* 1995;37(2):233–238. doi:10.1203/00006450-199502000-00018

16. Agren J, Sjörs G, Sedin G. Transepidermal water loss in infants born at 24 and 25 weeks of gestation. *Acta Paediatr.* 1998;87(11):1185–1190. doi:10.1080/080352598750031194

17. Nonato LB, Lund CH, Kalia YN, Guy RH. Transepidermal water loss in 24 and 25 weeks gestational age infants. *Acta Paediatr.* 2000;89(6):747–748. doi:10.1080/08035250075004418

18. Williams PR, Oh W. Effects of radiant warmer on insensible water loss in newborn infants. *Am J Dis Child.* 1974;128(4): 511–514. doi:10.1001/archpedi.1974.02110290081014

19. Baumgart S. Reduction of oxygen consumption, insensible water loss, and radiant heat demand with use of a plastic blanket for low-birth-weight infants under radiant warmers. *Pediatrics.* 1984;74(6):1022–1028.

20. Kim SM, Lee EY, Chen J, Ringer SA. Improved care and growth outcomes by using hybrid humidified incubators in very preterm infants. *Pediatrics.* 2010;125(1):e137–e145. doi:10.1542/peds.2008-2997

21. Hammarlund K, Nilsson GE, Oberg PA, Sedin G. Transepidermal water loss in newborn infants. II. Relation to activity and body temperature. *Acta Paediatr Scand.* 1979;68(3):371–376. doi:10.1111/j.1651-2227.1979.tb05022.x

22. Engle WD, Baumgart S, Schwartz JG, et al. Insensible water loss in the critically III neonate. Combined effect of radiant-warmer power and phototherapy. *Am J Dis Child.* 1981;135(6): 516–520. doi:10.1001/archpedi.1981.02130300016007

23. Oh W, Karecki H. Phototherapy and insensible water loss in the newborn infant. *Am J Dis Child.* 1972;124(2):230–232. doi:10.1001/archpedi.1972.02110140080010

24. Bertini G, Perugi S, Elia S, et al. Transepidermal water loss and cerebral hemodynamics in preterm infants: conventional versus LED phototherapy. *Eur J Pediatr.* 2008;167(1):37–42. doi:10.1007/s00431-007-0421-3

25. Riesenfeld T, Hammarlund K, Sedin G. Respiratory water loss in fullterm infants on their first day after birth. *Acta Paediatr Scand.* 1987;76(4):647–653. doi:10.1111/j.1651-2227.1987.tb10535.x

26. Riesenfeld T, Hammarlund K, Sedin G. Respiratory water loss in relation to gestational age in infants on their first day after birth. *Acta Paediatr.* 1995;84(9):1056–1059. doi:10.1111/j.1651-2227.1995.tb13824.x

27. Riesenfeld T, Hammarlund K, Sedin G. Respiratory water loss in relation to gestational age in infants on their first day after birth. *Acta Paediatr.* 1995;84(9):1056–1059. doi:10.1111/j.1651-2227.1995.tb13824.x

28. Omar SA, DeCristofaro JD, Agarwal BI, La Gamma EF. Effects of prenatal steroids on water and sodium homeostasis in extremely low birth weight neonates. *Pediatrics.* 1999;104(3 Pt 1): 482–488. doi:10.1542/peds.104.3.482

29. Ali R, Amlal H, Burnham CE, Soleimani M. Glucocorticoids enhance the expression of the basolateral Na+:HCO3- cotransporter in renal proximal tubules. *Kidney Int.* 2000;57(3):1063–1071. doi:10.1046/j.1523-1755.2000.00933.x

30. Baum M, Amemiya M, Dwarakanath V, et al. Glucocorticoids regulate NHE-3 transcription in OKP cells. *Am J Physiol.* 1996; 270(1Pt2):F164–F169. doi:10.1152/ajprenal.1996.270.1.F164

31. Omar SA, DeCristofaro JD, Agarwal BI, LaGamma EF. Effect of prenatal steroids on potassium balance in extremely low birth weight neonates. *Pediatrics.* 2000;106(3):561–567. doi:10.1542/peds.106.3.561

32. McCance RA, Young WF. The secretion of urine by newborn infants. *J Physiol.* 1941;99(3):265–282. doi:10.1113/jphysiol.1941.sp003900

33. Quigley R, Chakravarty S, Baum M. Antidiuretic hormone resistance in the neonatal cortical collecting tubule is mediated in part by elevated phosphodiesterase activity. *Am J Physiol Renal Physiol.* 2004;286(2):F317–F322. doi:10.1152/ajprenal.00122.2003

34. Edelman Jr CM. Normal kidney development. In: Edelman Jr CM, ed. *Pediatric Kidney Disease.* 2nd ed. Boston: Little, Brown and Company; 1992:3.

35. Arant BS. Neonatal adjustments to extrauterine life. In: Edelman CM, ed. *Pediatric Kidney Disease.* 2nd ed. Boston: Little, Brown and Company; 1992:1015.

36. Bueva A, Guignard JP. Renal function in preterm neonates. *Pediatr Res.* 1994;36(5):572–577. doi:10.1203/00006450-199411000-00005

37. Horster M. Embryonic epithelial membrane transporters. *Am J Physiol Renal Physiol.* 2000;279(6):F982–F996. doi:10.1152/ajprenal.2000.279.6.F982

38. Rodríguez Soriano J. Renal tubular acidosis: the clinical entity. *J Am Soc Nephrol*. 2002;13(8):2160–2170. doi:10.1097/01.asn.0000023430.92674.e5

39. Rodríguez-Soriano J. New insights into the pathogenesis of renal tubular acidosis—from functional to molecular studies. *Pediatr Nephrol*. 2000;14(12):1121–1136. doi:10.1007/s004670000407

40. Lorenz JM, Kleinman LI, Markarian K. Potassium metabolism in extremely low birth weight infants in the first week of life. *J Pediatr*. 1997;131(1 Pt 1):81–86. doi:10.1016/s0022-3476(97)70128-8

41. Iacobelli S, Guignard JP. Maturation of glomerular filtration rate in neonates and infants: an overview. *Pediatr Nephrol*. 2021;36(6):1439–1446. doi:10.1007/s00467-020-04632-1

42. Balakrishnan M, Tucker R, Stephens BE, Bliss JM. Blood urea nitrogen and serum bicarbonate in extremely low birth weight infants receiving higher protein intake in the first week after birth. *J Perinatol*. 2011;31(8):535–539. doi:10.1038/jp.2010.204

43. Thureen PJ, Melara D, Fennessey PV, Hay WW Jr. Effect of low versus high intravenous amino acid intake on very low birth weight infants in the early neonatal period. *Pediatr Res*. 2003;53(1):24–32. doi:10.1203/00006450-200301000-00008

44. Ridout E, Melara D, Rottinghaus S, Thureen PJ. Blood urea nitrogen concentration as a marker of amino-acid intolerance in neonates with birthweight less than 1250 g. *J Perinatol*. 2005;25(2):130–133. doi:10.1038/sj.jp.7211215

45. Paul IM, Schaefer EW, Miller JR, et al. Weight change nomograms for the first month after birth. *Pediatrics*. 2016;138(6):e20162625. doi:10.1542/peds.2016-2625

46. Baumgart S, Costarino AT. Water and electrolyte metabolism of the micropremie. *Clin Perinatol*. 2000;27(1):131–146, vi-vii. doi:10.1016/s0095-5108(05)70010-5

47. Monnikendam CS, Mu TS, Aden JK, et al. Dysnatremia in extremely low birth weight infants is associated with multiple adverse outcomes. *J Perinatol*. 2019;39(6):842–847. doi:10.1038/s41372-019-0359-0

48. Rees L, Brook CG, Shaw JC, Forsling ML. Hyponatraemia in the first week of life in preterm infants. Part I. Arginine vasopressin secretion. *Arch Dis Child*. 1984;59(5):414–422. doi:10.1136/adc.59.5.414

49. Moritz ML, Manole MD, Bogen DL, Ayus JC. Breastfeeding-associated hypernatremia: are we missing the diagnosis? *Pediatrics*. 2005;116(3):e343–e347. doi:10.1542/peds.2004-2647

50. Blum D, Brasseur D, Kahn A, Brachet E. Safe oral rehydration of hypertonic dehydration. *J Pediatr Gastroenterol Nutr*. 1986;5(2):232–235.

51. Späth C, Sjöström ES, Ahlsson F, et al. Sodium supply influences plasma sodium concentration and the risks of hyper- and hyponatremia in extremely preterm infants. *Pediatr Res*. 2017;81(3):455–460. doi:10.1038/pr.2016.264

52. Shaffer SG, Kilbride HW, Hayen LK, et al. Hyperkalemia in very low birth weight infants. *J Pediatr*. 1992;121(2):275–279. doi:10.1016/s0022-3476(05)81203-x

53. Mildenberger E, Versmold HT. Pathogenesis and therapy of non-oliguric hyperkalemia of the premature infant. *Eur J Pediatr*. 2002;161(8):415–422. doi:10.1007/s00431-002-0986-9

54. Lorenz JM, Kleinman LI, Markarian K. Potassium metabolism in extremely low birth weight infants in the first week of life. *J Pediatr*. 1997;131(1 Pt 1):81–86. doi:10.1016/s0022-3476(97)70128-8

55. Sato K, Kondo T, Iwao H, et al: Internal potassium shift in premature infants: cause of nonoliguric hyperkalemia. *J Pediatr*. 1995;126(1):109–113. doi:10.1016/s0022-3476(95)70511-2

Chapter 7

Pathophysiology and Management of Hyponatremia and Hypernatremia in the Neonate

Michael G. Michalopulos, MD, and Raymond Quigley, MD

Chapter Outline

Dysnatremias, hyponatremia and hypernatremia, are common in the neonatal intensive care unit. Recent studies indicate that these conditions can result in both short- and long-term morbidity and mortality.[1–3] This chapter will review the development of renal function with emphasis on the renal handling of water and sodium. We will then discuss the pathophysiology of water and sodium homeostasis that results in hyponatremia and hypernatremia. This will provide a framework for the workup and treatment of these disorders in the term and preterm neonate.

Development of Renal Function and Tubular Transport

The fetal kidney begins to function around the 10th to 11th week of gestation.[4] Although the kidney has its full complement of glomeruli at term, the function of the neonatal kidney continues to undergo development in its ability to filter the blood (glomerular filtration rate [GFR]) and modify the filtered fluid (tubular function).[4,5]

The GFR of a term neonate is only 30% of the normal adult rate when factored for body surface area.[6-10] The GFR in preterm infants is significantly lower than that of term infants.[8] The GFR increases during the first 12–18 months of life when it becomes approximately the same as the adult when factored for body surface area. The glomerular ultrafiltrate is then modified by the renal tubules to eventually form the final urine. The tubules reabsorb solutes including sodium, bicarbonate, glucose, and amino acids and secrete a number of solutes including potassium, acid and ammonium. The excretion rate of the primary nitrogenous waste product, urea, is determined by the GFR, which obligates a high filtration rate to excrete urea so the neonate can remain in nitrogen balance. The renal tubules then reabsorb a large amount of sodium and fluid to remain in balance.

RENAL TUBULAR SODIUM TRANSPORT

To excrete nitrogenous waste in the form of urea the mature adult kidneys filter approximately 150 L of blood per day. The renal tubules then reabsorb about 99% of the filtered load of water and solutes so that the final urine volume is on the order of 1–2 L per day. The key regulator of the reabsorbed fluid volume is sodium transport by the renal tubules.

Active transport of sodium is dependent on the sodium-potassium ATPase (Na-K-ATPase) located on the basolateral membrane of the cells throughout the nephron and utilizes energy from ATP to maintain a low intracellular sodium concentration.[11] There is an inwardly directed electrochemical gradient for sodium to enter the cell through the luminal membrane. The entry of sodium into the cell is driven by this gradient and is linked to other solutes for transport. As will be seen, the mechanism for entry of sodium through the luminal membrane varies throughout the different segments of the nephron.

PROXIMAL TUBULE SODIUM TRANSPORT

In the proximal tubule, the key transporter for luminal sodium entry is the sodium-hydrogen exchanger (Fig. 7.1).[12,13] The primary isoform of this transporter

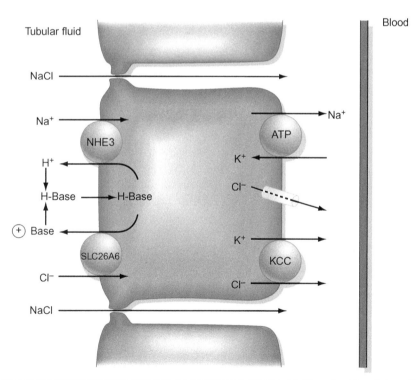

Fig. 7.1 Proximal tubule cell. The sodium-potassium ATPase on the basolateral membrane maintains a low intracellular sodium concentration. This sodium gradient is then used to secrete protons for the reabsorption of bicarbonate as well as the reabsorption of organic solutes such as glucose and amino acids. *KCC*, potassium-chloride cotransporter; *NHE3*, sodium-hydrogen exchanger-3; *SLC26A6*, chloride-base exchanger. (Courtesy of Bruce M. Koeppen.)

in the adult kidney is sodium-hydrogen exchanger-3 NHE3.[12,14] By linking the sodium entry to proton secretion, this transporter will increase the intracellular pH of the proximal tubule cell so there will be a gradient for sodium and bicarbonate exit through its basolateral membrane via the sodium-bicarbonate cotransporter, (NBC).[15]

In the luminal fluid of the proximal tubule, the proton combines with the filtered bicarbonate to form carbonic acid that is then converted to water and carbon dioxide in the presence of carbonic anhydrase.[12] Once the water and carbon dioxide enter the cell, they are converted back to carbonic acid that ionizes into a proton and bicarbonate. The proton can then be secreted and the bicarbonate is transported through the basolateral membrane and into the bloodstream.

Because the processes involved in the reabsorption of bicarbonate have finite rates, the entire process exhibits saturation kinetics and has a transport maximum.[16] When the filtered load of bicarbonate is below the transport maximum, all the filtered bicarbonate will be reabsorbed. If the filtered load exceeds the transport maximum, some of the filtered bicarbonate will be excreted. Because bicarbonate is an anion, it must be excreted with a cation such as sodium or potassium leading to volume depletion due to sodium loss and also to hypokalemia.[17]

Other sodium-coupled transporters on the luminal membrane include the sodium-glucose cotransporters (SGLT1 and SGLT2), sodium-phosphate cotransporter (NaPi2a), and sodium-amino acid cotransporters.[18–21] (The transport of amino acids is very complex and is beyond the scope of this chapter. Please see Broer[22,23] for further details.) These cotransporters account for only a small portion of the sodium that is reabsorbed but are responsible for reabsorbing almost the entire filtered load of glucose and amino acids. The amount of phosphate that is reabsorbed is dependent on the diet and comprises a very wide range of the filtered load. Thus, there is almost no glucose or amino acids in the final urine, but there can be a considerable amount of phosphate, depending on the dietary intake of phosphate.

Active, transcellular transport of sodium chloride occurs via the action of parallel transporters, NHE3 and the chloride-hydroxyl exchanger (Fig. 7.1).[13,24,25] As discussed previously, the sodium-hydrogen exchanger

raises the intracellular pH of the proximal tubule. This leads to a pH gradient that can be used to exchange intracellular base (hydroxyl ions) for luminal chloride ions. The hydrogen ion that is secreted combines with the hydroxyl ion to form water, and the sodium and chloride exit the cell via the basolateral membrane and into the bloodstream.

The actions of these transporters for the reabsorption of bicarbonate, glucose, and amino acids in the early proximal tubule will cause the luminal fluid in the distal portion of the proximal tubule to have a low bicarbonate concentration and a high chloride concentration (Fig. 7.2).[26] This chloride concentration gradient is then used to reabsorb NaCl and water by passive paracellular transport. The rate of reabsorption in this part of the nephron is dependent on the chloride concentration gradient that was generated as well as the paracellular permeability to chloride.[26]

Claudins, intercellular junction proteins, determine the paracellular permeability of the proximal tubule.[27] As will be discussed in the development of proximal tubule transport, the expression of these claudins changes during development and has a direct impact on the rate of transport of sodium chloride.

Development of Proximal Tubule Sodium Reabsorption

The plasma bicarbonate concentration of neonates is lower than that of older children and adults.[28] Direct measurement of the epithelial permeability to bicarbonate demonstrated a lower permeability in neonatal compared with adult rabbit proximal tubules.[29] Thus, lower active transport of bicarbonate in the neonatal tubule is the cause of the lower serum bicarbonate level in the neonate.

As the proximal tubule matures, the components of bicarbonate transport increase. Development of the Na-K ATPase activity parallels that of the basolateral surface area and provides the required energy for the secondary active secretion of protons through the luminal membrane.[30] This increase in the Na-K-ATPase provides the necessary energy for transporting bicarbonate as well as other filtered solutes such as glucose, phosphate and amino acids.[31]

The development of the luminal sodium hydrogen exchanger is more complex. The primary isoform in

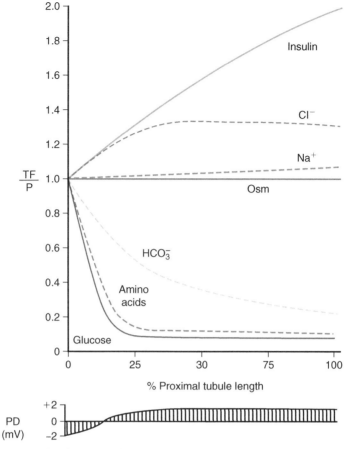

Fig. 7.2 Solute concentrations along the length of the proximal tubule. As fluid is reabsorbed, the concentration of infused insulin increases. The preferential reabsorption of bicarbonate leads to an increase in the luminal chloride concentration. *P, PD,* Potential Difference; *TF/P,* Tubular Fluid to Plasma ratio. (Reproduced with permission from Rector FC Jr. Sodium, bicarbonate, and chloride absorption by the proximal tubule. *Am J Physiol.* 1983;244(5):F461–F471.)

the adult kidney is NHE3.[12,14] Although the expression of NHE3 in neonatal rabbit proximal tubules is very low, the measured sodium-hydrogen exchange activity could not be explained by the negligible amount of NHE3 expressed.[32,33] The isoform responsible for this exchange activity in the neonatal tubules is NHE8.[34–36] This isoform is also expressed in adult proximal tubules but is in intracellular compartments, whereas in the neonatal tubules it is in the luminal membrane. This is evidence for an isoform switch for the luminal sodium-proton exchanger throughout development.

Developmental expression of NHE3 and NHE8 is under hormonal control. Glucocorticoids stimulate

the expression of NHE3[37,38] and also decrease the luminal expression of NHE8[39] and are one of the primary regulators of the development of transport of bicarbonate and sodium in the proximal tubule.

Although thyroid hormone has some effect on the maturational changes in the expression of NHE3 and NHE8, it has more significant effects on the paracellular transport of sodium chloride.[40,41] Proximal straight tubules from hypothyroid neonatal rabbits have a very low chloride permeability. Proximal straight tubules from hypothyroid animals that were treated with thyroid hormone have a chloride permeability that was not different from control animals.[41] Thus, the passive, paracellular transport in the proximal tubule also undergoes significant changes that appear to be affected by thyroid hormone.

Claudins 6, 9, and 13 have high expression in the neonatal tubules but not in the adult tubules.[42,43] These claudins were subsequently shown in a cell culture model to have effects on chloride permeability.[44] Thus, the mechanism of sodium chloride transport in the late proximal tubule has significant maturational changes that are stimulated in part by thyroid hormone.[45]

Proximal Tubule Water Permeability

The proximal tubule reabsorbs the bulk of the filtered load of sodium, chloride, and water in an isotonic fashion. The osmolality of the luminal fluid throughout the proximal tubule does not differ much from the osmolality of the blood. This isotonicity is maintained because of the high expression of aquaporin 1 (AQP1), the membrane water channel, in the luminal and basolateral membranes of the adult proximal tubule.[46,47] This high water permeability allows for the osmotic movement of water with the small solute concentration gradient generated by the active transport of sodium and other solutes.

Expression of AQP1 in the proximal tubule of the neonatal rabbit kidney is much lower than that of the adult proximal tubule.[48] In addition, water permeability measurements of vesicles made from proximal tubule luminal and basolateral membranes showed that the water permeability of these membranes is much lower in the neonatal tissue than the adult kidney tissue.[48,49] Thus, it appears that the water permeability of the neonatal proximal tubule should be much lower than the adult. However, direct measurements in isolated perfused rabbit proximal tubules showed that there is no difference in the water permeability between tubules from neonatal rabbits and adult rabbits.[50] This is explained by the fact that the intracellular compartment in the neonatal tubules is much smaller than that of the adult tubules and provides less resistance to the movement of water through the epithelium.[51] Thus, although the expression of AQP1 is lower in the neonatal proximal tubule, the epithelial water permeability remains high enough so that water could be reabsorbed with the solutes.[52]

Thin Descending and Thin Ascending Loops of Henle

Although transport of salt and water in the thin descending and ascending portions of the loop of Henle is primarily passive in nature, it is complex and its contribution to the medullary hypertonicity is incompletely understood.[53] The osmolality of the medullary interstitium is higher than that of the luminal fluid so there is an osmotic gradient for water reabsorption as the thin descending limb goes further into the medulla. Some, but not all, of the thin descending limbs of Henle express AQP1 so there is high water permeability in these segments. As water is reabsorbed, solute in the lumen becomes more concentrated so that when the fluid begins to ascend to the cortex, there is a gradient for passive sodium reabsorption from the lumen of the thin ascending limb of the loop of Henle.

The developing fetus has only short thin limbs of Henle. Shortly before birth, they begin to form the long loops of Henle that will eventually contribute to medullary hypertonicity. The molecular signals controlling this process have only recently been studied.[54,55] Defects in this process could contribute to the medullary hypoplasia seen in many forms of renal dysplasia.[56]

Thick Ascending Limb of Henle

The thick ascending limb of Henle (TAL) actively transports sodium from the luminal fluid to the bloodstream in a way that also causes many other ions to be reabsorbed as well (Fig. 7.3).[57,58] The primary active transporter is the Na-K-ATPase located in the basolateral membrane of the cell that maintains a very low intracellular sodium concentration. The luminal sodium-potassium-2-chloride cotransporter (NKCC2) utilizes this sodium concentration gradient to transport sodium, potassium, and two chloride ions into the cell. This transporter is electroneutral and does not directly affect the luminal membrane electric potential.

Potassium enters the thick ascending limb cells through both the basolateral membrane (via the Na-K-ATPase) and the luminal membrane (via NKCC2). Both membranes have potassium channels, known as renal outer medullary K channels (ROMK), for the recycling of potassium ions. Because of the luminal potassium recycling, there is a lumen positive electric potential

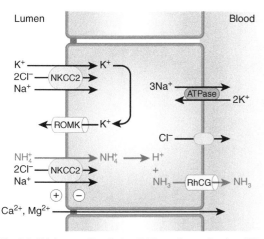

Fig. 7.3 Thick ascending limb cell. The sodium-potassium ATPase on the basolateral membrane provides the driving force for the entry of sodium through sodium-potassium-2-chloride cotransporter (NKCC2). The recycling of potassium through renal outer medullary K channels (ROMK) leads to the lumen positive electrical potential and contributes to the paracellular transport of cations. Defects in NKCC2, ROMK, the chloride channel CLC-NKB or in Barttin lead to Bartter syndrome. *RhCG,* Rhesus C Glycoprotein. (Scott F. Gilbert, Daniel E. Weiner, National Kidney Foundation Primer on Kidney Diseases, 8th Edition, Elsevier, 2023.)

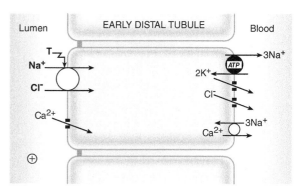

Fig. 7.4 Distal convoluted tubule cell. The sodium-potassium ATPase provides the driving force for sodium entry through NCC, the thiazide sensitive sodium-chloride cotransporter. Mutations in NCC lead to Gitelman syndrome. (Vincent W. Lee, Amanda Mather. *The Renal System.* 3rd ed., Elsevier; 2023.)

that leads to passive paracellular reabsorption of many cations including sodium, potassium, calcium, and magnesium. Thus, inhibition of transport of NKCC2 with loop diuretics such as furosemide and bumetanide results in increased excretion of not only sodium and potassium but also calcium and magnesium.

The thick ascending limb has no water channels on its luminal membrane but has AQP1 in the basolateral membrane so that the cell volume can respond to changes in interstitial osmolality.[57] In addition, the lipid composition of the luminal membrane is such that the water permeability is extremely low. As solute is actively reabsorbed from the lumen, the osmolality of the luminal fluid decreases and free water is generated. Thus, the thick ascending limb is considered part of the diluting segment of the nephron. Although neonatal transport of sodium chloride in the TAL is only about 20% of that of the adult TAL the normal newborn is still able to dilute its urine and avoid hyponatremia.[59]

Distal Convoluted Tubule

The distal convoluted tubule (DCT) continues reabsorbing sodium by an active mechanism driven by the Na-K-ATPase located on the basolateral membrane

(Fig. 7.4).[60,61] Sodium can then enter the cell down its electrochemical gradient through the luminal sodium-chloride cotransporter (NCC). The membranes of the DCT are similar to those of the TAL in that they have very low water permeability. This allows the DCT to continue to remove solute from the lumen, leaving behind the water, which will continue to dilute the tubular fluid and create free water. The TAL and DCT are collectively known as the diluting segment.

Collecting Duct

The cortical and medullary collecting ducts comprise several different cell types. The principal cells are involved in sodium reabsorption, potassium secretion, and water homeostasis, and the alpha and beta intercalated cells are involved in secretion of acid or base. We will focus on the principal cells.

As in the previous nephron segments, the collecting duct principal cells have Na-K ATPase on the basolateral membrane for maintaining a low intracellular sodium concentration (Fig. 7.5).[13,62] Sodium entry in this segment occurs through a channel instead of a cotransporter. Thus, the luminal transport of sodium is electrogenic and depends on the electrochemical gradient, not just the chemical gradient.

The primary hormonal regulator of sodium reabsorption in the collecting duct is aldosterone. The collecting duct principal cells have the mineralocorticoid receptor that responds to aldosterone to increase expression of the epithelial sodium channel (ENaC) as well as to increase

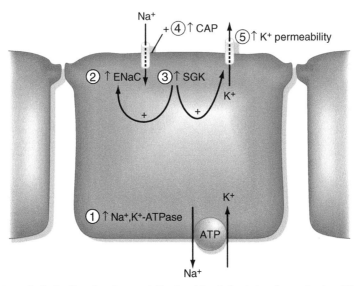

Fig. 7.5 Cortical collecting duct principal cell, sodium transport. The basolaterally located sodium-potassium ATPase maintains a low intracellular sodium concentration which allows for sodium to enter through the epithelial sodium channel (*ENaC*). Potassium is also secreted via renal outer medullary K channels. *NaP, SGK,* serum/glucocorticoid regulated kinase. (Courtesy of Bruce M. Koeppen.)

the Na-K-ATPase activity.[62] Because the mineralocorticoid receptor can bind cortisol and aldosterone, the enzyme, 11 beta hydroxy-steroid dehydrogenase (11BHSD) is present in the principal cells and is responsible for converting cortisol to cortisone, which cannot bind to the mineralocorticoid receptor inside the collecting duct principal cell.[63] Thus, the specificity of the mineralocorticoid receptor for aldosterone is due to the action of 11BHSD. Defects in the recycling of ENaC as well as the mineralocorticoid receptor or 11BHSD have large effects on the final amount of sodium that is reabsorbed. This can then lead to hypertension if sodium is retained or hypotension and hyponatremia if too much sodium is excreted.

The collecting duct principal cells are also responsible for the final regulation of water reabsorption (Fig. 7.6).[13,62] The basolateral membranes contain aquaporins 3 and 4 (AQP3 and 4) that are always present in the membrane. Aquaporin 2 (AQP2) is inserted into the apical membrane from endosomes when the tubule is stimulated by antidiuretic hormone (ADH) or arginine vasopressin (AVP). In the absence of ADH, AQP2 remains in the intracellular compartment and the water permeability of the luminal membrane of the tubule remains low. This allows for the free water that was generated in the diluting

segment to be excreted so that hyponatremia does not develop. Under conditions of dehydration or elevated serum osmolality, ADH is released from the posterior pituitary gland and binds to the V2 receptor (V2R) on the basolateral membrane of the tubule. This initiates a cascade of events that includes stimulation of adenylate cyclase and protein kinase A and insertion of the AQP2 containing endosomes in the luminal membrane. This then increases the tubule's water permeability and water will be reabsorbed, resulting in concentration of the urine. Defects in this pathway can result in the inability to appropriately concentrate or dilute the urine and can lead to dysnatremia.

Developmental Changes in Collecting Duct Sodium Transport

The collecting duct of the neonate has a lower rate of sodium transport than the adult collecting duct due to lower expression of sodium channel messenger RNA as well as posttranslational modifications.[64,65] In addition, the sodium channels that are present are more likely to be closed and thus not transport sodium.[66] This is more pronounced in preterm infants and can lead to sodium wasting and result in hyponatremia.

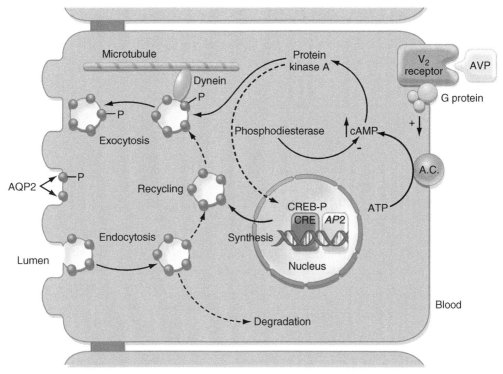

Fig. 7.6 Cortical collecting duct principal cell, water transport. Aquaporin 3 and aquaporin 4 water channels are constitutively present in the basolateral membrane. Aquaporin 2 (*AQP2*) is inserted into the luminal membrane in response to arginine vasopressin (*AVP*) binding to the vasopressin receptor (*V2R*). Mutations in V2R cause congenital nephrogenic diabetes insipidus as well as nephrogenic syndrome of inappropriate antidiuresis. *A.C.,* Adenylate Cyclase; *cAMP,* cyclic adenosine monophosphate; *P,* phosphate; *CREB-P,* cAMP Response Element Binding Protein; *CRE,* cAMP Response Element; *AQP2,* Aquaporin 2.   (Adapted from Brown D, Nielsen S. The cell biology of vasopressin action. In: Brenner BM, ed. *The Kidney.* 7th ed. Philadelphia: Saunders; 2004.)

Developmental Changes in Collecting Duct Water Transport

Neonates cannot concentrate their urine to the same degree as older children and adults. This is due in part to a lower osmotic gradient that is maintained in the interstitium of the medulla. There is also evidence that the response of the neonatal collecting duct to ADH is not as robust as the adult collecting duct.[67]

Initial experiments showed that one of the limiting factors in the response to ADH is an increase in prostaglandin secretion by the neonatal tubule.[68] When these prostaglandins were inhibited, the response of the collecting duct to produce cyclic adenosine monophosphate (CAMP) cAMP was improved. However, prostaglandin inhibition did not have an effect on the tubule water permeability response to ADH.[69]

Subsequent studies also examined the role of phosphodiesterase (PDE) in the limited neonatal tubule response to ADH. PDE will metabolize cAMP into 5'-AMP so that it is inactivated, thus limiting the response to ADH. A higher activity of PDE in the neonatal tubules would blunt the response to ADH. PDE activity was directly shown to be higher in the neonatal collecting ducts and once PDE was blocked, the water permeability response in the neonatal tubules was the same as the adult tubules.[70] Thus, PDE is probably the most significant factor in the limited response of the neonatal collecting duct to ADH.

Dysnatremias

Serum sodium concentration between 135 and 145 mEq/L is normal, or eunatremia. Hyponatremia, therefore, is defined as serum sodium < 135 mEq/L, and hyperna-tremia is defined as serum sodium > 145 mEq/L. Al-though serum sodium concentration is routinely mea-sured in most clinical laboratories, there are conditions that lead to inaccurate sodium measurements referred to as pseudohyponatremia and pseudohypernatre-mia.[71,72] To check for this, it is critical to obtain a se-rum osmolality in the initial workup of the patient. If the measured osmolality is normal or high when the serum sodium is low, then the patient most likely has "pseudohyponatremia." Conditions with elevated se-rum proteins or lipids can cause the laboratory mea-surement of sodium to be low. Although current labo-ratory techniques to measure sodium will minimize this effect, it is still possible to have pseudohyponatre-mia or pseudohypernatremia in these settings.[71,72] In addition, hyperglycemia will cause water to move from the intracellular compartment and dilute the sodium concentration leading to a condition referred to as factitious hyponatremia.[73] The following discus-sion will refer to patients with true dysnatremia.

The approach to patients with dysnatremia requires detailed information on the water and solute intake and losses. A good clinical history includes a detailed feeding history including the composition and amount of feeds and ensuring the caregivers can demonstrate appropriate formula mixing and feeding technique. Physical examination with attention to intravascular volume status is also key to the diagnosis and will help direct the treatment. Although there are many physical examination findings that suggest volume depletion, hypotension, tachycardia, dry mucus membranes, weak peripheral pulse, and skin turgor, assessing the intravascular volume in a patient can be very difficult. For example, generalized edema and ascites may be observed in a patient with nephrotic syndrome that has an increase in total body water but a decrease in the intravascular volume. We will also review the use of urinary electrolytes and serum and urine uric acid and urea levels that will help with this determination.

Hyponatremia

Hyponatremia is relatively common in neonates, par-ticularly in critically ill neonates with respiratory or neurologic complications as well as low birth weight, premature neonates.[74,75] Although many infants with mild hyponatremia may be asymptomatic, sodium is critical for the growth and development of the infant. Thus, hyponatremia should not be ignored. Infants, particularly preterm infants, with chronic hyponatre-mia are at risk for poor growth, neurocognitive delays, cerebral palsy, cerebral hemorrhage, and mortality.[74,75] Severe hyponatremia, with serum sodium < 120 mEq/L, is associated with high morbidity, particularly hyponatremic encephalopathy, and high mortality, ap-proaching 50%.[74,75]

Rapid correction of hyponatremia can result in central pontine myelinolysis, a devastating condition with poor neurological outcome.[76] In this syndrome, demyelination of white matter occurs. In addition, demyelination can occur outside of the central ner-vous system in a syndrome termed osmotic demyelin-ation syndrome. Although this was initially described in adults, it has also now been described in infants.[76,77]

Pathophysiology of Hyponatremia

Hyponatremia results from excessive free water in-take or impaired free water excretion. Thus, to under-stand the cause of hyponatremia, the physiology of free water excretion must be understood (reviewed in Gruskin et al.[73]).

The initial step in free water excretion is the filtra-tion of blood in the glomerulus. The filtered fluid must then be delivered distally to the diluting seg-ment (TAL and DCT) where free water is generated by removing solute from the filtrate and leaving the water behind in the tubular fluid. This dilute tubular fluid is then processed by the collecting duct before it exits the nephron. The final handling of water by the collecting duct is determined by its response to the presence or absence of ADH. To excrete free water, ADH action must be suppressed to prevent reabsorp-tion of water.

As we discuss the conditions that result in hypona-tremia, we will describe the mechanisms that are de-fective and result in hyponatremia. The differential diagnosis of hyponatremia can thus be divided into three broad categories:

1. Water intoxication (i.e., excessive water intake in the setting of normal kidney function).
2. Decreased distal delivery of fluid with subse-quent decreased generation of free water by the

diluting segment. Many of these conditions also cause nonosmotic secretion of ADH.

3. Free water retention in the collecting duct due to inappropriate action of ADH.

These will now be discussed in more detail.

WATER INTOXICATION

As discussed previously, the GFR of the neonate is 30% of the adult GFR when factored for body surface area.[6,9] This is the primary limiting factor for the neonate's ability to excrete a large free water load. The diluting segment is intact, and the neonate can suppress ADH to maximize the amount of free water to be excreted.[78] However, the amount of fluid that is filtered and delivered to the diluting segment can be inadequate and becomes the rate limiting step for free water excretion. Human breast milk and infant formulas are very hypotonic (Na concentration is ~10–20 mEq/L). However, the infant can excrete the ingested free water since the fat content of the meal will cause the infant to be satiated and the infant will stop drinking for some time. This allows the infant time to then excrete the ingested free water.

Formula that is inappropriately dilute can result in hyponatremia from water intoxication.[79] Since the fat content of the formula is also diluted, the infant does not become satiated and will then take in excessive amounts of free water. This can occur accidentally or voluntarily in situations where caregivers may be trying to maximize a supply of formula for more feedings, not knowing the risks it poses. Many times, the infant presents with seizures from the hyponatremia.[80] Therefore, when a formula-fed infant presents with hyponatremia, information about formula mixing is an important detail to obtain.

In terms of the workup for this condition, the urine osmolality is the key factor. Since the neonate's diluting segment functions well and the neonate can suppress ADH, the urine osmolality should be maximally dilute.[78] Thus, in a patient with hyponatremia, a urine osmolality of less than 100 mOsm/L is highly suggestive of water intoxication.

DECREASED DISTAL DELIVERY

The diluting segment of the nephron in neonates can generate free water and can produce a dilute urine. However, conditions that limit the distal delivery of the glomerular filtrate will not allow the neonate to excrete enough free water to prevent hyponatremia. The most common example of this is volume depletion. In this setting, the GFR might be slightly lower than normal, but the fraction of the filtrate reabsorbed by the proximal tubule is greatly increased.[81–84] Transport in the proximal tubule is also stimulated by the increased production of angiotensin II.[85–87] This is reflected in the fact that the neonate's blood urea nitrogen (BUN) increases out of proportion to the creatinine. Urea is passively reabsorbed in the proximal tubule and thus its concentration will increase in the neonate that is volume depleted. Uric acid handling by the tubule is very similar to that of urea. Thus, an elevated uric acid and increased BUN are suggestive of intravascular volume depletion.

Volume depletion occurs secondary to loss of sodium that leads to contraction of the extracellular volume. This can be either from extrarenal losses or from renal losses. In terms of the workup, the source of loss needs to be identified. In extrarenal losses, the kidney will attempt to retain sodium and thus the urine sodium and the fractional excretion of sodium (FENa) will be low. If the kidneys are responsible for the sodium loss, the urine sodium and FENa will be elevated. In older children and adults, the cutoff for the FENa is usually 0.01 (1%). However, in neonates, and preterm neonates, because sodium transport is not fully mature, the cutoff will be higher.[88]

In some circumstances, the FENa can be misleading because of excretion of a nonreabsorbable anion such as bicarbonate. The classic example is pyloric stenosis, where the infant becomes very alkalotic and the serum bicarbonate will exceed the transport maximum for proximal tubule reabsorption. In this setting, the bicarbonate will be excreted with sodium and potassium but the excretion of chloride will be very low. Thus, in some settings it is more relevant to examine the fractional secretion of chloride. The interpretation of the FENa has been recently reviewed in terms of its utility and limitations.[89,90]

Other conditions that lead to decreased distal delivery of fluid without having volume loss include congestive heart failure and third spacing of fluid such as nephrotic syndrome. In these conditions the hemodynamics of blood flow through the glomerulus are very similar to that of the neonate that is volume depleted. This will result in a larger fraction of the glomerular filtrate being reabsorbed by the proximal tubule with less being delivered to the diluting segment. As with volume depletion, the BUN and serum uric acid levels are generally elevated in this condition. Because the proximal tubule is reabsorbing a larger fraction of the filtered load of urea, the fractional excretion of urea is decreased. This can be a useful marker for assessing the renal perfusion in these patients.[91,92]

Many other conditions follow the same pathophysiologic pathway. Essentially any condition that leads to sodium and volume loss will mimic the condition of volume depletion from diarrhea. In addition, with significant volume loss, there will be an increase in the secretion of ADH.[93] This will also impede the ability to excrete free water. As discussed previously, the loss can be extrarenal or renal. We will first discuss the extrarenal losses of sodium.

Extrarenal Sodium Loss

Although infectious etiologies account for the bulk of the cases of gastrointestinal (GI) losses of sodium in older children, neonates can also have GI losses from congenital causes. These include congenital chloride diarrhea and congenital sodium diarrhea. Infants with congenital chloride diarrhea have a mutation in the intestinal chloride-hydroxyl exchanger that leads to GI losses of chloride.[94] They present with hypokalemic alkalosis. Congenital sodium diarrhea is a result of alterations in function of the sodium-proton exchanger in the intestines and results in GI losses of sodium.[95,96] These patients present with acidosis. Because the sodium loss is from the GI tract, the urine sodium will be low.

Another source of extrarenal sodium loss is from sweat ducts in patients with cystic fibrosis (CF), an autosomal recessive condition that results from mutations in the cystic fibrosis transmembrane regulator (*CFTR*) gene.[97] There are many genetic variants, with ΔF508 being the most common, and all result in abnormal CFTR protein expression. This protein is a chloride channel, and abnormalities result in excessive sodium and chloride loss in the sweat, which serves as the basis for diagnosis, with sweat chloride >60 mEq/L considered diagnostic.[97] CF is diagnosed via a newborn screen but it is important to note it can be missed on these screens. Therefore, in an infant

with hyponatremia and failure to thrive, CF should remain on the differential.

The increased salt losses can result in hyponatremia, hypochloremia, hypokalemia, and metabolic alkalosis.[98–100] In one center, about 16% of previously undiagnosed CF patients presented with such electrolyte derangements.[101] In these patients, hypokalemia and alkalosis occur due to the stimulation of the renin-aldosterone axis and subsequent tubular effects. There is recent evidence that the abnormal CFTR function in the kidney also limits the excretion of bicarbonate and will exacerbate the alkalosis.[102,103] This mimics Bartter syndrome, which is often considered in the differential diagnosis of these previously unidentified patients and is referred to as pseudo-Bartter syndrome of CF.[100] The urine electrolytes are key to differentiating these conditions. In Bartter syndrome, the urine sodium and chloride will be high, and in CF, these will be low.

Renal Sodium Loss

Losses of sodium from the kidneys can be the result of defects in the sodium transport mechanisms themselves or can result from defects in the hormonal regulation of these mechanisms. We will first describe the defects related to the primary mineralocorticoid, aldosterone.

Aldosterone Deficiency and Resistance Disorders

Aldosterone is produced in the zona glomerulosa of the adrenal cortex and is the main mineralocorticoid steroid hormone in humans.[104] Its primary functions are to regulate extracellular volume via sodium reabsorption and to regulate serum potassium.[104] It binds to mineralocorticoid receptors in the DCT and cortical collecting duct, signaling messenger RNA transcription, production, and eventual cellular expression of ENaC.[104,105] This allows for sodium reabsorption from the tubular fluid and the increased electrochemical gradient promotes potassium secretion via the ROMK in the principal cells and hydrogen secretion via a proton pump (H$^+$-ATPase) in the alpha intercalated cells. The net result is sodium retention, potassium excretion, hydrogen ion excretion, and volume expansion.

ENaC is also found in the lung, colon, sweat glands, and salivary glands, which will be addressed later.[106]

Alterations of this mechanism disrupt sodium homeostasis. Although inhibition, downregulation, or failure of this pathway results in hyponatremia, excessive aldosterone action and upregulation of this pathway do not induce hypernatremia. The excess sodium reabsorption will lead to volume expansion and hypertension, but water retention and thirst will maintain a normal sodium concentration. There are a few disorders that result in disruption of this pathway that are of clinical significance in the neonate.

Congenital adrenal hyperplasia (CAH) is a group of autosomal recessive disorders with impaired adrenal steroid production.[107,108] Although the many enzymes necessary for normal production of mineralocorticoids, glucocorticoids, and sex steroids share some pathways, defects in these enzymes can result in different phenotypes.[108] The most common form of CAH, which accounts for approximately 95% of cases, is due to 21-hydroxylase deficiency and classically results in renal salt wasting.[107,108] The 21-hydroxylase enzyme is necessary to cleave the precursor hormones progesterone and 17-hydroxyprogesterone into deoxycorticosterone and 11-deoxycortisol, respectively, which are then further metabolized into aldosterone and cortisol.[108] Deficiency of this enzyme results in impaired aldosterone and cortisol production, and testosterone is produced in excess.[108] The classic disease manifestation includes excessive virilization, which can result in ambiguous genitalia in female patients.[108]

The diagnosis of 21-hydroxylase deficiency should be considered in infants with hyponatremia, dehydration, hypotension, acidosis, and ambiguous genitalia. It can be confirmed with genetic studies, but one would find serum aldosterone levels to be absent and levels of serum 17-OH hydroxyprogesterone to be elevated.[108,109] This condition is screened for on standard newborn panels in the United States and many other countries.[109] Treatment for this condition involves salt supplementation and regular administration of exogenous hormones with hydrocortisone and fludrocortisone.[109] Treatment should be done in consultation with a pediatric endocrinologist.

Although the clinical findings of CAH result from aldosterone deficiency, there are aldosterone-resistant disorders, referred to as pseudohypoaldosteronism (PHA), which result in similar electrolyte disturbances. Ultimately, the clinical findings in these conditions result from mineralocorticoid resistance, and aldosterone levels are quite elevated.[106]

The two forms that lead to hyponatremia are renal PHA type I and systemic PHA type I.[106] PHA type II, referred to as Gordon's syndrome, generally does not present with hyponatremia and will not be discussed.[110] It is important to note these PHA conditions are uncommon and have variable phenotypic manifestations, but sodium excretion due to mineralocorticoid resistance is consistent.

Renal type I PHA is inherited in an autosomal dominant pattern and results in renal tubular sodium wasting.[105,106] The defect is a mutation in the NR3C2 gene that results in a nonfunctional mineralocorticoid receptor.[105] Most patients present early in life with dehydration and the expected electrolyte abnormalities of hyponatremia, hyperkalemia, and acidosis.[105] These patients can typically be managed with sodium supplementation and potassium restriction.[106] Although many patients do not require prolonged sodium supplementation, they will often need continued treatment for hyperkalemia.[105,106] A sweat chloride test will be normal in these patients.[105]

Systemic type I PHA is an autosomal recessive disorder and involves mutations in one of the three subunit genes SCNN1A, SCNN1B, or SCNN1Γ of ENaC.[105] Because ENaC is also expressed in the lung, colon, salivary glands, and sweat glands, mutations in this channel result in a systemic phenotype. Patients with systemic type I PHA are generally affected more severely than patients with renal PHA type I and frequently suffer severe electrolyte disturbances due to salt loss in the stool, sweat, urine, and saliva.[105] Clinically, these patients often appear with failure to thrive, vomiting, diarrhea, electrolyte abnormalities, and lower respiratory tract infections due to the defective ENaC in the lungs.[105] They can mimic CF clinically, and a sweat chloride test will often be positive.[105,106] Genetic analysis can confirm the diagnosis of systemic PHA type I. Treatment generally involves sodium supplementation, often in higher amounts than in renal type I PHA, low potassium diet, and potassium-lowering agents such as sodium polystyrene sulfonate (Kayexalate).[105,106]

All neonates have a transient aldosterone resistance at birth, regardless of gestational age and health.[111] Neonatal levels of renin and aldosterone are markedly elevated, ranging 6–10 times the normal adult ranges.[111] The underlying mechanism is likely due to decreased mineralocorticoid receptor expression early in life, which has been found to increase as the infant matures as well as immaturity of the renal tubules.[5,111] Generally, this transient resistance on its own does not cause hyponatremia but when it occurs with other conditions or factors, it can potentiate hyponatremia. Recent studies have shown that sodium losses in these infants require some degree of supplementation for growth.[112,113]

Urinary tract pathologies can also result in transient aldosterone resistance. Pyelonephritis, obstructive uropathies, and other congenital malformations of the urinary tract have been documented to do so.[114–116] These infants, when compared with healthy controls, will have increased fractional excretion of sodium, and elevated aldosterone levels.[115] The same electrolyte and metabolic disturbances occur in these conditions as they do in others with aldosterone deficient disorders, but in these cases the effect is transient and will often correct.[116] Therefore, in infants with the typical abnormal laboratory values hypoaldosteronism, clinicians should suspect and evaluate for urinary tract infections, obstruction, and other congenital urologic malformations.

Salt Losing Tubulopathies

A number of defects in tubule transport systems of the TAL and the DCT result in renal salt wasting and hyponatremia. Mutations in several of the transporters in the TAL cause Bartter syndrome, characterized by polyuria and hypokalemic alkalosis.[117] The first one that was identified was NKCC2 so this has been termed Bartter syndrome type 1.[118] The next defect that was identified was in ROMK, which is one of the causes of antenatal Bartter syndrome and polyhydramnios.[119] Neonates with this form of Bartter syndrome will often be hyperkalemic instead of hypokalemic because the secretion of potassium in the cortical collecting duct CCD will be limited due to the lack of functional potassium channels in the cortical collecting duct CCD of the neonate.

As the infant matures and the maxi-K channel expression increases, they will eventually manifest the typical hypokalemic alkalosis.[120,121]

The typical patient with Bartter syndrome will have hypercalciuria and will develop nephrocalcinosis. However, in type 3 Bartter syndrome, caused by mutations in the chloride channel (CLC-NKB), there are variable amounts of calciuria due to the fact that the calcium channel is also present in the DCT.[122] Type 4 Bartter syndrome is caused by mutations in Barttin, an accessory protein for the chloride channel. Because Barttin is also found in the inner ear, these patients will also have sensorineural deafness.[123,124]

Although most forms of Bartter syndrome are chronic and lifelong, a transient form of Bartter syndrome has been described recently that is caused by mutations in the gene melanoma-associated antigen D2 (*MAGED-D2*) that is found on the X chromosome.[125,126] Mutations were also found in a number of fetuses that were associated with polyhydramnios and fetal death. Thus, the authors were unable to characterize the phenotype of the fetus except for the fact that the fetuses were male. It is not clear how this gene defect affects the thick ascending limb and why it is transient in nature.[126]

Gitelman et al. described a group of patients with hypokalemic alkalosis that were similar to patients with Bartter syndrome.[127,128] The key difference was that the patients Gitelman et al. described had hypocalciuria instead of hypercalciuria, which patients with typical Bartter syndrome had. It was subsequently shown that these patients had a mutation in the thiazide-sensitive transporter NCC.[129] They are usually not as severely affected as patients with Bartter syndrome, and many times they are found incidentally when electrolytes are measured.

Syndrome of Inappropriate Antidiuretic Hormone

ADH is generated and secreted from the hypothalamic-pituitary axis, released from the posterior pituitary, binds to the V2 receptor in the distal nephron, and stimulates translocation of the AQP2 water channels from the cytosol and into the tubular luminal membrane of the collecting duct.[90] The net effect is free water retention and concentration of the urine.

Under normal conditions, the secretion of ADH is controlled by the plasma osmolality.[90]

In syndrome of inappropriate antidiuretic hormone (SIADH) there is a pathologic stimulus for secretion of ADH.[93,130] The patient has hypotonic hyponatremia, with serum osmolality < 275 mOsm/kg, inappropriately high urine osmolality of >100 mOsm/kg and a clinical examination of either euvolemia or hypervolemia.[127] Features are consistent with volume expansion and include a low plasma uric acid, low BUN, and increased fractional excretion of sodium, uric acid, and urea.[127] The low urate level is not due to a dilution effect; rather, it is due to decreased proximal tubule reabsorption of urate.[130,131] Urinary sodium losses are elevated and the initial description of SIADH was a severe sodium wasting syndrome.[130,132] Atrial natriuretic peptide, which induces natriuresis, is upregulated in volume overload states, including SIADH.[133] ADH levels are elevated or inappropriately normal.

SIADH has many causes and is often transient.[130] Increased intracranial pressure, interventricular hemorrhages, subarachnoid and subdural hemorrhages, meningitis, encephalitis, and other central nervous system infections all can serve as insults for excess ADH and are somewhat common in neonates.[130] Lower respiratory tract infections, atelectasis, and pneumothoraxes have all been documented to cause SIADH in neonates.[130,134] Hypothyroidism has been associated with SIADH, so thyroid hormone levels should be measured.[135]

Treatment of SIADH involves correction of the offending agent and water restriction. Patients generally respond well to fluid restriction below traditional "maintenance levels."[130] Sometimes, sodium supplementation is used but is not the preferred initial management. In symptomatic hyponatremia with seizures, 3% NaCl should be administered to cause a small increase in serum sodium, which will often stop the seizures.[130] Vaptans, V2 receptor antagonists that block ADH binding to its receptor, can be used in chronic cases of increased ADH secretion.[130] Fluid balance and sodium levels can shift rapidly with response to this blockade and need to be monitored closely.[130] At this time, tolvaptan is the only approved oral agent for the treatment of SIADH, but these studies were for adults. More studies will be necessary to determine the appropriate dosage, dosing intervals, and safety for children and neonates, but it remains an interesting potential therapeutic option.

Nephrogenic Syndrome of Inappropriate Antidiuresis

Although SIADH is the result of excessive ADH secretion, a renal form of inappropriate antidiuresis that is independent of ADH has been recently described.[136] This is due to an X-linked recessive genetic condition called nephrogenic syndrome of inappropriate antidiuresis (NSIAD) and clinically mimics SIADH except that ADH levels will be low or undetectable.[136,137] In these cases, the *AVPR2* gene, which codes for the V2 receptor, has a gain of function mutation resulting in constitutive activation of the V2 receptor. Since the osmoreceptors are unaffected, the body will inhibit ADH secretion as the osmolality lowers,[136,137] Sequencing of the *AVPR2* gene yields the diagnosis. Recently, another cause of NSIAD was described. These patients were found to have mutations in the G-protein that couples the V2R with adenylate cyclase.[138,139]

Patients with NSIAD can be treated with fluid restriction, but this can prove challenging in infants as proper nutrition is of critical importance for their overall health. Oral urea supplementation, which is an osmotic diuretic and simultaneously reduces natriuresis, has been used successfully.[137] This form of therapy has been shown to be safe, increases serum sodium levels, is nonnephrotoxic, and allows for optimal nutritional intake while the infant remains on a liquid only diet.[137] More trials are needed regarding oral urea use.

Hypernatremia

Hypernatremia is generally due to inadequate intake of free water or from excessive loss of free water. Although it is rarely due to excessive intake of sodium, this has occurred in the setting of accidental salt poisoning.[140,141] Many of these patients died or had severe neurologic sequelae.[140] Hypernatremia is associated with seizures, bradycardia, renal failure, intracranial hemorrhage, pontine myelinolysis, vascular thrombosis, and disseminated intravascular coagulopathy.[142] It will cause fluid shifts from the intracellular space into the extracellular space to equilibrate the osmotic gradient, leading to cellular shrinkage. This cellular shrinkage, when it occurs acutely in the cerebral hemisphere, results in tearing of the bridging veins and intracranial hemorrhage.[142] The brain will form idiogenic osmoles to help correct the cell volume of the neurons.[143] Thus, correction of hypernatremia, particularly chronic hypernatremia, should occur slowly, with no more than 10–12 mEq/L per day, which is an average of 0.5 mEq/L correction per hour. Rapid correction has adverse outcomes such as cerebral edema.[142]

When assessing a patient with hypernatremia, a number of factors must be determined. First, the free water deficit should be calculated. This is the amount of water that is required to decrease the serum sodium to a desired concentration and is calculated: free water deficit (L) = 0.7 × current weight (kg) × [(current serum sodium/desired serum sodium) − 1].[144] Second, one needs to determine if the patient has an isotonic fluid loss as in vomiting or diarrhea. This might need replacement with an isotonic fluid to replenish the extracellular fluid space. Third, the source of the free water loss needs to be determined. As will be seen, there can be extrarenal loss of free water or the free water can be renally excreted.

To evaluate whether the free water loss is from the kidney or if it is extrarenal, the urine osmolality and urine chemistries should be measured. In the setting of extrarenal losses, the kidneys will be maximally concentrating the urine. However, if the kidneys are the source of free water loss, the urine will be inappropriately dilute. In some circumstances, there might be an osmolar diuresis that causes the urine osmolality to be high, but the electrolyte free water clearance is also high indicating loss of free water.[145]

Renal Free Water Loss: Central and Nephrogenic Diabetes Insipidus

Diabetes insipidus (DI) is a urine concentrating defect that results in polyuria, dehydration, hypernatremia, and inappropriately dilute urine.[146] When evaluating this condition, studies to obtain include urine and serum sodium and osmolalities and serum vasopressin levels. Patients with untreated DI will have laboratory findings of hypernatremia, serum osmolality of >290 mOsm/L, and an inappropriately dilute urine with an osmolality that is generally <300 mOsm/L.[146]

DI can be central, which is due to lack of production of ADH, or nephrogenic, which is due to tubular unresponsiveness to ADH. Both present the same

clinically but have different management considerations. Determination of what type of DI the patient has is evaluating the response to exogenous vasopressin. If following its administration, the patient's urine output decreases, urine osmolality increases, and serum osmolality decreases, this indicates that the collecting tubules have a normal response to vasopressin and the patient has central DI (CDI). Alternatively, if exogenous vasopressin is administered and there is no change in urine output, serum sodium, serum osmolality, and urine osmolality, the renal tubules have a defective response to vasopressin, thus providing the diagnosis of nephrogenic DI (NDI). Serum ADH levels can be measured and should be absent in patients with CDI and should be high in patients with NDI.

Central DI occurs in infants with defects in the hypothalamus-pituitary axis including genetic defects, autoimmune conditions, congenital midline and midbrain defects, structural brain anomalies such as tumors (especially germinomas), Langerhans cell histiocytosis, after both bacterial and viral meningitis, following cerebral infarction, with intraventricular hemorrhage or other traumatic brain injuries, and idiopathically.[146,147] There have been reports of transient CDI in premature infants, especially those who have brain malformations, but these are uncommon.[146] Once CDI is diagnosed, there should be further head imaging with a brain MRI and other workup to determine the underlying cause. Treatment for CDI is regular administration of exogenous vasopressin. Recently, thiazide diuretics have been used to help in the treatment of small infants with CDI that rely on a liquid diet.[148,149]

NDI, is due to the collecting tubules inability to respond to vasopressin.[150] The same clinical syndrome of polyuria, dilute urine osmolality, hypernatremia, dehydration, and high serum osmolality will still occur. Genetic mutations in *AVPR2* and *AQP2* genes are almost always associated with congenital NDI.[147] The *AVPR2* gene is located on the X-chromosome, inherited in an X-linked recessive pattern, codes for the V2 receptor, and is the most frequently mutated gene, with over 90% of patients with congenital NDI having one of over 300 mutations at this locus.[147] Being X-linked recessive, it is mostly found in male infants. It can occur in female infants if both parents were to have the same mutation, if skewed inactivation of the normal X-chromosome occurs, or in female infants with Turner's syndrome.[147] Some female carriers of the mutation have been shown to have polyuria and are considered partial NDI, but the majority do not develop any significant syndrome.[151] The *AQP2* gene is found on chromosome 12 and codes for the AQP2 tetramer; mutations in this gene are often loss-of-function mutations.[150] Generally, this is an autosomal recessive condition, but cases of autosomal dominant inheritance have been described.[150]

NDI can be acquired. Noninherited forms of NDI have been documented to be transient, provided the underlying insult is corrected. Hypokalemia and hypercalciuria are both associated with decreased AQP2 expression, independent of vasopressin activity.[152,153] Interestingly, Bartter syndrome, an inherited tubular wasting disorder, and apparent mineralocorticoid excess can cause the necessary electrolyte derangements for NDI.[150] Obstructive uropathy is another important cause of NDI. The increased hydrostatic pressure on the ipsilateral collecting tubules from the obstruction has an inhibitory effect on apical AQP2 expression and can persist for up to 30 days following resolution of the obstruction.[150] Lastly, lithium toxicity is known to cause nephrogenic DI. Lithium enters the apical ENaC sodium channels, has been shown to reduce apical *AQP2* expression, and, chronically, leads to epithelial remodeling of the collecting ducts and reduced principal cells.[154,155] Although lithium is not used in infants, it both crosses the placental barrier and is expressed in limited amounts in breastmilk and therefore can be serologically evident in infants born to and breastfed by lithium-ingesting mothers.[156,157] Amiloride, which inhibits ENaC, has been used successfully to reduce lithium reabsorption and promote lithium excretion.[158]

Thiazide diuretics are effective in treating NDI and are the current mainstay of therapy. Thiazide diuretics decrease sodium reabsorption in the distal tubule by inhibiting NCC in the DCT, thus favoring sodium and water loss.[150,159] The initial natriuresis results in volume depletion but after regular thiazide administration, patients with NDI experienced decreased natriuresis, a significant reduction in urine output, increased urine osmolality, and decreased serum osmolality.[160] It is hypothesized this paradoxical reaction results from increased compensatory proximal tubule reabsorption of sodium and water in response to the initial volume loss.[160] Recent studies also show that there is increased expression of NCC, ENaC, and AQP2.[161]

Extrarenal Free Water Loss

The more extremes of prematurity are associated with an underdeveloped infant in a multisystem way. Notably, the body's largest organ, the skin, is underkeratinized and thus becomes is highly permeable to water, serving as a source of insensible fluid loss in these patients.[162] AQP3 is expressed in abundance on the basal layer of the epidermis on premature neonates, thereby allowing increased passage of water from the dermis to the epidermis, which then evaporates and increases free water loss.[75] Physiologically, it is comparable to the excessive fluid losses and dehydration in burn patients, who have severe disruption of their skin. Hypernatremia is quite common in preterm neonates with up to 40% of infants born less than 28 weeks' gestation and weighing less than 1250 g and as many as 69% of infants less than 27 weeks' gestation all developing hypernatremia.[162] Infants with substantial abdominal wall defects such as gastroschisis and omphaloceles also experience increased transepidermal water loss and are at higher risk for hypernatremia.[162] High humidity incubators, with up to 60%–80% humidity, can minimize these losses in infants and should be employed routinely for the extremely preterm infants.

Some centers have utilized placing a semipermeable polyurethane membrane to reduce the transepidermal free water losses. One center in Rome applied the membrane to the infants chest, abdomen, back, and extremities within the first 6 hours of life and left them in place for a minimum of 2 weeks and compared these infants to demographically similar infants who had no membranes applied. Overall, the intervention group had fewer episodes of hypernatremia, reduced weight loss, increased incidence of hyponatremia, and greater urine output compared with the control group.[162] Overall, weight loss was reduced by 3.8% in the intervention group compared with the control further supporting less fluid losses in these patients.[162] Although this study found success in minimizing water loss and hypernatremia in premature infants with application of a semipermeable membrane, this should only occur in experienced centers and with skilled nursing and careful monitoring of daily weights, sodium levels, and urine output as hyponatremia could occur.

Feeding Insufficiency

Although most of the neonatal dehydration hypernatremia stems from difficulties with breastfeeding, formula feeding can also present with challenges. Formula mixing can be unfamiliar or confusing to new parents and, if mixed in incorrect ratios, can result in an overly concentrated solute load, less free water, and subsequent hypernatremic dehydration. Rarely, some premature infants or cardiac patients who are on fortified and highly concentrated formulas and may have intrinsic renal disease due to prematurity or poor perfusion can also develop dehydrated hypernatremia.

After their birth, it is physiologic for neonates to diurese and lose a significant portion of their weight as free water losses. Generally, 7%–10% weight loss is considered normal in the first week of life; the infant should regain it in the coming weeks. Excessive weight loss is defined as more than 10% of the birth weight being lost in the within the first week of life and indicates dehydration and malnutrition.[75] Approximately 15% of all breastfed neonates will experience severe weight loss in the first week, and one third of them will have hypernatremia on laboratory findings.[75]

REFERENCES

1. Moritz ML, Ayus JC. Hyponatremia in preterm neonates: not a benign condition. *Pediatrics*. 2009;124(5):e1014–e1016. doi:10.1542/peds.2009-1869
2. Boskabadi H, Akhondian J, Afarideh M, et al. Long-term neurodevelopmental outcome of neonates with hypernatremic dehydration. *Breastfeed Med*. 2017;12:163–168. doi:10.1089/bfm.2016.0054
3. Baraton L, Ancel PY, Flamant C, Orsonneau JL, Darmaun D, Roze JC. Impact of changes in serum sodium levels on 2-year neurologic outcomes for very preterm neonates. *Pediatrics*. 2009;124(4):e655–e661. doi:10.1542/peds.2008-3415
4. Gomez RA, Sequeira Lopez ML, Fernandez L, Chernavvsky DR, Norwood VF. The maturing kidney: development and susceptibility. *Ren Fail*. 1999;21(3–4):283–291. doi:10.3109/08860229909085090
5. Gattineni J, Baum M. Developmental changes in renal tubular transport-an overview. *Pediatr Nephrol*. 2015;30(12):2085–2098. doi:10.1007/s00467-013-2666-6
6. Filler G. A step forward towards accurately assessing glomerular filtration rate in newborns. *Pediatr Nephrol*. 2015;30(8):1209–1212. doi:10.1007/s00467-014-3014-1
7. Abitbol CL, DeFreitas MJ, Strauss J. Assessment of kidney function in preterm infants: lifelong implications. *Pediatr Nephrol*. 2016;31(12):2213–2222. doi:10.1007/s00467-016-3320-x
8. Wilhelm-Bals A, Combescure C, Chehade H, Daali Y, Parvex P. Variables of interest to predict glomerular filtration rate in preterm newborns in the first days of life. *Pediatr Nephrol*. 2020;35(4):703–712. doi:10.1007/s00467-019-04257-z
9. Iacobelli S, Guignard JP. Maturation of glomerular filtration rate in neonates and infants: an overview. *Pediatr Nephrol*. 2021;36(6):1439–1446. doi:10.1007/s00467-020-04632-1
10. Rubin MI, Bruck E, Rapoport M, Snively M, McKay H, Baumler A. Maturation of renal function in childhood: clearance studies. *J Clin Invest*. 1949;28(5 Pt 2):1144–1162. doi:10.1172/JCI102149
11. Palmer LG, Schnermann J. Integrated control of Na transport along the nephron. *Clin J Am Soc Nephrol*. 2015;10(4):676–687. doi:10.2215/CJN.12391213
12. Curthoys NP, Moe OW. Proximal tubule function and response to acidosis. *Clin J Am Soc Nephrol*. 2014;9(9):1627–1638. doi:10.2215/CJN.10391012
13. Koeppen B. Solute and water transport. *Berne & Levy Physiology*. 8th ed. Elsevier; 2023.
14. Brant SR, Bernstein M, Wasmuth JJ, et al. Physical and genetic mapping of a human apical epithelial Na+/H+ exchanger (NHE3) isoform to chromosome 5p15.3. *Genomics*. 1993;15(3):668–672. doi:10.1006/geno.1993.1122
15. Romero MF, Boron WF. Electrogenic Na+/HCO3- cotransporters: cloning and physiology. *Annu Rev Physiol*. 1999;61:699–723. doi:10.1146/annurev.physiol.61.1.699
16. Quigley R. Proximal renal tubular acidosis. *J Nephrol*. 2006;19(Suppl 9):S41–S45.
17. Galla JH. Metabolic alkalosis. *J Am Soc Nephrol*. 2000;11(2):369–375. doi:10.1681/ASN.V112369
18. Hummel CS, Lu C, Loo DD, Hirayama BA, Voss AA, Wright EM. Glucose transport by human renal Na+/D-glucose cotransporters SGLT1 and SGLT2. *Am J Physiol Cell Physiol*. 2011;300(1):C14–C21. doi:10.1152/ajpcell.00388.2010
19. Vallon V, Platt KA, Cunard R, et al. SGLT2 mediates glucose reabsorption in the early proximal tubule. *J Am Soc Nephrol*. 2011;22(1):104–112. doi:10.1681/ASN.2010030246
20. Biber J, Hernando N, Forster I, Murer H. Regulation of phosphate transport in proximal tubules. *Pflugers Arch*. 2009;458(1):39–52. doi:10.1007/s00424-008-0580-8
21. Virkki LV, Biber J, Murer H, Forster IC. Phosphate transporters: a tale of two solute carrier families. *Am J Physiol Renal Physiol*. 2007;293(3):F643–F654. doi:10.1152/ajprenal.00228.2007
22. Broer S. Apical transporters for neutral amino acids: physiology and pathophysiology. *Physiology (Bethesda)*. 2008;23:95–103. doi:10.1152/physiol.00045.2007
23. Broer S. Amino acid transport across mammalian intestinal and renal epithelia. *Physiol Rev*. 2008;88(1):249–286. doi:10.1152/physrev.00018.2006
24. Berry CA, Rector FC Jr. Electroneutral NaCl absorption in the proximal tubule: mechanisms of apical Na-coupled transport. *Kidney Int*. 1989;36(3):403–411. doi:10.1038/ki.1989.209
25. Aronson PS. Ion exchangers mediating Na+, HCO3 - and Cl- transport in the renal proximal tubule. *J Nephrol*. 2006;19(Suppl 9):S3–S10.

26. Rector FC Jr. Sodium, bicarbonate, and chloride absorption by the proximal tubule. *Am J Physiol.* 1983;244(5):F461–F471. doi:10.1152/ajprenal.1983.244.5.F461

27. Muto S. Physiological roles of claudins in kidney tubule paracellular transport. *Am J Physiol Renal Physiol.* 2017;312(1):F9–F24. doi:10.1152/ajprenal.00204.2016

28. Schwartz GJ, Haycock GB, Edelmann CM Jr, Spitzer A. Late metabolic acidosis: a reassessment of the definition. *J Pediatr.* 1979;95(1):102–107. doi:10.1016/s0022-3476(79)80098-0

29. Quigley R, Baum M. Developmental changes in rabbit juxtamedullary proximal convoluted tubule bicarbonate permeability. *Pediatr Res.* 1990;28(6):663–666. doi:10.1203/00006450-199012000-00024

30. Schwartz GJ, Evan AP. Development of solute transport in rabbit proximal tubule. III. Na-K-ATPase activity. *Am J Physiol.* 1984;246(6 Pt 2):F845–F852. doi:10.1152/ajprenal.1984.246.6.F845

31. Schwartz GJ, Evan AP. Development of solute transport in rabbit proximal tubule. I. HCO-3 and glucose absorption. *Am J Physiol.* 1983;245(3):F382–F390. doi:10.1152/ajprenal.1983.245.3.F382

32. Baum M, Quigley R. Maturation of proximal tubular acidification. *Pediatr Nephrol.* 1993;7(6):785–791. doi:10.1007/BF01213361

33. Baum M, Quigley R. Ontogeny of proximal tubule acidification. *Kidney Int.* 1995;48(6):1697–1704. doi:10.1038/ki.1995.467

34. Goyal S, Vanden Heuvel G, Aronson PS. Renal expression of novel Na+/H+ exchanger isoform NHE8. *Am J Physiol Renal Physiol.* 2003;284(3):F467–F473. doi:10.1152/ajprenal.00352.2002

35. Becker AM, Zhang J, Goyal S, et al. Ontogeny of NHE8 in the rat proximal tubule. *Am J Physiol Renal Physiol.* 2007;293(1):F255–F261. doi:10.1152/ajprenal.00400.2006

36. Joseph C, Twombley K, Gattineni J, Zhang Q, Dwarakanath V, Baum M. Acid increases NHE8 surface expression and activity in NRK cells. *Am J Physiol Renal Physiol.* 2012;302(4):F495–F503. doi:10.1152/ajprenal.00331.2011

37. Gupta N, Tarif SR, Seikaly M, Baum M. Role of glucocorticoids in the maturation of the rat renal Na+/H+ antiporter (NHE3). *Kidney Int.* 2001;60(1):173–181. doi:10.1046/j.1523-1755.2001.00784.x

38. Baum M, Quigley R. Prenatal glucocorticoids stimulate neonatal juxtamedullary proximal convoluted tubule acidification. *Am J Physiol.* 1991;261(5 Pt 2):F746–F752. doi:10.1152/ajprenal.1991.261.5.F746

39. Joseph C, Gattineni J, Dwarakanath V, Baum M. Glucocorticoids reduce renal NHE8 expression. *Physiol Rep.* 2013;1(2):1–10.

40. Gattineni J, Sas D, Dagan A, Dwarakanath V, Baum M. Effect of thyroid hormone on the postnatal renal expression of NHE8. *Am J Physiol Renal Physiol.* 2008;294(1):F198–F204. doi:10.1152/ajprenal.00332.2007

41. Baum M, Quigley R. Thyroid hormone modulates rabbit proximal straight tubule paracellular permeability. *Am J Physiol Renal Physiol.* 2004;286(3):F477–F482. doi:10.1152/ajprenal.00248.2003

42. Abuazza G, Becker A, Williams SS, et al. Claudins 6, 9, and 13 are developmentally expressed renal tight junction proteins. *Am J Physiol Renal Physiol.* 2006;291(6):F1132–F1141. doi:10.1152/ajprenal.00063.2006

43. Haddad M, Lin F, Dwarakanath V, Cordes K, Baum M. Developmental changes in proximal tubule tight junction proteins. *Pediatr Res.* 2005;57(3):453–457. doi:10.1203/01.PDR.0000151354.07752.9B

44. Sas D, Hu M, Moe OW, Baum M. Effect of claudins 6 and 9 on paracellular permeability in MDCK II cells. *Am J Physiol Regul Integr Comp Physiol.* 2008;295(5):R1713–R1719. doi:10.1152/ajpregu.90596.2008

45. Baum M. Developmental changes in proximal tubule NaCl transport. *Pediatr Nephrol.* 2008;23(2):185–194. doi:10.1007/s00467-007-0569-0

46. Preston GM, Carroll TP, Guggino WB, Agre P. Appearance of water channels in Xenopus oocytes expressing red cell CHIP28 protein. *Science.* 1992;256(5055):385–387. doi:10.1126/science.256.5055.385

47. Agre P, Preston GM, Smith BL, et al. Aquaporin CHIP: the archetypal molecular water channel. *Am J Physiol.* 1993;265(4 Pt 2):F463–F476. doi:10.1152/ajprenal.1993.265.4.F463

48. Quigley R, Harkins EW, Thomas PJ, Baum M. Maturational changes in rabbit renal brush border membrane vesicle osmotic water permeability. *J Membr Biol.* 1998;164(2):177–185. doi:10.1007/s002329900403

49. Quigley R, Gupta N, Lisec A, Baum M. Maturational changes in rabbit renal basolateral membrane vesicle osmotic water permeability. *J Membr Biol.* 2000;174(1):53–58. doi:10.1007/s002320001031

50. Quigley R, Baum M. Developmental changes in rabbit juxtamedullary proximal convoluted tubule water permeability. *Am J Physiol.* 1996;271(4 Pt 2):F871–F876. doi:10.1152/ajprenal.1996.271.4.F871

51. Quigley R, Baum M. Water transport in neonatal and adult rabbit proximal tubules. *Am J Physiol Renal Physiol.* 2002;283(2):F280–285. doi:10.1152/ajprenal.00341.2001

52. Quigley R, Mulder J, Baum M. Ontogeny of water transport in the rabbit proximal tubule. *Pediatr Nephrol.* 2003;18(11):1089–1094. doi:10.1007/s00467-003-1241-y

53. Dantzler WH, Layton AT, Layton HE, Pannabecker TL. Urine-concentrating mechanism in the inner medulla: function of the thin limbs of the loops of Henle. *Clin J Am Soc Nephrol.* 2014;9(10):1781–1789. doi:10.2215/CJN.08750812

54. Kim YM, Kim WY, Nam SA, et al. Role of Prox1 in the transforming ascending thin limb of Henle's loop during mouse kidney development. *PLoS One.* 2015;10(5):e0127429. doi:10.1371/journal.pone.0127429

55. Cha JH, Kim YH, Jung JY, Han KH, Madsen KM, Kim J. Cell proliferation in the loop of Henle in the developing rat kidney. *J Am Soc Nephrol.* 2001;12(7):1410–1421. doi:10.1681/ASN.V1271410

56. Song R, Yosypiv IV. Development of the kidney medulla. *Organogenesis.* 2012;8(1):10–7. doi:10.4161/org.19308

57. Mount DB. Thick ascending limb of the loop of Henle. *Clin J Am Soc Nephrol.* 2014;9(11):1974–1986. doi:10.2215/CJN.04480413

58. Gilbert S, Weiner D Eds. *National Kidney Foundation Primer on Kidney Diseases.* 8th ed. Elsevier; 2022.

59. Horster M. Loop of Henle functional differentiation: in vitro perfusion of the isolated thick ascending segment. *Pflugers Arch.* 1978;378(1):15–24. doi:10.1007/BF00581953

60. Subramanya AR, Ellison DH. Distal convoluted tubule. *Clin J Am Soc Nephrol.* 2014;9(12):2147–2163. doi:10.2215/CJN.05920613

61. Lee V, Mather A. *The Renal System.* Systems of the Body Series. Elsevier; 2022.

62. Pearce D, Soundararajan R, Trimpert C, Kashlan OB, Deen PM, Kohan DE. Collecting duct principal cell transport processes and their regulation. *Clin J Am Soc Nephrol.* 2015;10(1): 135–146. doi:10.2215/CJN.05760513

63. White PC, Mune T, Agarwal AK. 11 beta-Hydroxysteroid dehydrogenase and the syndrome of apparent mineralocorticoid excess. *Endocr Rev.* 1997;18(1):135–156. doi:10.1210/edrv.18.1.0288

64. Vehaskari VM. Ontogeny of cortical collecting duct sodium transport. *Am J Physiol.* 1994;267(1 Pt 2):F49–F54. doi:10.1152/ajprenal.1994.267.1.F49

65. Vehaskari VM, Hempe JM, Manning J, Aviles DH, Carmichael MC. Developmental regulation of ENaC subunit mRNA levels in rat kidney. *Am J Physiol.* 1998;274(6):C1661–C1666. doi:10.1152/ajpcell.1998.274.6.C1661

66. Satlin LM, Palmer LG. Apical Na+ conductance in maturing rabbit principal cell. *Am J Physiol.* 1996;270(3 Pt 2):F391–F397. doi:10.1152/ajprenal.1996.270.3.F391

67. Bonilla-Felix M. Development of water transport in the collecting duct. *Am J Physiol Renal Physiol.* 2004;287(6):F1093–F101. doi:10.1152/ajprenal.00119.2004

68. Bonilla-Felix M, John-Phillip C. Prostaglandins mediate the defect in AVP-stimulated cAMP generation in immature collecting duct. *Am J Physiol.* 1994;267(1 Pt 2):F44–F48. doi:10.1152/ajprenal.1994.267.1.F44

69. Bonilla-Felix M, Vehaskari VM, Hamm LL. Water transport in the immature rabbit collecting duct. *Pediatr Nephrol.* 1999;13(2):103–107. doi:10.1007/s004670050572

70. Quigley R, Chakravarty S, Baum M. Antidiuretic hormone resistance in the neonatal cortical collecting tubule is mediated in part by elevated phosphodiesterase activity. *Am J Physiol Renal Physiol.* 2004;286(2):F317–F322. doi:10.1152/ajprenal.00122.2003

71. Chow E, Fox N, Gama R. Effect of low serum total protein on sodium and potassium measurement by ion-selective electrodes in critically ill patients. *Br J Biomed Sci.* 2008;65(3): 128–131. doi:10.1080/09674845.2008.11732815

72. King RI, Mackay RJ, Florkowski CM, Lynn AM. Electrolytes in sick neonates—which sodium is the right answer? *Arch Dis Child Fetal Neonatal Ed.* 2013;98(1):F74–F76. doi:10.1136/archdischild-2011-300929

73. Gruskin AB, Baluarte HJ, Prebis JW, Polinsky MS, Morgenstern BZ, Perlman SA. Serum sodium abnormalities in children. *Pediatr Clin North Am.* 1982;29(4):907–932. doi:10.1016/s0031-3955(16)34220-1

74. Marcialis MA, Dessi A, Pintus MC, Irmesi R, Fanos V. Neonatal hyponatremia: differential diagnosis and treatment. *J Matern Fetal Neonatal Med.* 2011;24(Suppl 1):75–79. doi:10.3109/14767058.2011.607667

75. Marcialis MA, Dessi A, Pintus MC, Marinelli V, Fanos V. Hyponatremia and hypernatremia in the newborn: in medio stat virtus. *Front Biosci (Elite Ed).* 2012;4:132–140. doi:10.2741/364

76. Martin RJ. Central pontine and extrapontine myelinolysis: the osmotic demyelination syndromes. *J Neurol Neurosurg Psychiatry.* 2004;75(Suppl 3):iii22–iii28. doi:10.1136/jnnp.2004.045906

77. Bansal LR, Zinkus T. Osmotic demyelination syndrome in children. *Pediatr Neurol.* 2019;97:12–17. doi:10.1016/j.pediatrneurol.2019.03.018

78. Aperia A, Broberger O, Herin P, Thodenius K, Zetterstrom R. Postnatal control of water and electrolyte homeostasis in

pre-term and full-term infants. *Acta Paediatr Scand Suppl.* 1983;305:61–65. doi:10.1111/j.1651-2227.1983.tb09861.x

79. O'Connor RE. Water intoxication with seizures. *Ann Emerg Med.* 1985;14(1):71–73. doi:10.1016/s0196-0644(85)80740-x

80. Crumpacker RW, Kriel RL. Voluntary water intoxication in normal infants. *Neurology.* 1973;23(11):1251–1255. doi:10.1212/wnl.23.11.1251

81. Brenner BM, Bennett CM, Berliner RW. The relationship between glomerular filtration rate and sodium reabsorption by the proximal tubule of the rat nephron. *J Clin Invest.* 1968;47(6):1358–1374. doi:10.1172/JCI105828

82. Brenner BM, Berliner RW. Relationship between extracellular volume and fluid reabsorption by the rat nephron. *Am J Physiol.* 1969;217(1):6–12. doi:10.1152/ajplegacy.1969.217.1.6

83. Brenner BM, Falchuk KH, Keimowitz RI, Berliner RW. The relationship between peritubular capillary protein concentration and fluid reabsorption by the renal proximal tubule. *J Clin Invest.* 1969;48(8):1519–1531. doi:10.1172/JCI106118

84. Falchuk KH, Brenner BM, Tadokoro M, Berliner RW. Oncotic and hydrostatic pressures in peritubular capillaries and fluid reabsorption by proximal tubule. *Am J Physiol.* 1971;220(5): 1427–1433. doi:10.1152/ajplegacy.1971.220.5.1427

85. Quan A, Baum M. Endogenous production of angiotensin II modulates rat proximal tubule transport. *J Clin Invest.* 1996;97(12):2878–2882. doi:10.1172/JCI118745

86. Quan A, Baum M. Endogenous angiotensin II modulates rat proximal tubule transport with acute changes in extracellular volume. *Am J Physiol.* 1998;275(1):F74–F78. doi:10.1152/ajprenal.1998.275.1.F74

87. Quan A, Baum M. Regulation of proximal tubule transport by endogenously produced angiotensin II. *Nephron.* 2000;84(2): 103–110. doi:10.1159/000045556

88. Bueva A, Guignard JP. Renal function in preterm neonates. *Pediatr Res.* 1994;36(5):572–577. doi:10.1203/00006450-199411000-00005

89. Seethapathy H, Fenves AZ. Fractional excretion of sodium (FENa): an imperfect tool for a flawed question. *Clin J Am Soc Nephrol.* 2022;17(6):777–778. doi:10.2215/CJN.04750422.

90. Abdelhafez M, Nayfeh T, Atieh A, et al. Diagnostic performance of fractional excretion of sodium for the differential diagnosis of acute kidney injury: a systematic review and meta-analysis. *Clin J Am Soc Nephrol.* 2022;17(6):785–797. doi:10.2215/CJN.14561121

91. Berger AA, Mawson TL, Dejam A. Fractional excretion of urate for diuresis management in heart failure and cardiorenal syndrome. *JACC Case Rep.* 2021;3(7):1051–1054. doi:10.1016/j.jaccas.2020.12.035

92. Pepin MN, Bouchard J, Legault L, Ethier J. Diagnostic performance of fractional excretion of urea and fractional excretion of sodium in the evaluations of patients with acute kidney injury with or without diuretic treatment. *Am J Kidney Dis.* 2007;50(4):566–573. doi:10.1053/j.ajkd.2007.07.001

93. Schrier RW, Goldberg JP. The physiology of vasopressin release and the pathogenesis of impaired water excretion in adrenal, thyroid, and edematous disorders. *Yale J Biol Med.* 1980;53(6):525–541.

94. Di Meglio L, Castaldo G, Mosca C, et al. Congenital chloride diarrhea clinical features and management: a systematic review. *Pediatr Res.* 2021;90(1):23–29. doi:10.1038/s41390-020-01251-2

95. Janecke AR, Heinz-Erian P, Muller T. Congenital sodium diarrhea: a form of intractable diarrhea, with a link to

inflammatory bowel disease. *J Pediatr Gastroenterol Nutr.* 2016;63(2):170–176. doi:10.1097/MPG.0000000000001139

96. Janecke AR, Heinz-Erian P, Yin J, et al. Reduced sodium/ proton exchanger NHE3 activity causes congenital sodium diarrhea. *Hum Mol Genet.* 2015;24(23):6614–6623. doi:10. 1093/hmg/ddv367

97. Rowe SM, Miller S, Sorscher EJ. Cystic fibrosis. *N Engl J Med.* 2005;352(19):1992–2001. doi:10.1056/NEJMra043184

98. Beckerman RC, Taussig LM. Hypoelectrolytemia and metabolic alkalosis in infants with cystic fibrosis. *Pediatrics.* 1979; 63(4):580–583.

99. Guimaraes EV, Schettino GC, Camargos PA, Penna FJ. Prevalence of hyponatremia at diagnosis and factors associated with the longitudinal variation in serum sodium levels in infants with cystic fibrosis. Editors Scott Gilbert and Daniel. Weiner *J Pediatr.* 2012;161(2):285–289. doi:10.1016/ j.jpeds.2012.01.052

100. Faraji-Goodarzi M. Pseudo-Bartter syndrome in children with cystic fibrosis. *Clin Case Rep.* 2019;7(6):1123–1126. doi:10. 1002/ccr3.2180

101. Ballestero Y, Hernandez MI, Rojo P, et al. Hyponatremic dehydration as a presentation of cystic fibrosis. *Pediatr Emerg Care.* 2006; 22(11):725–727. doi:10.1097/01.pec.0000245170.31343.bb

102. Berg P, Jeppesen M, Leipziger J. Cystic fibrosis in the kidney: new lessons from impaired renal HCO3- excretion. *Curr Opin Nephrol Hypertens.* 2021;30(4):437–443. doi:10.1097/MNH. 0000000000000725

103. Berg P, Svendsen SL, Sorensen MV, Schreiber R, Kunzelmann K, Leipziger J. The molecular mechanism of CFTR- and secretin-dependent renal bicarbonate excretion. *J Physiol.* 2021;599(12):3003–3011. doi:10.1113/JP281285

104. Williams GH. Aldosterone biosynthesis, regulation, and classical mechanism of action. *Heart Fail Rev.* 2005;10(1):7–13. doi:10.1007/s10741-005-2343-3

105. Gopal-Kothandapani JS, Doshi AB, Smith K, et al. Phenotypic diversity and correlation with the genotypes of pseudohypoaldosteronism type 1. *J Pediatr Endocrinol Metab.* 2019;32(9): 959–967. doi:10.1515/jpem-2018-0538

106. Amin N, Alvi NS, Barth JH, et al. Pseudohypoaldosteronism type 1: clinical features and management in infancy. *Endocrinol Diabetes Metab Case Rep.* 2013;2013:130010. doi:10.1530/ EDM-13-0010

107. White PC. Aldosterone synthase deficiency and related disorders. *Mol Cell Endocrinol.* 2004;217(1-2):81–87. doi:10.1016/j. mce.2003.10.013

108. El-Maouche D, Arlt W, Merke DP. Congenital adrenal hyperplasia. *Lancet.* 2017;390(10108):2194–2210. doi:10.1016/ S0140-6736(17)31431-9

109. Speiser PW. Prenatal and neonatal diagnosis and treatment of congenital adrenal hyperplasia. *Horm Res.* 2007;68(Suppl 5):90–92. doi:10.1159/000110586

110. Casas-Alba D, Vila Cots J, Monfort Carretero L, et al. Pseudohypoaldosteronism types I and II: little more than a name in common. *J Pediatr Endocrinol Metab.* 2017;30(5):597–601. doi:10.1515/jpem-2016-0467

111. Martinerie L, Viengchareun S, Meduri G, Kim HS, Luther JM, Lombes M. Aldosterone postnatally, but not at birth, is required for optimal induction of renal mineralocorticoid receptor expression and sodium reabsorption. *Endocrinology.* 2011;152(6):2483–2491. doi:10.1210/en.2010-1460

112. Isemann B, Mueller EW, Narendran V, Akinbi H. Impact of early sodium supplementation on hyponatremia and growth in premature infants: a randomized controlled trial. *JPEN J Parenter Enteral Nutr.* 2016;40(3):342–349. doi:10. 1177/0148607114558303

113. Segar JL, Grobe CC, Grobe JL. Maturational changes in sodium metabolism in periviable infants. *Pediatr Nephrol.* 2021;36(11):3693–3698. doi:10.1007/s00467-021-05119-3

114. Gil-Ruiz MA, Alcaraz AJ, Maranon RJ, Navarro N, Huidobro B, Luque A. Electrolyte disturbances in acute pyelonephritis. *Pediatr Nephrol.* 2012;27(3):429–433. doi:10.1007/s00467-011-2020-9

115. Rodriguez-Soriano J, Vallo A, Oliveros R, Castillo G. Transient pseudohypoaldosteronism secondary to obstructive uropathy in infancy. *J Pediatr.* 1983;103(3):375–380. doi:10.1016/ s0022-3476(83)80406-5

116. Delforge X, Kongolo G, Cauliez A, Braun K, Haraux E, Buisson P. Transient pseudohypoaldosteronism: a potentially severe condition affecting infants with urinary tract malformation. *J Pediatr Urol.* 2019;15(3):265 e1–265 e7. doi:10.1016/j.jpurol.2019.03.002

117. Bartter FC, Pronove P, Gill JR Jr, Maccardle RC. Hyperplasia of the juxtaglomerular complex with hyperaldosteronism and hypokalemic alkalosis. A new syndrome. *Am J Med.* 1962;33:811–828. doi:10.1016/0002-9343(62)90214-0

118. Simon DB, Karet FE, Hamdan JM, DiPietro A, Sanjad SA, Lifton RP. Bartter's syndrome, hypokalaemic alkalosis with hypercalciuria, is caused by mutations in the Na-K-2Cl cotransporter NKCC2. *Nat Genet.* 1996;13(2):183–188. doi: 10.1038/ng0696-183

119. Simon DB, Karet FE, Rodriguez-Soriano J, et al. Genetic heterogeneity of Bartter's syndrome revealed by mutations in the K+ channel, ROMK. *Nat Genet.* 1996;14(2):152–156. doi: 10.1038/ng1096-152

120. Woda CB, Miyawaki N, Ramalakshmi S, et al. Ontogeny of flow-stimulated potassium secretion in rabbit cortical collecting duct: functional and molecular aspects. *Am J Physiol Renal Physiol.* 2003;285(4):F629–F639. doi:10.1152/ajprenal.00191.2003

121. Satlin LM. Developmental regulation of expression of renal potassium secretory channels. *Curr Opin Nephrol Hypertens.* 2004;13(4):445–450. doi:10.1097/01.mnh.0000133979.17311.21

122. Simon DB, Bindra RS, Mansfield TA, et al. Mutations in the chloride channel gene, CLCNKB, cause Bartter's syndrome type III. *Nat Genet.* 1997;17(2):171–178. doi:10.1038/ng1097-171

123. Birkenhager R, Otto E, Schurmann MJ, et al. Mutation of BSND causes Bartter syndrome with sensorineural deafness and kidney failure. *Nat Genet.* 2001;29(3):310–314. doi:10. 1038/ng752

124. Jeck N, Reinalter SC, Henne T, et al. Hypokalemic salt-losing tubulopathy with chronic renal failure and sensorineural deafness. *Pediatrics.* 2001;108(1):E5. doi:10.1542/ peds.108.1.e5

125. Laghmani K, Beck BB, Yang SS, et al. Polyhydramnios, transient antenatal Bartter's syndrome, and MAGED2 mutations. *N Engl J Med.* 2016;374(19):1853–1863. doi:10.1056/NEJMoa1507629

126. Quigley R, Saland JM. Transient antenatal Bartter's syndrome and X-linked polyhydramnios: insights from the genetics of a rare condition. *Kidney Int.* 2016;90(4):721–723. doi:10.1016/j. kint.2016.07.031

127. Gitelman HJ, Graham JB, Welt LG. A new familial disorder characterized by hypokalemia and hypomagnesemia. *Trans Assoc Am Physicians.* 1966;79:221–235.

128. Gitelman HJ, Graham JB, Welt LG. A familial disorder characterized by hypokalemia and hypomagnesemia. *Ann N Y Acad Sci.* 1969;162(2):856–864. doi:10.1111/j.1749-6632.1969.tb13015.x

129. Simon DB, Nelson-Williams C, Bia MJ, et al. Gitelman's variant of Bartter's syndrome, inherited hypokalaemic alkalosis, is caused by mutations in the thiazide-sensitive Na-Cl cotransporter. *Nat Genet.* 1996;12(1):24–30. doi:10.1038/ng0196-24

130. Peri A, Pirozzi N, Parenti G, Festuccia F, Mene P. Hyponatremia and the syndrome of inappropriate secretion of antidiuretic hormone (SIADH). *J Endocrinol Invest.* 2010;33(9):671–682. doi:10.1007/BF03346668

131. Decaux G, Musch W. Clinical laboratory evaluation of the syndrome of inappropriate secretion of antidiuretic hormone. *Clin J Am Soc Nephrol.* 2008;3(4):1175–1184. doi:10.2215/CJN.04431007

132. Schwartz WB, Bennett W, Curelop S, Bartter FC. A syndrome of renal sodium loss and hyponatremia probably resulting from inappropriate secretion of antidiuretic hormone. *Am J Med.* 1957;23(4):529–542. doi:10.1016/0002-9343(57)90224-3

133. Kamoi K, Ebe T, Kobayashi O, et al. Atrial natriuretic peptide in patients with the syndrome of inappropriate antidiuretic hormone secretion and with diabetes insipidus. *J Clin Endocrinol Metab.* 1990;70(5):1385–1390. doi:10.1210/jcem-70-5-1385

134. Paxson CL Jr, Stoerner JW, Denson SE, Adcock EW 3rd, Morriss FH Jr. Syndrome of inappropriate antidiuretic hormone secretion in neonates with pneumothorax or atelectasis. *J Pediatr.* 1977;91(3):459–463. doi:10.1016/s0022-3476(77)81325-5

135. Asami T, Uchiyama M. Sodium handling in congenitally hypothyroid neonates. *Acta Paediatr.* 2004;93(1):22–24. doi:10.1080/08035250310007259

136. Feldman BJ, Rosenthal SM, Vargas GA, et al. Nephrogenic syndrome of inappropriate antidiuresis. *N Engl J Med.* 2005;352(18):1884–1890. doi:10.1056/NEJMoa042743

137. Bardanzellu F, Pintus MC, Masile V, Fanos V, Marcialis MA. Focus on neonatal and infantile onset of nephrogenic syndrome of inappropriate antidiuresis: 12 years later. *Pediatr Nephrol.* 2019;34(5):763–775. doi:10.1007/s00467-018-3922-6

138. Miyado M, Fukami M, Takada S, et al. Germline-derived gain-of-function variants of Gsα-coding *GNAS* gene identified in nephrogenic syndrome of inappropriate antidiuresis. *J Am Soc Nephrol.* 2019;30(5):877–889. doi:10.1681/ASN.2018121268

139. Bichet DG, Granier S, Bockenhauer D. GNAS: a new nephrogenic cause of inappropriate antidiuresis. *J Am Soc Nephrol.* 2019;30(5):722–725. doi:10.1681/ASN.2019020143

140. Finberg L, Kiley J, Luttrell CN. Mass accidental salt poisoning in infancy. A study of a hospital disaster. *JAMA.* 1963;184:187–190. doi:10.1001/jama.1963.03700160063009

141. Miller NL, Finberg L. Peritoneal dialysis for salt poisoning. Report of a case. *N Engl J Med.* 1960;263:1347–1450. doi:10.1056/NEJM196012292632607

142. Sarin A, Thill A, Yaklin CW. Neonatal hypernatremic dehydration. *Pediatr Ann.* 2019;48(5):e197–e200. doi:10.3928/19382359-20190424-01

143. Lee JH, Arcinue E, Ross BD. Brief report: organic osmolytes in the brain of an infant with hypernatremia. *N Engl J Med.* 1994;331(7):439–442. doi:10.1056/NEJM199408183310704

144. Adrogue HJ, Madias NE. Hypernatremia. *N Engl J Med.* 2000;342(20):1493–1499. doi:10.1056/NEJM200005183422006

145. Shah SR, Bhave G. Using electrolyte free water balance to rationalize and treat dysnatremias. *Front Med (Lausanne).* 2018;5:103. doi:10.3389/fmed.2018.00103

146. Patti G, Ibba A, Morana G, et al. Central diabetes insipidus in children: diagnosis and management. *Best Pract Res Clin Endocrinol Metab.* 2020;34(5):101440. doi:10.1016/j.beem.2020.101440

147. Kasim N, Bagga B, Diaz-Thomas A. Intracranial pathologies associated with central diabetes insipidus in infants. *J Pediatr Endocrinol Metab.* 2018;31(9):951–958. doi:10.1515/jpem-2017-0300

148. Raisingani M, Palliyil Gopi R, Shah B. Use of chlorothiazide in the management of central diabetes insipidus in early infancy. *Case Rep Pediatr.* 2017;2017:2407028. doi:10.1155/2017/2407028

149. Al Nofal A, Lteif A. Thiazide diuretics in the management of young children with central diabetes insipidus. *J Pediatr.* 2015;167(3):658–661. doi:10.1016/j.jpeds.2015.06.002

150. Bockenhauer D, Bichet DG. Pathophysiology, diagnosis and management of nephrogenic diabetes insipidus. *Nat Rev Nephrol.* 2015;11(10):576–5-88. doi:10.1038/nrneph.2015.89

151. Sasaki S, Chiga M, Kikuchi E, Rai T, Uchida S. Hereditary nephrogenic diabetes insipidus in Japanese patients: analysis of 78 families and report of 22 new mutations in AVPR2 and AQP2. *Clin Exp Nephrol.* 2013;17(3):338–344. doi:10.1007/s10157-012-0726-z

152. Marples D, Frokiaer J, Dorup J, Knepper MA, Nielsen S. Hypokalemia-induced downregulation of aquaporin-2 water channel expression in rat kidney medulla and cortex. *J Clin Invest.* 1996;97(3):1960–1968. doi:10.1172/JCI118628

153. Hebert SC, Brown EM, Harris HW. Role of the Ca(2+)-sensing receptor in divalent mineral ion homeostasis. *J Exp Biol.* 1997;200(Pt 2):295–302.

154. Walker RJ, Weggery S, Bedford JJ, McDonald FJ, Ellis G, Leader JP. Lithium-induced reduction in urinary concentrating ability and urinary aquaporin 2 (AQP2) excretion in healthy volunteers. *Kidney Int.* 2005;67(1):291–294. doi:10.1111/j.1523-1755.2005.00081.x

155. Christensen BM, Marples D, Kim YH, Wang W, Frokiaer J, Nielsen S. Changes in cellular composition of kidney collecting duct cells in rats with lithium-induced NDI. *Am J Physiol Cell Physiol.* 2004;286(4):C952–C964. doi:10.1152/ajpcell.00266.2003

156. Newport DJ, Viguera AC, Beach AJ, Ritchie JC, Cohen LS, Stowe ZN. Lithium placental passage and obstetrical outcome: implications for clinical management during late pregnancy. *Am J Psychiatry.* 2005;162(11):2162–2170. doi:10.1176/appi.ajp.162.11.2162

157. Viguera AC, Newport DJ, Ritchie J, et al. Lithium in breast milk and nursing infants: clinical implications. *Am J Psychiatry.* 2007;164(2):342–345. doi:10.1176/ajp.2007.164.2.342

158. Kortenoeven ML, Li Y, Shaw S, et al. Amiloride blocks lithium entry through the sodium channel thereby attenuating the resultant nephrogenic diabetes insipidus. *Kidney Int.* 2009;76(1):44–53. doi:10.1038/ki.2009.91

159. Akbari P, Khorasani-Zadeh A. Thiazide diuretics. *StatPearls.* 2022. https://www.ncbi.nlm.nih.gov/books/NBK532918/

160. Loffing J. Paradoxical antidiuretic effect of thiazides in diabetes insipidus: another piece in the puzzle. *J Am Soc Nephrol.* 2004;15(11):2948–2950. doi:10.1097/01.ASN.0000146568.82353.04

161. Kim GH, Lee JW, Oh YK, et al. Antidiuretic effect of hydrochlorothiazide in lithium-induced nephrogenic diabetes insipidus is associated with upregulation of aquaporin-2, Na-Cl cotransporter, and epithelial sodium channel. *J Am Soc Nephrol.* 2004;15(11):2836–2843. doi:10.1097/01.ASN.0000143476.93376.04

162. Cardiello V, Zecca E, Corsello M, et al. Semipermeable membranes and hypernatremic dehydration in preterms. A randomized-controlled trial. *Early Hum Dev.* 2018;119:4550. doi:10.1016/j.earlhumdev.2018.03.002

Chapter 8

Genetic Causes of Congenital Anomalies of the Kidney and Urinary Tract

Thomas Hays, MD, PhD

Chapter Outline

Introduction

Congenital anomalies of the kidneys and urinary tract (CAKUT) encompass many heterogenous anomalies of the kidney, ureter, bladder, and urethra (Fig. 8.1). CAKUT is the leading cause of kidney disease and of renal failure in children.[1] The prevalence of CAKUT is estimated by population studies to lie between 0.1% and 2%, with higher prevalence in preterm infants.[2-4] CAKUT has a complex etiology with environmental and genetic risk factors identified. Ongoing research demonstrates that a growing portion of CAKUT is attributable to genetic disorders. These estimates vary widely by diagnostic method and the population studied. Large studies using genomic microarrays have found copy number variants (CNVs) in 5%–15% of cases of CAKUT.[5-10] A significant portion of CAKUT is also caused by single-gene disorders diagnosed by

genome-wide sequencing. Studies of large cohorts of individuals with CAKUT have demonstrated that 10%–20% have single-gene disorders.[11-14] An unknown portion of CAKUT may be attributable to yet undescribed genetic diseases, as well as polygenic or epigenetic mechanisms.[15]

Many of the implications of CAKUT to neonatal clinical management are unclear and are an active area of research. Intriguing questions and controversies exist in the diagnosis and management of CAKUT, specifically with regards to its genetic basis (Box 8.1). To frame these questions, this chapter reviews evidence for the genetic basis of CAKUT, the genetic regulation of renal development, and the spectrum of clinical disease. This chapter concludes with a discussion of future directions of research through which these questions may be

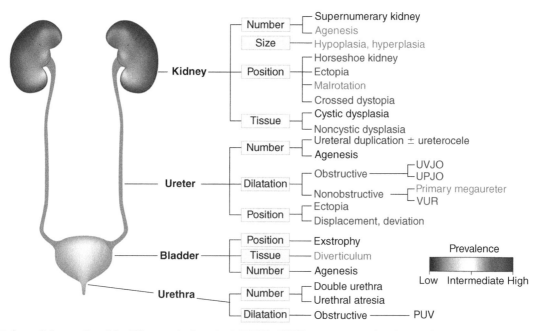

Fig. 8.1 Congenital anomalies of the kidneys and urinary tract (*CAKUT*). CAKUT encompasses a broad array of anomalies affecting the kidney, ureter, bladder, or urethra. These anomalies vary widely in prevalence. *PUV,* posterior urethral valves; *UPJO,* ureteropelvic junction obstruction; *UVJO,* ureterovesical junction obstruction; *VUR,* vesicoreteral reflux. (From Khan K, Ahram DK, Liu YP, et al. Multidisciplinary approaches for elucidating genetics and molecular pathogenesis of urinary tract malformations. *Kidney Int.* 2022;101(3):473–484. doi: 10.1016/j.kint.2021.09.034.)

BOX 8.1 QUESTIONS AND CONTROVERSIES REGARDING THE GENETIC BASIS OF CONGENITAL ANOMALIES OF THE KIDNEYS AND URINARY TRACT

Recent advances in genomic sequencing and basic science have dramatically expanded our understanding of the genetic contribution to congenital anomalies of the kidneys and urinary tract (CAKUT). However, several areas remain unresolved.

1. **What is the missing heritability of CAKUT?** Many genetic disorders cause CAKUT, yet these explain a fraction of cases. Compelling evidence indicates that a larger portion of CAKUT is heritable or genetically influenced. Novel methods are needed to explain this gap.

2. **What are the clinical benefits of genetic testing?** CAKUT can be the heralding feature of syndromic disease that manifests later in life. Reduced cost and improved quality of care have been demonstrated for genetic testing in other congenital diseases. Clinical trials are needed to assess the full risks and benefits of genome-wide testing in CAKUT.

3. **How can genetic testing be more equitable?** Genome-wide sequencing is now recommended as first-line testing for congenital anomalies such as CAKUT.

However, testing is not universally available. Improved health-care approaches are needed to establish how to improve care in underserved communities. Inclusive population genomic studies are also needed to better understand the genetic basis of CAKUT in people of diverse backgrounds.

4. **What is the clinical significance of nonspecific anomalies?** Many forms of CAKUT, such as unilateral renal agenesis, duplicated collecting system, or urinary tract dilation, are associated with highly variable impacts on health. Often they are benign, but they are also associated with progression to renal failure. Genetic testing may help stratify the significance of such anomalies. Studies involving screening, longitudinal follow-up, and genome-wide testing are needed, particularly in high-risk groups such as in infants admitted to the neonatal intensive care unit, to clarify the implications of anomalies.

answered. This chapter is intended to be a resource for training and practicing neonatologists, nephrologists, pediatricians, and geneticists, as well as for researchers studying the renal system and its genetic architecture.

Evidence for Genetic Basis

CAKUT, like all diseases, is caused by a combination of genetic and environmental factors. The precise balance of genetic and environmental contribution to CAKUT is unknown. Teratogen exposure, high or low levels of retinoic acid, and gestational diabetes each account for a small portion of CAKUT.[16,17] A growing body of evidence demonstrates that a portion of CAKUT is also caused by mendelian disorders, such as DiGeorge syndrome.[18] Interestingly, factors traditionally described as environmental may themselves be genetically influenced.[19] For example, preterm delivery, an "environmental" factor associated with arrest of nephrogenesis and renal hypoplasia,[20] is itself a phenotype heavily influenced by genetic factors.[21] Thus, even with a complete understanding of the etiology of CAKUT, quantifying its exact genetic contribution depends upon a somewhat arbitrary delineation. With this caveat in mind, a large body of literature has described the portion of CAKUT with genetic causes.

TWINS

One of the foundational approaches to measure the heritability of traits is to assess concordance in twins. Twin studies assume that monozygotic and dizygotic twins share similar environments. Traits found to be more frequently concordant in monozygotic twins are therefore more likely to be genetically influenced.[22] Twin studies and related family studies demonstrate high rates of concordance and familial clustering of multiple forms of CAKUT, therefore demonstrating a significant contribution of genetic factors to CAKUT etiology.[23–27]

MENDELIAN INHERITANCE

Further evidence of a genetic basis comes from studies of rare families with mendelian inheritance of CAKUT.[15,28] Segregation in these families usually demonstrates autosomal dominant inheritance of disease. Analysis of these families is often complicated by incomplete penetrance and variable expressivity of CAKUT phenotypes. Penetrance refers to whether an individual

with a given genetic change manifests with a phenotype, whereas expressivity refers to different phenotypes found in individuals with the same genetic changes.[29] In the context of CAKUT, individuals with the same genetic disorders may or may not manifest with renal anomalies (incomplete penetrance); and those individuals who do manifest renal anomalies may express different forms of CAKUT (variable expressivity). Despite this complexity, studies of affected families using classical genetics methods identified canonical CAKUT genes including *HNF1B*, *EYA1*, *PAX2*.[30–32] Familial cases represent a very small portion of CAKUT. The rarity of familial CAKUT has been hypothesized to occur due to reduced reproductive fitness in affected individuals, greater contribution to CAKUT on a population level from de novo variants, recessive disorders, polygenic and epigenetic mechanisms, as well as environmental factors.[15,16,33,34]

SINGLE-GENE DISORDERS

The expanded use of genome-wide sequencing has demonstrated that approximately 10%–20% of individuals with CAKUT have single-gene disorders.[11–14,35] Several genes are frequently implicated in genome-wide studies. These include genes in the RET and WNT signaling pathways, as well as novel genes, such as *GREB1L*, which encodes a poorly characterized transcription factor associated with development of the brain, heart, and kidney.[11–15,28,35,36] Interestingly, although these genes are repeatedly found associated with CAKUT, they each account for a small fraction of genetic diagnoses. Indeed, rather than having just these few genes responsible for CAKUT, many genes are found in genome-wide studies of CAKUT. To date, approximately 50 CAKUT genes have been identified.[15]

COPY NUMBER VARIANTS AND ANEUPLOIDY

In addition to single and oligonucleotide variants, structural genomic disorders and aneuploidy cause a significant portion of CAKUT. A large study of adults with CAKUT found that 4% of individuals had known pathogenic CNVs and another 2% had novel, putatively pathogenic CNVs.[9] Caruana et al. similarly found that as much as 10% of CAKUT in children could be attributable to CNVs.[7] Fetal studies have identified aneuploidy in 13% and CNVs in 4%–15% of CAKUT cases.[10,37–39] As with genome-wide sequencing, using microarray-based studies, a small number of disorders are repeatedly found associated with CAKUT, but these each account for a small portion of disease. Disorders commonly found in individuals with CAKUT include CNVs at the loci 22q11 (associated with DiGeorge syndrome), 4p (Wolf-Hirschhorn syndrome), and 17q12 (renal cysts and diabetes [RCAD] syndrome).[7,9]

In addition to human genetics research, studies using basic animal models have been instrumental in determining the genetic basic of CAKUT.[40] The novel CAKUT gene *DSTYK* was implicated in familial studies, then validated when its phenotype was recapitulated in knockout zebrafish and mouse models.[41] Similar approaches discovered the novel CAKUT gene *GREB1L* and found that *CRKL* is the gene within the 22q11 locus likely responsible for renal anomalies in DiGeorge syndrome.[18,42,43] In addition to confirming genetic findings, research in animals allows direct investigation of the mechanisms of disease pathogenesis. Much of what has been learned about the molecular regulation of renal development comes from such animal models.

Renal Development

The renal system forms through a complex, developmental interplay between multiple cellular lineages, regulated by many transcriptional and signaling pathways. From approximately 6 to 36 weeks of gestation the metanephros develops into the kidney.[20] The development of the metanephros itself depends upon the development and regression of the pronephros and mesonephros.[44] The metanephros then develops through reciprocal signaling between the ureteric bud and the metanephric mesenchyme in a process known as branching morphogenesis. Through this process, the treelike structure of the renal pelvis, major and minor calyces, and smaller collecting ducts emerges. While this is taking place, the cells of the metanephric mesenchyme also divide and differentiate to form the nephron in a process known as nephrogenesis.[20] Concurrent with branching morphogenesis and nephrogenesis, the early kidney also begins migrating cranially, and the tract of the ureters, bladder, and urethra continues to develop.[45]

Manifestations of CAKUT often correspond to disruptions at specific time points in renal development. Disruptions that occur prior to 4–6 weeks are associated with renal agenesis; disruptions after 4–6 weeks are associated with renal hypoplasia; disruptions after 6–8 weeks are associated with renal ectopy, dysplasia, and obstructive uropathies.[45]

Much of our understanding of the molecular regulation of renal development comes from study in model organisms such as the mouse. This work has demonstrated that RET signaling is necessary for nephrogenesis, particularly in regulating the interaction between the ureteric bud and metanephric mesenchyme.[20,46] The genes *BMP4, HNF1B, EYA1*, and *RET* participate in this pathway and are each associated with autosomal dominant forms of CAKUT.[31,32,46,47] Likewise, genes involved in WNT signaling regulate ureteric budding.[20] Variants in the WNT pathway genes *WNT4* and *SIX2* are also found in autosomal dominant CAKUT.[47–50]

Genes involved in CAKUT often have complex and overlapping roles within renal development. Thus, individuals with the same genetic disease may develop variable forms of CAKUT. For example, the murine orthologs of *PAX2* and *PAX8* have partially redundant roles in formation of the mouse kidney.[51] Pathogenic variants in these genes cause renal agenesis, but with variable penetrance.[52,53] Similarly, individuals with variants in *HNF1B* may manifest with renal agenesis, hypoplasia, dysplasia, or cystic disease.[54] Finally, genes associated with CAKUT are often involved in the development of other organs as well. Individuals presenting with CAKUT often have extrarenal manifestations, such as disease affecting the heart, brain, or liver.[55]

Spectrum of Congenital Anomalies of the Kidney and Urinary Tract

CAKUT can be grouped into the following categories: solitary or bilaterally absent kidney (SBK), ectopy or fusion (EF), renal hypoplasia or dysplasia (RHD), and urinary tract malformations or dilation (UTD). Several complex and rare forms of CAKUT, such as prune belly syndrome, do not fit easily into one category. These categories have clinical and research utility, as entities within each category often have similar pathogenic mechanisms and clinical implications. However, these categories have significant overlap. For example, the diagnosis of a solitary kidney may represent primary agenesis of one kidney, the resorption of a severely dysplastic kidney, or a pelvic kidney not detected on ultrasound. Likewise, a urinary tract malformation may result in isolated dilation of the renal pelvis or in dysplastic changes within the renal parenchyma. The categorization of CAKUT is particularly challenging when viewed through a genomic lens. CAKUT arising from genetic disorders has an unusually high degree of complexity in terms of phenotype and penetrance. Individuals with the same genetic disorder may have no clinically apparent disease, a minor renal anomaly, or a catastrophic congenital syndrome.[56] Furthermore, individuals with similar presentations of CAKUT are often found to have many different genetic disorders.[56] Thus, although these categorizations of CAKUT provide some usefulness in clinical practice and research, it is important to keep in mind their limitations.

SOLITARY OR BILATERALLY ABSENT KIDNEY

Renal agenesis arises from a failure preceding the formation of the metanephros in the sixth week of gestation. It can be unilateral or bilateral, with the bilateral form a virtually lethal diagnosis. Bilateral renal agenesis is a rare phenomenon, which is estimated to affect less than one in a thousand pregnancies.[57,58] Affected infants are born not only with absent renal function, but also with pulmonary hypoplasia resulting from Potter sequence.[58] The true prevalence of solitary kidney is unknown as it is often an incidental finding. Population studies estimate its prevalence at between 1 in 3000 and 1 in 10,000 live births.[2,3,59] A solitary kidney may arise from unilateral agenesis or a severe form of RHD leading to involution and resorbtion.[60,61]

The clinical implications of a solitary kidney are unclear. Given that it is often an incidental finding, and based on studies in small cohorts, it had been described as a benign condition.[62,63] However, emerging evidence indicates a heightened risk of chronic kidney disease (CKD) and progression to renal failure in individuals with solitary kidneys.[64–66]

Multiple lines of evidence support a genetic basis of SBK. In individuals with a solitary kidney, one-third have additional forms of CAKUT, such as renal dysplasia, and one-third also have extrarenal manifestations.[61] These diffuse anomalies suggest underlying genetic anomalies. Syndromic forms of bilateral renal agenesis have also been described including the branchio-oto-renal syndrome and Fraser syndrome and in recently described cases associated with variants in GREB1L.[42,43,67–69] Rare, disruptive CNVs are also more common in individuals with SBK.[5] Interestingly, of the CNVs associated with SBK, deletions predominate over duplications.[9] Genes commonly responsible for SBK include many of the genes that regulate early renal development, such as HNF1B, PAX2, EYA1, and DSTYK.[20,64] Although these genes are repeatedly found in studies of SBK, they still represent a minority of cases, reflecting the genetic complexity of the disease.

Genetic diagnoses have the potential to inform better care for individuals with solitary kidneys. Although there is not yet consensus on the implications for renal *function* in individuals with solitary kidneys and underlying genetic disorders, there are other implications to these individuals. Many of the extrarenal manifestations associated with unilateral renal agenesis are not apparent until later in life. For example, variants affecting HNF1B are among the most common genetic diagnoses made in SBK.[9,13,70] HNF1B encodes a transcription factor that functions early in the RET signaling pathway.[20] Pathogenic variants in HNF1B cause not only renal agenesis, but also the broader renal cysts and diabetes (RCAD) syndrome.[71,72] In addition to SBK and other forms of CAKUT, this syndrome is associated with manifestations not apparent until later in life such as developmental delays, maturity-onset diabetes, epilepsy, and progression to renal failure. Thus, what might present as an isolated finding on prenatal ultrasound of a solitary kidney may in fact represent this syndromic process. Importantly, the extrarenal manifestations of RCAD are modifiable with surveillance and referral to specialists.[35] These cases are likely rare, but to individuals with such a genetic disorder, there is a large potential clinical and counseling benefit. This phenomenon, in which CAKUT can be the presenting feature of a syndromic disease, is a common theme across many forms of CAKUT. Because of the associated lethality with bilateral renal agenesis, a genetic diagnosis provides little utility for affected infants. However, the diagnosis can be helpful to provide clarity to parents, enable reproductive planning, and to facilitate testing of relatives.[73]

ECTOPY/FUSION

Several anomalies affect the location of the kidneys. The most common of these are renal ectopy, in which fetal migration of the kidney from the pelvis is disrupted, and renal fusion, in which disrupted migration of both kidneys leads to their connection. Less commonly, crossed fused ectopy occurs in which one kidney migrates ectopically and fuses with the contralateral kidney. These anomalies are rare, estimated to occur in approximately 1 in 1000–10,000 individuals.[2,74] Ectopy is sometimes misdiagnosed as solitary kidney, as ectopic kidneys can be more difficult to detect by ultrasound.[74] The clinical impact of EF anomalies is unclear as there are limited prospective studies. However, multiple studies have found significant rates of CKD and renal failure in individuals with EF.[65,75–77] EF is often found in association with other forms of CAKUT, as well as extrarenal anomalies.[75,78,79] EF is also found as a component of rare genetic syndromes including Treacher Collins, Mayer-Rokitansky-Kuster-Hauser, and Goldenhar syndromes, as well as in individuals with common aneuploidies.[75,80] Associated anomalies, evidence of renal dysfunction, and descriptions of rare syndromic cases indicate that EF may be linked to underlying dysfunction of the renal parenchyma. Further research, particularly genome-wide sequencing efforts, are needed to explore the genetic architecture of these anomalies and to analyze the risk of renal dysfunction in cases of EF when individuals are stratified by the presence of genetic disorders.

RENAL HYPODYSPLASIA

RHD represents a particularly broad category of CAKUT. In renal hypoplasia, kidneys develop with an overall preserved structure but with a reduced number of nephrons. Renal dysplasia refers to any abnormalities of the renal parenchyma, such as scarring, cysts, or disorganization.[45] Hypoplasia and dysplasia frequently occur together. Their diagnostic classification is largely based on renal ultrasound, which can often be nonspecific, particularly in advanced disease. Severely small, scarred kidneys with cystic changes can be seen on ultrasound in several disease processes, with very different etiologies. SBK is often categorized within RHD; however, given its unique clinical characteristics it is described here as a separate entity. Congenital RHD is generally a result of disruption of normal development after 4–6 weeks of fetal life. It often occurs as a result of pathology in the developing renal parenchyma; however, it can also be the result of obstruction of the distal collecting system or the vasculature serving the kidneys.[20]

RHD occurs in nearly 1 in 100 live births.[2,81,82] It accounts for 23% of all congenital anomalies.[83] And RHD is a leading cause of CKD and renal failure in children.[84,85] The most severe form of RHD, multicystic dysplastic kidneys (MCDK), is characterized by numerous, noncommunicating cysts, separated by dysplastic tissue, and atretic ureters.[45] MCDK occurs in approximately 1 in 4000 births.[86] It is frequently associated with congenital anomalies of the contralateral kidney such as obstructive uropathies.[86] MCDK frequently progresses to renal failure, in large part depending on the structure and function of the contralateral kidney.[60,65,87]

Multiple other forms of RHD with varying degrees of clinical severity also exist. Several have relatively well-defined courses associated with specific signs. These include cystic disease and tubular dysgenesis (described later). These well-characterized disease processes also have well-characterized associations with a small number of genes and less phenotypic variability than other forms of CAKUT. Finally, RHD includes a broad array of nonspecific processes with unclear clinical implications. In general, the risk of CKD progression in these diseases is proportional to the number of affected nephrons.[88,89]

CYSTIC CILIOPATHIES

These diseases are among the best-characterized genetic nephropathies. They involve components of the primary cilium or the centrosome complex, which regulate cell cycle.[90] Ciliopathies are often considered as a distinct entity from CAKUT given that they usually present later in life; however, ciliopathies, even autosomal dominant polycystic kidney disease (ADPKD), can present perinatally and with phenotypes similar to other forms of CAKUT.[91]

ADPKD is the most common heritable nephropathy, affecting approximately 1 in 1000 individuals.[92] Nearly all cases of ADPKD are caused by pathogenic variants in two genes: *PKD1* and *PKD2*.[55] ADPKD has a relatively predictable clinical course usually characterized by progressive renal dysfunction in late adulthood.[55] The diagnosis is typically made by history and imaging, without the need for genetic testing.[93] Genetic testing is recommended to evaluate cases with atypical presentations, particular those presenting congenitally, and to assist in kidney donor evaluation.[94,95] Interestingly, cases presenting perinatally often involve multiple genetic changes, such as multiple hypomorphic variants in *PKD1* or variants in *PKD1* and an additional gene.[95] For example, CNVs in which portions of *PKD1* and the adjacent gene *TSC2* are affected cause a contiguous deletion syndrome characterized by aggressive, infantile disease.[96] Thus genetic testing in these atypical presentations can be valuable for prognostic counseling and to determine clinical monitoring.

Autosomal recessive polycystic kidney disease (ARPKD) is less common and more severe than ADPKD. The disease usually presents in the perinatal period, with multiple small cysts throughout the kidney, loss of corticomedullary borders, and kidneys that rapidly enlarge.[97,98] It is associated with a high rate of mortality, both from renal failure in infancy, as well from Potter sequence.[98] It is also associated with a progressive, dysplastic disease of the liver referred to as Caroli disease.[98] Many cases of ARPKD are found to have pathogenic variants in *PKHD1* or *DZIPL1*.[99,100] However, variants in multiple other genes are also found.[101] Given this complexity, as well as the difficulty in interpreting *PKHD1* variants, there is not yet a consensus for first-tier genetic testing in the diagnosis of ARPKD, and it remains an area of active research.[101,102] These research efforts are particularly exciting given the possibility of genetic testing to direct tailored therapy, such as vasopressin antagonists, for infantile polycystic disease.[103,104]

Nephronophthisis involves renal cysts at the corticomedullary junction and usually does not present clinically until later childhood.[105] Like other ciliopathies, it can present congenitally in its most severe form.[106,107] It is often associated with anomalies affecting the skeleton, heart, eyes, and brain, often as one of several well-characterized syndromes including Bardet-Biedel, Joubert, and Meckel-Gruber syndromes.[107] Nephronophthisis is associated with more than 20 genes with autosomal recessive inheritance.[105,107] Extrarenal manifestations, such as neurocognitive impairment, may not present until later childhood but can be anticipated with a genetic diagnosis.[107]

TUBULAR DYSGENESIS

In addition to ciliopathies, there are other forms of RHD with distinct clinical characteristics and genetic associations. Tubular dysgenesis is a rare disease in which the proximal tubules fail to develop. It causes nearly uniform lethality secondary to Potter sequence. Tubular dysgenesis is caused by autosomal recessive variants in genes functioning within the renin-angiotensin-aldosterone system.[108] Determining the genetic basis of this disease demonstrated the molecular mechanism by which inhibitors of the renin-angiotensin-aldosterone system cause renal teratogenesis. Like other forms of lethal CAKUT, prompt genetic diagnosis is crucial to families for management of pregnancies, determining goals of care, and planning future pregnancies.

TUBEROUS SCLEROSIS

Tuberous sclerosis is a well-characterized disease caused by variants in *TSC1* and *TSC2*, and with autosomal dominant inheritance.[109] In addition to affecting the brain, heart, and skin, it includes variably penetrant tumors of the kidney.[110,111] The renal lesions are angiomyolipomas and less commonly renal cysts with the potential for malignant transformation. Tuberous sclerosis is often not considered as a form of CAKUT; however, it uncommonly presents as a severe congenital cystic disease, and thus is included here.[96,112]

RENAL CYSTS AND DIABETES SYNDROME

HNF1B, discussed previously for its role in renal agenesis, is also responsible for the cysts found in RCAD, which is characterized by highly variable renal cysts, progressively worsening CKD, and diabetes onset in the second to third decade of life.[71,72] Unlike other renal cystic diseases, RCAD is not caused by a component of the primary cilium or centromere, but rather by a transcription factor regulating renal development. Cystic disease in RCAD is highly variable, ranging from a few cysts to MCDK.[56,113] It is not yet clear whether identifying specific genetic disruptions in *HNF1B* can predict the degree of cystic disease and CKD progression; however, identifying disruptions in *HNF1B* does establish the risk of diabetes, which might not be otherwise anticipated.[113]

NONSPECIFIC FORMS OF RENAL HYPOPLASIA OR DYSPLASIA

In addition to these relatively well-characterized processes, RHD often manifests as nonspecific structural changes of the renal parenchyma including isolated hypoplasia or nonspecific dysplastic changes. These nonspecific manifestations of RHD share many of the genetic associations described in syndromic disease. Pathogenic variants in *HNF1B*, *PAX2*, *EYA1*, and *DSTYK*, as well as approximately 50 other genes, are often found in isolated RHD.[15,28] Pathogenic CNVs, particularly deletions as opposed duplications, are also often found in individuals with RHD.[9]

The classical descriptions of a dysplastic kidney refer to a globally and heterogeneously echogenic kidney, often accompanied by cortical cysts, hypoplastic, and often accompanied by collapse of the ureter and/or renal artery.[87,114] Renal dysplasia is often associated with a distal obstruction of the ipsilateral urinary tract. As with MCDK, the clinical significance is largely dependent upon the structure and function of the contralateral kidney.[60,65,87] Dysplastic kidneys are often accompanied by other anomalies including the well-defined variable phenotype that encompasses vertebral, anorectal, cardiac, tracheoesophageal, renal, and limb anomalies (commonly referred to as VACTERL association). These constellations can include partial aspects of syndromic CAKUT (e.g., RCAD or Kabuki syndrome). Genomic research increasingly demonstrates that many canonical syndromes and single-gene disorders can present with isolated, mild forms of RHD and with variable penetration.[95,115–119]

Bilateral renal hypoplasia is often found in infants born prematurely, as well as those born with intrauterine growth restriction.[4,120] Nephrogenesis does not complete until approximately 36 weeks of gestation.[20] Preterm birth or intrauterine growth restriction can arrest or slow this process, resulting in kidneys with reduced nephron number, but with preservation of the overall structure.[121] Impairment of nephrogenesis in these infants is also associated with microscopic alternations in nephron structure.[122] These factors likely contribute to the increased lifetime risk of renal impairment.[120] Preterm infants have many other risk factors for renal disease including nephrotoxic drug exposures, hypoxic insults, and an increased burden of critical illness.[123,124] Genetic disorders may also indirectly contribute to such forms of CAKUT by contributing to prematurity. The interaction and prevalence of genetic disorders and CAKUT in preterm infants are both unknown and are active areas of investigation.

The true spectrum of RHD is unclear. Less severe anomalies found on imaging, such as decreased corticomedullary differentiation, or simple cysts, are generally considered nonspecific findings rather than RHD.[125–127] However, studies of families with variably penetrant, syndromic CAKUT reveal that affected individuals sometimes have such minor anomalies as

well as reduced renal function.[118] Broad population studies, combined with population genomics, are required to determine the spectrum of renal dysplasia, its genetic background, and clinical significance.

URINARY TRACT MALFORMATIONS OR DILATION

A large, heterogenous group of anomalies affect the urinary tract and are associated with dilation. These include obstructive lesions of the collecting system, ureter, bladder, and urethra, as well as malformations that variably are associated with dilation of the urinary tract, such as a duplicated collecting system (DCS). The clinical impacts of UTD anomalies vary widely. Duplications are a common autopsy finding, with often no apparent relevance in life; others may have implications for renal function.[128,129] In contrast to this variability in urinary tract duplications, many individuals with posterior urethral valves (PUV) progress to renal failure.[65] Despite this heterogeneity, broadly grouping UTD anomalies highlights shared prognostic features and underlying genetic contributions. There is a strong association of CNVs with UTD. Intriguingly, reciprocal CNVs are often observed in which deletions at a given locus are associated with SBK and RHD, whereas duplications are associated with UTD.[9] The pathogenic implications of this "mirroring phenomenon" are unclear, though it has also been observed in congenital brain anomalies.[9,130,131]

ANOMALIES OF THE RENAL PELVIS AND URETER

Dilation of the renal pelvis is detected on prenatal ultrasound in approximately 1%–2% of fetuses.[132] It is often a transient finding, particularly in the perinatal period.[133] Its classification is complicated by overlapping, nonspecific terms including pelviectasis, pyelectasis, caliectasis, and hydronephrosis. A unified, multidisciplinary nomenclature was recently proposed to simplify classification of congenital UTD, stratified by degree of dilation, associated anomalies, and gestational age.[133] The term "hydronephrosis" is generally reserved for severe dilation of the renal pelvis.[134] The clinical implications of congenital hydronephrosis are unclear, particularly as it can be a transient finding.[135] However, it is often found in association with other forms of CAKUT, particularly ipsilateral distal urinary tract anomalies, and is also associated with aneuploidy.[135–138] Like hydronephrosis, persistent dilation of the ureter is a nonspecific anomaly. It can be referred to as hydroureter or megaureter, though these terms are generally reserved for cases associated with obstruction or severe dilation, respectively.[133,139,140] Ureteropelvic junction obstruction is a more specific clinical entity, with a stronger genetic association. It is bilateral in 10% of cases, supporting the hypothesis that it arises from a developmental disruption.[141] It is variably found in syndromic CAKUT arising from multiple single-gene defects, including *JAG1, PAX2, DHCR7,* and *NFIA*.[142,143] Individuals with ureteropelvic junction obstruction also often have multiple pathogenic CNVs.[9]

DCS is one of the most frequently encountered forms of CAKUT, with prevalence estimated to be as high as 1% to 5%.[128,129] DCS is often an incidental finding, without clear clinical implication.[129] There is evidence of a genetic etiology to DCS. It is overrepresented in relatives of individuals with other forms of CAKUT.[25] And DCS has been described in multiple forms of syndromic CAKUT.[144–146] Pathogenic CNVs, particularly genomic deletion syndromes, are significantly overrepresented in individuals with DCS. DCS can exist as a partial or complete duplication of the collecting system and ureter. When two ureters are present, one is often ectopically inserted into the bladder and prone to reflux, obstruction, and loss of renal function.[129,147]

Vesicoureteral reflux (VUR) refers to retrograde flow of urine from the bladder into the ureters. VUR is associated with ascending bacterial infections, renal scarring, and reflux nephropathy.[148–150] However, prognosis is challenging, as even advanced VUR is observed to spontaneously resolve in some cases and has a variable association with renal parenchymal damage and dysfunction later in later.[151] There is strong evidence for the genetic basis of VUR. Monozygotic twins are frequently concordant for VUR, and VUR often clusters in families.[23,24] Multiple genetic loci have been implicated as contributing to VUR, including known pathogenic CNVs.[9,152–154] It is unclear what mediates the variable degree of reflux nephropathy. Possible explanations include disruption of fetal nephrogenesis from the physical effect of reflux, pleiotropic effects on the genetic regulation of renal development, as well as the possibility that genetic factors mediate how kidneys heal from injury caused by reflux.[155,156]

ANOMALIES OF THE BLADDER AND URETHRA

Anomalies of the bladder and urethra are also a large group of heterogenous anomalies that include the

bladder exstrophy-epispadias complex (BEEC), hypospadias, and PUV. In BEEC the uroepithelium is contiguous with the skin, open to the environment, and often partially prolapsed through an abdominal wall defect. In its most extreme form a primitive cloaca persists, including the bladder and distal hind gut. Minor forms consist of epispadias, or small openings along the urethra or bladder.[157] BEEC is rare, found in 1 in 30,000 births.[158] Maternal folic acid deficiency may contribute to its pathogenesis.[159] Although most cases are sporadic, it is more common in first-degree relatives.[160] Twin studies also demonstrate evidence of high heritability of BEEC.[158] Recent human studies with animal model validation demonstrated that variants in *WNT3* and the WNT signaling pathway cause BEEC.[161] And although BEEC is usually isolated, rare syndromic cases including deafness were found to be associated with a duplication at the 22q11 locus.[162–164] Variants in ISL1, a transcription factor with broad embryologic roles, may also contribute to BEEC.[165]

Hypospadias is more common, found in approximately 5 per 1000 male infants.[166] It is also usually an isolated anomaly, though it can be a component of rare genetic syndromes, which also include developmental delays.[167] Genome-wide association studies found that variants in several developmental genes, including the CAKUT gene *EYA1*, are strongly associated with hypospadias.[168] PUV occurs in approximately 1 in 4000 male infants.[169] It is nearly always sporadic, and associated anomalies are usually directly sequential (proximal obstructive uropathy or Potter sequence).[169] Despite the relative lack of syndromic or familial descriptions, cohorts with PUV are found to have a significantly higher burden of CNVs, including CNVs associated with other forms of CAKUT.[9]

Future Directions

Despite the increasing body of data supporting the genetic basis of CAKUT, there are unresolved questions regarding this genetic basis (Box 8.1). Potential ways in which these challenges may be navigated are presented next.

MISSING HERITABILITY

There is significant evidence for the genetic basis of CAKUT including familial clustering and associations with syndromic anomalies. However, genome-wide studies have identified genetic disorders in only 10%–25% of CAKUT. Although this is more than known environmental factors account for, it is less than would be expected based on studies of the heritability of CAKUT. This gap has been referred to as the "missing heritability."[15] Closing this gap will rely upon novel methods of genomic and transcriptional analysis. Noncoding variants that regulate gene expression have been shown to account for a portion of the missing heritability in congenital heart disease (CHD).[170] Discovery of these variants in CHD was dependent upon genome (rather than exome) sequencing, machine learning algorithms, and transcriptional profiling. Similar approaches combining transcriptomics and genomics will likely be required to identify the noncoding variants that contribute to CAKUT.[171,172] Elucidating the role of complex structural changes in DNA will also depend on novel platforms that are able to sequence longer fragments of DNA.[173]

CLINICAL BENEFITS OF GENETIC TESTING

Perhaps the greatest potential benefit of genetic testing in CAKUT is to treat, manage, or prevent syndromic processes, particularly neurodevelopmental delays. Pediatric kidney disease has a well-described association with neurocognitive impairment, the cause of which has been speculated to be related to the burden of medical illness, effects of treatment, and disruption of education.[174] However, there are likely genetic contributions as well. Verbitsky et al. investigated a cohort of 400 children with CKD (most caused by CAKUT) for the presence of CNVs. They found that carriers of pathogenic CNVs had significantly lower IQ and executive function.[175] Genetic disorders likely account for a substantial portion of the neurocognitive delays in children with kidney disease. Neurocognitive impairment likely arises from pleiotropic effects of genes necessary for the development of the brain and kidney. Early intervention's role in ameliorating developmental delays is one of the great success stories in modern pediatrics; however, its success depends upon implementation in the first years of life.[176] Genetic testing of children with CAKUT early in life has the potential to identify those with genetic disorders that predispose to developmental delay and facilitate early intervention. Given this possible benefit, there is an urgent need to evaluate whether genetic testing early in life can improve the neurocognitive outcomes of children with CAKUT.

Genome-wide sequencing has also been demonstrated to support clinical decision making and reproductive planning for families of children with a variety of congenital diseases including CHD and developmental delay.[177] Dramatic clinical benefits have been demonstrated in the use of rapid genomic sequencing for infants with critical illness.[178–180] Given this evidence, exome or genome sequencing is now recommended as a first-line test for infants with congenital anomalies, including CAKUT.[181] There are many potential benefits to genomic sequencing in CAKUT.[35] CAKUT is the leading cause of pediatric CKD and renal failure, and severe anomalies confer a high risk of death in infancy.[182] Given this burden of illness, there is an urgent need to test strategies to improve the care of infants with CAKUT. However, little research has been done to assess clinical benefits of genetic testing, or the extent to which benefits may be offset by risks. Randomized controlled trials are needed to quantify changes in short-term morbidity and mortality and neurocognitive outcomes, particularly for cases presenting in pregnancy or in the neonatal intensive care unit.

Research is also needed to better understand how parents are affected by genetic testing of their children. Tremblay et al. retrospectively found evidence that parents of children undergoing genetic testing for development delays received inadequate genetic counseling and that results often failed to meet expectations.[183] However, in a prospective study of parents of critically ill infants undergoing genomic testing, Cakici et al. found that 97% of parents perceived at least some benefit from testing.[184] The discrepancy between these findings highlights the critical need for trained genetic counsellors to provide appropriate pre- and posttest counseling.[35,185–187] In a field advancing as rapidly as genomic medicine, improved strategies are also needed to educate physicians.[188–190] Finally, research is needed to address the genomic literacy of patients and their families.[191,192]

EQUITABLE GENETIC TESTING

Genetic testing, like many aspects of medical care, disproportionately benefits privileged communities. There are many factors that contribute to this. Utilization of genetic testing can be limited by low proficiency in English, poor literacy and numeracy, and low education.[191,192] Minority communities sometimes report distrust or fear of how genetic information will be used.[193,194] Genetic testing is not uniformly covered and reimbursed by insurance providers.[195,196] Medicare and Medicaid cover genome-wide testing for some diseases but not yet for broad indications.[197] Access to genetic testing and counseling is also limited, particularly in low-income countries.[198–200]

To facilitate equitable genetic testing, research efforts are needed in several areas. Tools are needed to assess genetic literacy and tailor genetic counseling.[191] Genetic education strategies are needed to directly target underserved communities.[201] The Undiagnosed Disease Network, and similar efforts worldwide, provide genetic testing at no cost, but these efforts are limited.[198,202] Broader, innovative strategies are urgently needed to expand access to genetic testing.

There is also an urgent need for genomic data that reflect diverse human populations. Diagnosing genetic disorders depends in part on evaluating the frequency of variants in individuals against population controls.[203] However, genomic research has disproportionately focused on people of Western European ancestry and failed to gather data representative of broader populations.[204] Lack of diverse population data hinders not only genetic diagnosis but also our understanding of disease pathogenesis. The extent to which the molecular pathogenesis of CAKUT differs in individuals from different backgrounds is not known. The National Institutes of Health–funded program All of Us was founded to establish a diverse, representative genomic database from more than one million Americans.[205] All of Us aims to dramatically improve our understanding of genomics in diverse populations. In addition, CAKUT research efforts must make deliberate efforts to recruit more inclusively.

CLINICAL SIGNIFICANCE OF NONSPECIFIC ANOMALIES

As reviewed previously, many forms of CAKUT have unclear clinical implications, particularly when found in isolation. Research is needed to identify the determinants of these outcomes. The presence of genetic disorders may explain this variability but only in part. Answering this question has important implications for living related kidney donation and in the risk-benefit calculations for nephrotoxic exposures.[206] It is also unclear how the presence of renal anomalies confers risk of unappreciated syndromic illnesses in populations at risk. For example, preterm infants experience high rates of death and critical illness.[207,208] Genetic disorders have been shown to contribute significantly to critical illness in term infants.[36,209–224] As discussed previously, individuals with CAKUT are at increased risk of having genetic disorders. The extent to which renal anomalies may represent the heralding feature of underlying syndromic illnesses has not been investigated. Intriguingly, the presence of CAKUT, whether in isolation or as a syndromic process, may confer increased risk of death and critical illness in preterm infants.[4] Further research and prospective studies are needed to explore this possibility.

Conclusion

CAKUT encompasses a heterogenous group of anomalies, which range widely in their clinical implications—some have no health impact, and others lead to progression to renal failure. There is also a wide range of associated extrarenal manifestations including CHD, developmental delays, and deficits in hearing and vision. Extrarenal manifestations are often not apparent until later in childhood or adulthood. A unifying feature of all forms of CAKUT is a strong contribution of genetic disorders. Approximately 10%–25% of individuals with CAKUT have underlying genetic disorders. Diagnosing these genetic disorders may help predict the variable clinical outcomes found in CAKUT. Genomic and transcriptomic studies are needed to fully map out the landscape of single/oligonucleotide variants and structural genomic changes that cause CAKUT. Prospective studies are needed to determine whether genetic diagnoses can clarify the importance of nonspecific anomalies, lead to improved neonatal intensive care unit outcomes, and improved neurocognitive outcomes. Improved strategies are needed to make the benefits of genetic testing available to historically underserved communities. These unresolved issues represent daunting challenges. However, the field of genomic medicine continues to advance rapidly. Novel testing strategies, breakthroughs in our fundamental understanding of renal development, and multidisciplinary collaboration from geneticists, genetic counselors, neonatologists, nephrologists, and basic scientists have tremendous potential to improve the welfare of infants and families affected by CAKUT.

REFERENCES

1. Smith JM, Stablein DM, Munoz R, Hebert D, McDonald RA. Contributions of the Transplant Registry: the 2006 annual report of the North American Pediatric Renal Trials and Collaborative Studies (NAPRTCS). *Pediatr Transplant.* 2007;11(4):366–373. doi:10.1111/j.1399-3046.2007.00704

2. Caiulo VA, Caiulo S, Gargasole C, et al. Ultrasound mass screening for congenital anomalies of the kidney and urinary tract. *Pediatr Nephrol.* 2012;27(6):949–953. doi:10.1007/s00467-011-2098-0

3. Wiesel A, Queisser-Luft A, Clementi M, Bianca S, Stoll C. Prenatal detection of congenital renal malformations by fetal ultrasonographic examination: an analysis of 709,030 births in 12 European countries. *Eur J Med Genet.* 2005;48(2):131–144. doi:10.1016/j.ejmg.2005.02.003

4. Hays T, Thompson MV, Bateman DA, et al. The prevalence and clinical significance of congenital anomalies of the kidney and urinary tract in preterm infants. *JAMA Netw Open.* 2022;5(9):e2231626. doi:10.1001/jamanetworkopen.2022.31626

5. Westland R, Verbitsky M, Vukojevic K, et al. Copy number variation analysis identifies novel CAKUT candidate genes in children with a solitary functioning kidney. *Kidney Int.* 2015;88(6):1402–1410. doi:10.1038/ki.2015.239

6. Sanna-Cherchi S, Kiryluk K, Burgess KE, et al. Copy-number disorders are a common cause of congenital kidney malformations. *Am J Hum Genet.* 2012;91(6):987–997. doi:10.1016/j.ajhg.2012.10.007

7. Caruana G, Wong MN, Walker A, et al. Copy-number variation associated with congenital anomalies of the kidney and urinary tract. *Pediatr Nephrol.* 2015;30(3):487–495. doi:10.1007/s00467-014-2962-9

8. Siomou E, Mitsioni AG, Giapros V, Bouba I, Noutsopoulos D, Georgiou I. Copy-number variation analysis in familial nonsyndromic congenital anomalies of the kidney and urinary tract: evidence for the causative role of a transposable element-associated genomic rearrangement. *Mol Med Rep.* 2017;15(6):3631–3636. doi:10.3892/mmr.2017.6462

9. Verbitsky M, Westland R, Perez A, et al. The copy number variation landscape of congenital anomalies of the kidney and urinary tract. *Nat Genet.* 2019;51(1):117–127. doi:10.1038/s41588-018-0281-y

10. Cai M, Lin N, Su L, et al. Copy number variations associated with fetal congenital kidney malformations. *Mol Cytogenet.* 2020;13:11. doi:10.1186/s13039-020-00481-7

11. Groopman EE, Marasa M, Cameron-Christie S, et al. Diagnostic utility of exome sequencing for kidney disease. *N Engl J Med.* 2019;380(2):142–151. doi:10.1056/nejmoa1806891

12. Rao J, Liu X, Mao J, et al. Genetic spectrum of renal disease for 1001 Chinese children based on a multicenter registration system. *Clin Genet.* 2019;96(5):402–410. doi:10.1111/cge.13606

13. Thomas R, Sanna-Cherchi S, Warady BA, Furth SL, Kaskel FJ, Gharavi AG. HNF1B and PAX2 mutations are a common cause of renal hypodysplasia in the CKiD cohort. *Pediatr Nephrol.* 2011;26(6):897–903. doi:10.1007/s00467-011-1826-9

14. Ahn YH, Lee C, Kim NKD, et al. Targeted exome sequencing provided comprehensive genetic diagnosis of congenital anomalies of the kidney and urinary tract. *J Clin Med.* 2020;9(3):751. doi:10.3390/jcm9030751

15. Khan K, Ahram DK, Liu YP, et al. Multidisciplinary approaches for elucidating genetics and molecular pathogenesis of urinary tract malformations. *Kidney Int.* 2022;101(3):473–484. doi:10.1016/j.kint.2021.09.034

16. Nicolaou N, Renkema KY, Bongers EMHF, Giles RH, Knoers NVAM. Genetic, environmental, and epigenetic factors involved in CAKUT. *Nat Rev Nephrol.* 2015;11(12):720–731. doi:10.1038/nrneph.2015.140

17. Lee LMY, Leung CY, Tang WWC, et al. A paradoxical teratogenic mechanism for retinoic acid. *Proc Natl Acad Sci U S A.* 2012;109(34):13668–13673. doi:10.1073/pnas.1200872109

18. Lopez-Rivera E, Liu YP, Verbitsky M, et al. Genetic drivers of kidney defects in the DiGeorge syndrome. *N Engl J Med.* 2017;376(8):742–754. doi:10.1056/NEJMoa1609009

19. Plomin R, Bergeman CS. The nature of nurture: genetic influence on "environmental" measures. *Behav Brain Sci.* 1991;14(3):373–386. doi:10.1017/S0140525X00070278

20. Smyth IM, Cullen-McEwen LA, Combes AN, O'Brien LL, Black MJ, Bertram JF. Development of the kidney: morphology and mechanisms. In: Polin R, Abman S, Rowitch D, Benitz WE, eds. *Fetal and Neonatal Physiology.* 6th ed. Elsevier; 2022: 941–954.

21. Zhang G, Feenstra B, Bacelis J, et al. Genetic associations with gestational duration and spontaneous preterm birth. *N Engl J Med.* 2017;377(12):1156–1167. doi:10.1056/NEJMoa1612665

22. Falconer DS, Mackay TF. *Introduction to Quantitative Genetics.* 4th ed. Benjamin-Cummings; 1996.

23. Kaefer M, Curran M, Treves ST, et al. Sibling vesicoureteral reflux in multiple gestation births. *Pediatrics.* 2000;105(4 Pt 1):800–804. doi:10.1542/peds.105.4.800

24. Connolly LP, Treves ST, Connolly SA, et al. Vesicoureteral reflux in children: incidence and severity in siblings. *J Urol.* 1997;157(6):2287–2290. doi:10.1016/s0022-5347(01)64764-5

25. Bulum B, Özçakar ZB, Ustüner E, et al. High frequency of kidney and urinary tract anomalies in asymptomatic first-degree relatives of patients with CAKUT. *Pediatr Nephrol.* 2013;28(11):2143–2147. doi:10.1007/s00467-013-2530-8

26. Carter CO, Evans K, Pescia G. A family study of renal agenesis. *J Med Genet.* 1979;16(3):176–188. doi:10.1136/jmg.16.3.176

27. Roodhooft AM, Birnholz JC, Holmes LB. Familial nature of congenital absence and severe dysgenesis of both kidneys. *N Engl J Med.* 1984;310(21):1341–1345. doi:10.1056/NEJM198405243102101

28. Vivante A, Kohl S, Hwang D-Y, Dworschak GC, Hildebrandt F. Single-gene causes of congenital anomalies of the kidney and urinary tract (CAKUT) in humans. *Pediatr Nephrol.* 2014;29(4):695–704. doi:10.1007/s00467-013-2684-4

29. Jarvik GP, Evans JP. Mastering genomic terminology. *Genet Med.* 2017;19(5):491–492. doi:10.1038/gim.2016.139

30. Sanyanusin P, Schimmenti LA, McNoe LA, et al. Mutation of the PAX2 gene in a family with optic nerve colobomas, renal anomalies and vesicoureteral reflux. *Nat Genet.* 1995;9(4):358–364. doi:10.1038/ng0495-358

31. Lindner TH, Njolstad PR, Horikawa Y, Bostad L, Bell GI, Sovik O. A novel syndrome of diabetes mellitus, renal dysfunction and genital malformation associated with a partial deletion of the pseudo-POU domain of hepatocyte nuclear factor-1beta. *Hum Mol Genet.* 1999;8(11):2001–2008.

32. Abdelhak S, Kalatzis V, Heilig R, et al. A human homologue of the Drosophila eyes absent gene underlies branchio-oto-renal (BOR) syndrome and identifies a novel gene family. *Nat Genet.* 1997;15(2):157–164. doi:10.1038/ng0297-157

33. Capone VP, Morello W, Taroni F, Montini G. Genetics of congenital anomalies of the kidney and urinary tract: the current state of play. *Int J Mol Sci.* 2017;18(4):796. doi:10.3390/ijms18040796

34. Westland R, Sanna-Cherchi S. Recessive mutations in CAKUT and VACTERL association. *Kidney Int.* 2014;85(6):1253–1255. doi:https://doi.org/10.1038/ki.2013.495

35. Hays T, Groopman EE, Gharavi AG. Genetic testing for kidney disease of unknown etiology. *Kidney Int.* 2020;98(3):590–600. doi:10.1016/j.kint.2020.03.031

36. Kingsmore SF, Cakici JA, Clark MM, et al. A randomized, controlled trial of the analytic and diagnostic performance of singleton and trio, rapid genome and exome sequencing in ill infants. *Am J Hum Genet.* 2019;105(4):1–15. doi:10.1016/j.ajhg.2019.08.009

37. Nicolaides KH, Cheng HH, Abbas A, Snijders RJ, Gosden C. Fetal renal defects: associated malformations and chromosomal defects. *Fetal Diagn Ther.* 1992;7(1):1–11. doi:10.1159/000263642

38. Li S, Han X, Wang Y, et al. Chromosomal microarray analysis in fetuses with congenital anomalies of the kidney and urinary tract: a prospective cohort study and meta-analysis. *Prenat Diagn.* 2019;39(3):165–174. doi:10.1002/pd.5420

39. Donnelly JC, Platt LD, Rebarber A, Zachary J, Grobman WA, Wapner RJ. Association of copy number variants with specific ultrasonographically detected fetal anomalies. *Obstet Gynecol.* 2014;124(1):83–90. doi:10.1097/AOG.0000000000000336

40. Kuure S, Sariola H. Mouse models of congenital kidney anomalies BT—animal models of human birth defects. In: Liu A, ed. Springer Singapore; 2020:109–136. doi:10.1007/978-981-15-2389-2_5

41. Sanna-Cherchi S, Sampogna RV, Papeta N, et al. Mutations in DSTYK and dominant urinary tract malformations. *N Engl J Med.* 2013;369(7):621–629. doi:10.1056/NEJMoa1214479

42. Sanna-Cherchi S, Khan K, Westland R, et al. Exome-wide association study identifies GREB1L mutations in congenital lidney malformations. *Am J Hum Genet.* 2017;101(5):789–802. doi: 10.1016/j.ajhg.2017.09.018.

43. De Tomasi L, David P, Humbert C, et al. Mutations in GREB1L cause bilateral kidney agenesis in humans and mice. *Am J Hum Genet.* 2017;101(5):803–814. doi:10.1016/j.ajhg.2017.09.026

44. Saxén L, Sariola H. Early organogenesis of the kidney. *Pediatr Nephrol.* 1987;1(3):385–392. doi:10.1007/BF00849241

45. Murugapoopathy V, Gupta IR. A primer on congenital anomalies of the kidneys and urinary tracts (CAKUT). *Clin J Am Soc Nephrol.* 2020;15(5):723–731. doi:10.2215/CJN.12581019

46. van der Ven AT, Vivante A, Hildebrandt F. Novel insights into the pathogenesis of monogenic congenital anomalies of the kidney and urinary tract. *J Am Soc Nephrol.* 2018;29(1):36–50. doi:10.1681/ASN.2017050561

47. Weber S, Taylor JC, Winyard P, et al. SIX2 and BMP4 mutations associate with anomalous kidney development. *J Am Soc Nephrol.* 2008;19(5):891–903. doi:10.1681/ASN.2006111282

48. Biason-Lauber A, Konrad D, Navratil F, Schoenle EJ. A WNT4 mutation associated with Müllerian-duct regression and virilization in a 46,XX woman. *N Engl J Med.* 2004;351(8):792–798. doi:10.1056/NEJMoa040533

49. Mandel H, Shemer R, Borochowitz ZU, et al. SERKAL syndrome: an autosomal-recessive disorder caused by a loss-of-function mutation in WNT4. *Am J Hum Genet.* 2008;82(1):39–47. doi:10.1016/j.ajhg.2007.08.005

50. Vivante A, Mark-Danieli M, Davidovits M, et al. Renal hypodysplasia associates with a WNT4 variant that causes aberrant canonical WNT signaling. *J Am Soc Nephrol.* 2013;24(4):550–558. doi:10.1681/ASN.2012010097

51. Bouchard M, Souabni A, Mandler M, Neubüser A, Busslinger M. Nephric lineage specification by Pax2 and Pax8. *Genes Dev.* 2002;16(22):2958–2970. doi:10.1101/gad.240102

52. Bower M, Salomon R, Allanson J, et al. Update of PAX2 mutations in renal coloboma syndrome and establishment of a locus-specific database. *Hum Mutat.* 2012;33(3):457–466. doi:10.1002/humu.22020

53. Meeus L, Gilbert B, Rydlewski C, et al. Characterization of a novel loss of function mutation of PAX8 in a familial case of congenital hypothyroidism with in-place, normal-sized thyroid. *J Clin Endocrinol Metab.* 2004;89(9):4285–4291. doi:10.1210/jc.2004-0166

54. Bellanné-Chantelot C, Chauveau D, Gautier J-F, et al. Clinical spectrum associated with hepatocyte nuclear factor-1beta mutations. *Ann Intern Med.* 2004;140(7):510–517. doi:10.7326/0003-4819-140-7-200404060-00009

55. Hildebrandt F. Genetic kidney diseases. *Lancet.* 2010;375(9722):1287–1295. doi:10.1016/S0140-6736(10)60236-X

56. Sanna-Cherchi S, Westland R, Ghiggeri GM, Gharavi AG. Genetic basis of human congenital anomalies of the kidney and urinary tract. *J Clin Invest.* 2018;128(1):4–15. doi: 10.1172/jci95300.

57. Isaksen CV, Eik-Nes SH, Blaas HG, Torp SH. Fetuses and infants with congenital urinary system anomalies: correlation between prenatal ultrasound and postmortem findings. *Ultrasound Obstet Gynecol.* 2000;15(3):177–185. doi:10.1046/j.1469-0705.2000.00065

58. Huber C, Shazly SA, Blumenfeld YJ, Jelin E, Ruano R. Update on the prenatal diagnosis and outcomes of fetal bilateral renal agenesis. *Obstet Gynecol Surv.* 2019;74(5):298–302. doi:10.1097/OGX.0000000000000670

59. Laurichesse Delmas H, Kohler M, Doray B, et al. Congenital unilateral renal agenesis: prevalence, prenatal diagnosis, associated anomalies. Data from two birth-defect registries. *Birth Defects Res.* 2017;109(15):1204–1211. doi:10.1002/bdr2.1065

60. Hayes WN, Watson AR. Unilateral multicystic dysplastic kidney: does initial size matter? *Pediatr Nephrol.* 2012;27(8):1335–1340. doi:10.1007/s00467-012-2141-9

61. Westland R, Schreuder MF, Ket JCF, van Wijk JAE. Unilateral renal agenesis: a systematic review on associated anomalies and renal injury. *Nephrol Dial Transplant.* 2013;28(7):1844–1855. doi:10.1093/ndt/gft012

62. Wilson BE, Davies P, Shah K, Wong W, Taylor CM. Renal length and inulin clearance in the radiologically normal single kidney. *Pediatr Nephrol.* 2003;18(11):1147–1151. doi:10.1007/s00467-003-1244-8

63. Vu K-H, Van Dyck M, Daniels H, Proesmans W. Renal outcome of children with one functioning kidney from birth. A study of 99 patients and a review of the literature. *Eur J Pediatr.* 2008;167(8):885–890. doi:10.1007/s00431-007-0612-y

64. Westland R, Schreuder MF, van Goudoever JB, Sanna-Cherchi S, van Wijk JAE. Clinical implications of the solitary functioning kidney. *Clin J Am Soc Nephrol.* 2014;9(5):978–986. doi:10.2215/CJN.08900813

65. Sanna-Cherchi S, Ravani P, Corbani V, et al. Renal outcome in patients with congenital anomalies of the kidney and urinary tract. *Kidney Int.* 2009;76(5):528–533. doi:10.1038/ki.2009.220

66. Alfandary H, Haskin O, Goldberg O, et al. Is the prognosis of congenital single functioning kidney benign? A population-based study. *Pediatr Nephrol.* 2021;36(9):2837–2845. doi:10.1007/s00467-021-04980-6

67. Online Mendelian Inheritance in Man, OMIM®. Johns Hopkins University, Baltimore, MD. MIM Number: 113650. https://www.omim.org/entry/113650

68. Online Mendelian Inheritance in Man, OMIM®. Johns Hopkins University, Baltimore, MD. MIM Number: 219000. https://www.omim.org/entry/219000

69. Arora V, Khan S, El-Hattab AW, et al. Biallelic pathogenic GFRA1 variants cause autosomal recessive bilateral renal agenesis. *J Am Soc Nephrol.* 2021;32(1):223–228. doi:10.1681/ASN.2020040478

70. Verbitsky M, Sanna-Cherchi S, Fasel DA, et al. Genomic imbalances in pediatric patients with chronic kidney disease. *J Clin Invest.* 2015;125(5):2171–2178. doi:10.1172/JCI80877

71. Mefford HC, Clauin S, Sharp AJ, et al. Recurrent reciprocal genomic rearrangements of 17q12 are associated with renal disease, diabetes, and epilepsy. *Am J Hum Genet.* 2007; 81(5):1057–1069. doi:10.1086/522591

72. Rasmussen M, Vestergaard EM, Graakjaer J, et al. 17q12 deletion and duplication syndrome in Denmark—a clinical cohort of 38 patients and review of the literature. *Am J Med Genet A.* 2016;170(11):2934–2942. doi:10.1002/ajmg.a.37848

73. Hays T, Wapner RJ. Genetic testing for unexplained perinatal disorders. *Curr Opin Pediatr.* 2021;33:195–202. doi:10.1097/MOP.0000000000000999

74. Yuksel A, Batukan C. Sonographic findings of fetuses with an empty renal fossa and normal amniotic fluid volume. *Fetal Diagn Ther.* 2004;19(6):525–532. doi:10.1159/000080166

75. van den Bosch CMA, van Wijk JAE, Beckers GMA, van der Horst HJR, Schreuder MF, Bökenkamp A. Urological and nephrological findings of renal ectopia. *J Urol.* 2010;183(4): 1574–1578. doi:10.1016/j.juro.2009.12.041

76. Kang M, Kim YC, Lee H, et al. Renal outcomes in adult patients with horseshoe kidney. *Nephrol Dial Transplant.* 2021;36(3): 498–503. doi:10.1093/ndt/gfz217

77. Yavuz S, Kıyak A, Sander S. Renal outcome of children with horseshoe kidney: a single-center experience. *Urology.* 2015; 85(2):463–466. doi:10.1016/j.urology.2014.10.010

78. Murphy JJ, Altit G, Zerhouni S. The intrathoracic kidney: should we fix it? *J Pediatr Surg.* 2012;47(5):970–973. doi:10.1016/j.jpedsurg.2012.01.056

79. Je B-K, Kim HK, Horn PS. Incidence and spectrum of renal complications and extrarenal diseases and syndromes in 380 children and young adults with horseshoe kidney. *AJR Am J Roentgenol.* 2015;205(6):1306–1314. doi:10.2214/AJR.15.14625

80. Limwongse C, Clarren SK, Cassidy SB. Syndromes and malformations of the urinary tract. *Pediatr Nephrol.* 2004;4:427–452.

81. Birth Defects Monitoring Program (BDMP)/Commission on Professional and Hospital Activities (CPHA) surveillance data, 1988-1991. *Teratology.* 1993;48(6):658–675. doi:10.1002/tera.1420480608

82. Livera LN, Brookfield DS, Egginton JA, Hawnaur JM. Antenatal ultrasonography to detect fetal renal abnormalities: a prospective screening programme. *BMJ.* 1989;298(6685):1421–1423. doi:10.1136/bmj.298.6685.1421

83. Dolk H, Loane M, Garne E. The prevalence of congenital anomalies in Europe. *Adv Exp Med Biol.* 2010;686:349–364. doi:10.1007/978-90-481-9485-8_20

84. Fathallah-Shaykh SA, Flynn JT, Pierce CB, et al. Progression of pediatric CKD of nonglomerular origin in the CKiD cohort. *Clin J Am Soc Nephrol.* 2015;10(4):571–577. doi:10.2215/CJN.07480714

85. Ardissino G, Daccò V, Testa S, et al. Epidemiology of chronic renal failure in children: data from the ItalKid project. *Pediatrics.* 2003;111(4 Pt 1):e382–e387. doi:10.1542/peds.111.4.e382

86. Schreuder MF, Westland R, van Wijk JAE. Unilateral multicystic dysplastic kidney: a meta-analysis of observational studies on the incidence, associated urinary tract malformations and the contralateral kidney. *Nephrol Dial Transplant.* 2009;24(6): 1810–1818. doi:10.1093/ndt/gfn777

87. Winyard P, Chitty LS. Dysplastic kidneys. *Semin Fetal Neonatal Med.* 2008;13(3):142–151. doi:10.1016/j.siny.2007.10.009

88. Keller G, Zimmer G, Mall G, Ritz E, Amann K. Nephron number in patients with primary hypertension. *N Engl J Med.* 2003;348(2):101–108. doi:10.1056/NEJMoa020549

89. Eriksson JG, Salonen MK, Kajantie E, Osmond C. Prenatal growth and CKD in older adults: longitudinal findings from the Helsinki Birth Cohort Study, 1924-1944. *Am J Kidney Dis.* 2018;71(1):20–26. doi:10.1053/j.ajkd.2017.06.030

90. Hildebrandt F, Otto E. Cilia and centrosomes: a unifying pathogenic concept for cystic kidney disease? *Nat Rev Genet.* 2005;6(12):928–940. doi:10.1038/nrg1727

91. Garel J, Lefebvre M, Cassart M, et al. Prenatal ultrasonography of autosomal dominant polycystic kidney disease mimicking recessive type: case series. *Pediatr Radiol.* 2019;49(7):906–912. doi:10.1007/s00247-018-4325-3

92. Torres VE, Harris PC. Autosomal dominant polycystic kidney disease: the last 3 years. *Kidney Int.* 2009;76(2):149–168. doi:10.1038/ki.2009.128

93. Pei Y, Hwang Y-H, Conklin J, et al. Imaging-based diagnosis of autosomal dominant polycystic kidney disease. *J Am Soc Nephrol.* 2015;26(3):746–753. doi:10.1681/ASN.2014030297

94. Cornec-Le Gall E, Alam A, Perrone RD. Autosomal dominant polycystic kidney disease. *Lancet.* 2019;393(10174):919–935. doi:10.1016/S0140-6736(18)32782-X

95. Cornec-Le Gall E, Torres VE, Harris PC. Genetic complexity of autosomal dominant polycystic kidney and liver diseases. *J Am Soc Nephrol.* 2018;29(1):13–23. doi:10.1681/ASN.2017050483

96. Brook-Carter PT, Peral B, Ward CJ, et al. Deletion of the TSC2 and PKD1 genes associated with severe infantile polycystic kidney disease—a contiguous gene syndrome. *Nat Genet.* 1994;8(4):328–332. doi:10.1038/ng1294-328

97. Boal DK, Teele RL. Sonography of infantile polycystic kidney disease. *AJR Am J Roentgenol.* 1980;135(3):575–580. doi:10.2214/ajr.135.3.575

98. Hartung EA, Guay-Woodford LM. Autosomal recessive polycystic kidney disease: a hepatorenal fibrocystic disorder with pleiotropic effects. *Pediatrics.* 2014;134(3):e833–e845. doi:10.1542/peds.2013-3646

99. Bergmann C, Senderek J, Windelen E, et al. Clinical consequences of PKHD1 mutations in 164 patients with autosomal-recessive polycystic kidney disease (ARPKD). *Kidney Int.* 2005;67(3): 829–848. doi:10.1111/j.1523-1755.2005.00148

100. Guay-Woodford LM, Desmond RA. Autosomal recessive polycystic kidney disease: the clinical experience in North America. *Pediatrics.* 2003;111(5 Pt 1):1072–1080. doi:10.1542/peds.111.5.1072

101. Guay-Woodford LM, Bissler JJ, Braun MC, et al. Consensus expert recommendations for the diagnosis and management of autosomal recessive polycystic kidney disease: report of an international conference. *J Pediatr.* 2014;165(3):611–617. doi:10.1016/j.jpeds.2014.06.015

102. Alzarka B, Morizono H, Bollman JW, Kim D, Guay-Woodford LM. Design and implementation of the hepatorenal fibrocystic disease core center clinical database: a centralized resource for characterizing autosomal recessive polycystic kidney disease and other hepatorenal fibrocystic diseases. *Front Pediatr.* 2017;5:80. doi:10.3389/fped.2017.00080

103. Gilbert RD, Evans H, Olalekan K, Nagra A, Haq MR, Griffiths M. Tolvaptan treatment for severe neonatal autosomal-dominant polycystic kidney disease. *Pediatr Nephrol.* 2017;32(5):893–896. doi:10.1007/s00467-017-3584-9

104. Janssens P, Weydert C, De Rechter S, Wissing KM, Liebau MC, Mekahli D. Expanding the role of vasopressin antagonism in

polycystic kidney diseases: from adults to children? *Pediatr Nephrol.* 2018;33(3):395–408. doi:10.1007/s00467-017-3672-x

105. König J, Kranz B, König S, et al. Phenotypic spectrum of children with nephronophthisis and related ciliopathies. *Clin J Am Soc Nephrol.* 2017;12(12):1974–1983. doi:10.2215/CJN.01280217

106. Gagnadoux MF, Bacri JL, Broyer M, Habib R. Infantile chronic tubulo-interstitial nephritis with cortical microcysts: variant of nephronophthisis or new disease entity? *Pediatr Nephrol.* 1989;3(1):50–55. doi:10.1007/BF00859626

107. Srivastava S, Molinari E, Raman S, Sayer JA. Many genes—one disease? Genetics of nephronophthisis (NPHP) and NPHP-associated disorders. *Front Pediatr.* 2017;5:287–287. doi:10.3389/fped.2017.00287

108. Gribouval O, Gonzales M, Neuhaus T, et al. Mutations in genes in the renin-angiotensin system are associated with autosomal recessive renal tubular dysgenesis. *Nat Genet.* 2005;37(9):964–968. doi:10.1038/ng1623

109. Crino PB, Nathanson KL, Henske EP. The tuberous sclerosis complex. *N Engl J Med.* 2006;355(13):1345–1356. doi:10.1056/NEJMra055323

110. Schwartz RA, Fernández G, Kotulska K, Józ'wiak S. Tuberous sclerosis complex: advances in diagnosis, genetics, and management. *J Am Acad Dermatol.* 2007;57(2):189–202. doi:10.1016/j.jaad.2007.05.004

111. Curatolo P, Bombardieri R, Jozwiak S. Tuberous sclerosis. *Lancet.* 2008;372(9639):657–668. doi:10.1016/S0140-6736(08)61279-9

112. Murakami A, Gomi K, Tanaka M, et al. Unilateral glomerulocystic kidney disease associated with tuberous sclerosis complex in a neonate. *Pathol Int.* 2012;62(3):209–215. doi:10.1111/j.1440-1827.2011.02777

113. Izzi C, Dordoni C, Econimo L, et al. Variable expressivity of HNF1B nephropathy, from renal cysts and diabetes to medullary sponge kidney through tubulo-interstitial kidney disease. *Kidney Int Rep.* 2020;5(12):2341–2350. doi:10.1016/j.ekir.2020.09.042

114. Dias T, Sairam S, Kumarasiri S. Ultrasound diagnosis of fetal renal abnormalities. *Best Pract Res Clin Obstet Gynaecol.* 2014;28(3):403–415. doi:10.1016/j.bpobgyn.2014.01.009

115. Baldridge D, Spillmann RC, Wegner DJ, et al. Phenotypic expansion of KMT2D-related disorder: beyond Kabuki syndrome. *Am J Med Genet A.* 2020;182(5):1053–1065. doi:10.1002/ajmg.a.61518

116. Stokman MF, Renkema KY, Giles RH, Schaefer F, Knoers NVAM, van Eerde AM. The expanding phenotypic spectra of kidney diseases: insights from genetic studies. *Nat Rev Nephrol.* 2016;12(8):472–483. doi:10.1038/nrneph.2016.87

117. Bierhals T, Maddukuri SB, Kutsche K, Girisha KM. Expanding the phenotype associated with 17q12 duplication: case report and review of the literature. *Am J Med Genet A.* 2013;161A(2):352–359. doi:10.1002/ajmg.a.35730

118. Belge H, Dahan K, Cambier J-F, et al. Clinical and mutational spectrum of hypoparathyroidism, deafness and renal dysplasia syndrome. *Nephrol Dial Transplant.* 2017;32(5):830–837. doi:10.1093/ndt/gfw271

119. Bergman JEH, Janssen N, Hoefsloot LH, Jongmans MCJ, Hofstra RMW, van Ravenswaaij-Arts CMA. CHD7 mutations and CHARGE syndrome: the clinical implications of an expanding phenotype. *J Med Genet.* 2011;48(5):334–342. doi:10.1136/jmg.2010.087106

120. White SL, Perkovic V, Cass A, et al. Is low birth weight an antecedent of CKD in later life? A systematic review of observational studies. *Am J Kidney Dis.* 2009;54(2):248–261. doi:10.1053/j.ajkd.2008.12.042

121. Rodríguez MM, Gómez AH, Abitbol CL, Chandar JJ, Duara S, Zilleruelo GE. Histomorphometric analysis of postnatal glomerulogenesis in extremely preterm infants. *Pediatr Dev Pathol.* 2004;7(1):17–25. doi:10.1007/s10024-003-3029-2

122. Sutherland MR, Gubhaju L, Moore L, et al. Accelerated maturation and abnormal morphology in the preterm neonatal kidney. *J Am Soc Nephrol.* 2011;22(7):1365–1374. doi:10.1681/ASN.2010121266

123. Charlton JR, Boohaker L, Askenazi D, et al. Late onset neonatal acute kidney injury: results from the AWAKEN Study. *Pediatr Res.* 2019;85(3):339–348. doi:10.1038/s41390-018-0255-x

124. Jetton JG, Boohaker LJ, Sethi SK, et al. Incidence and outcomes of neonatal acute kidney injury (AWAKEN): a multicentre, multinational, observational cohort study. *Lancet Child Adolesc Health.* 2017;1(3):184–194. doi:10.1016/S2352-4642(17)30069-X

125. Blazer S, Zimmer EZ, Blumenfeld Z, Zelikovic I, Bronshtein M. Natural history of fetal simple renal cysts detected in early pregnancy. *J Urol.* 1999;162(3 Pt 1):812–814. doi:10.1097/00005392-199909010-00066

126. Lee VS, Kaur M, Bokacheva L, et al. What causes diminished corticomedullary differentiation in renal insufficiency? *J Magn Reson Imaging.* 2007;25(4):790–795. doi:10.1002/jmri.20878

127. Chaumoitre K, Brun M, Cassart M, et al. Differential diagnosis of fetal hyperechogenic cystic kidneys unrelated to renal tract anomalies: a multicenter study. *Ultrasound Obstet Gynecol.* 2006;28(7):911–917. doi:10.1002/uog.3856

128. Decter RM. Renal duplication and fusion anomalies. *Pediatr Clin North Am.* 1997;44(5):1323–1341. doi:10.1016/s0031-3955(05)70559-9

129. Williams H. Renal revision: from lobulation to duplication—what is normal? *Arch Dis Child Educ Pract Ed.* 2007;92(5):ep152-ep158. doi:10.1136/adc.2007.126680

130. Golzio C, Willer J, Talkowski ME, et al. KCTD13 is a major driver of mirrored neuroanatomical phenotypes of the 16p11.2 copy number variant. *Nature.* 2012;485(7398):363–367. doi:10.1038/nature11091

131. Golzio C, Katsanis N. Genetic architecture of reciprocal CNVs. *Curr Opin Genet Dev.* 2013;23(3):240–248. doi:10.1016/j.gde.2013.04.013

132. Hamilton BE, Martin JA, Ventura SJ. Births: preliminary data for 2012. *Natl Vital Stat Rep.* 2013;62(3):1–20.

133. Nguyen HT, Benson CB, Bromley B, et al. Multidisciplinary consensus on the classification of prenatal and postnatal urinary tract dilation (UTD classification system). *J Pediatr Urol.* 2014;10(6):982–998. doi:10.1016/j.jpurol.2014.10.002

134. Zanetta VC, Rosman BM, Bromley B, et al. Variations in management of mild prenatal hydronephrosis among maternal-fetal medicine obstetricians, and pediatric urologists and radiologists. *J Urol.* 2012;188(5):1935–1939. doi:10.1016/j.juro.2012.07.011

135. Lee RS, Cendron M, Kinnamon DD, Nguyen HT. Antenatal hydronephrosis as a predictor of postnatal outcome: a meta-analysis. *Pediatrics.* 2006;118(2):586–593. doi:10.1542/peds.2006-0120

136. Havutcu AE, Nikolopoulos G, Adinkra P, Lamont RF. The association between fetal pyelectasis on second trimester ultrasound scan and aneuploidy among 25,586 low risk unselected women. *Prenat Diagn.* 2002;22(13):1201–1206. doi:10.1002/pd.490

137. Coco C, Jeanty P. Isolated fetal pyelectasis and chromosomal abnormalities. *Am J Obstet Gynecol.* 2005;193(3 Pt 1):732–738. doi:10.1016/j.ajog.2005.02.074

138. Corteville JE, Dicke JM, Crane JP. Fetal pyelectasis and Down syndrome: is genetic amniocentesis warranted? *Obstet Gynecol.* 1992;79(5 (Pt 1):770–772.

139. Holzman SA, Braga LH, Zee RS, et al. Risk of urinary tract infection in patients with hydroureter: an analysis from the Society of Fetal Urology Prenatal Hydronephrosis Registry. *J Pediatr Urol.* 2021;17(6):775–781. doi:10.1016/j.jpurol.2021.09.001

140. Dekirmendjian A, Braga LH. Primary non-refluxing megaureter: analysis of risk factors for spontaneous resolution and surgical intervention. *Front Pediatr.* 2019;7:126. doi:10.3389/fped.2019.00126

141. Duong HP, Piepsz A, Collier F, et al. Predicting the clinical outcome of antenatally detected unilateral pelviureteric junction stenosis. *Urology.* 2013;82(3):691–696. doi:10.1016/j.urology.2013.03.041

142. Uy N, Reidy K. Developmental genetics and congenital anomalies of the kidney and urinary tract. *J Pediatr Genet.* 2016;5(1):51–60. doi:10.1055/s-0035-1558423

143. Chen F. Genetic and developmental basis for urinary tract obstruction. *Pediatr Nephrol.* 2009;24(9):1621–1632. doi:10.1007/s00467-008-1072-y

144. Rieke JM, Zhang R, Braun D, et al. SLC20A1 is involved in urinary tract and urorectal development. *Front Cell Dev Biol.* 2020;8:567. doi:10.3389/fcell.2020.00567

145. Okur V, LeDuc CA, Guzman E, Valivullah ZM, Anyane-Yeboa K, Chung WK. Homozygous noncanonical splice variant in LSM1 in two siblings with multiple congenital anomalies and global developmental delay. *Cold Spring Harb Mol Case Stud.* 2019;5(3):a004101. doi:10.1101/mcs.a004101

146. Johnston JJ, Gropman AL, Sapp JC, et al. The phenotype of a germline mutation in PIGA: the gene somatically mutated in paroxysmal nocturnal hemoglobinuria. *Am J Hum Genet.* 2012;90(2):295–300. doi:10.1016/j.ajhg.2011.11.031

147. Elder JS, Peters CA, Arant BS Jr, et al. Pediatric Vesicoureteral Reflux Guidelines Panel summary report on the management of primary vesicoureteral reflux in children. *J Urol.* 1997;157(5):1846–1851.

148. Mattoo TK, Chesney RW, Greenfield SP, et al. Renal Scarring in the Randomized Intervention for Children with Vesicoureteral Reflux (RIVUR) trial. *Clin J Am Soc Nephrol.* 2016;11(1):54–61. doi:10.2215/CJN.05210515

149. Shaikh N, Ewing AL, Bhatnagar S, Hoberman A. Risk of renal scarring in children with a first urinary tract infection: a systematic review. *Pediatrics.* 2010;126(6):1084–1091. doi:10.1542/peds.2010-0685

150. Shaikh N, Craig JC, Rovers MM, et al. Identification of children and adolescents at risk for renal scarring after a first urinary tract infection: a meta-analysis with individual patient data. *JAMA Pediatr.* 2014;168(10):893–900. doi:10.1001/jamapediatrics.2014.637

151. Sjöström S, Sillén U, Bachelard M, Hansson S, Stokland E. Spontaneous resolution of high grade infantile vesicoureteral reflux. *J Urol.* 2004;172(2):694–698; discussion 699. doi:10.1097/01.ju.0000130747.89561.cf

152. Verbitsky M, Krithivasan P, Batourina E, et al. Copy number variant analysis and genome-wide association study identify loci with large effect for vesicoureteral reflux. *J Am Soc Nephrol.* 2021;32(4):805–820. doi:10.1681/ASN.2020050681

153. Darlow JM, Dobson MG, Darlay R, et al. A new genome scan for primary nonsyndromic vesicoureteric reflux emphasizes high genetic heterogeneity and shows linkage and association with various genes already implicated in urinary tract development. *Mol Genet Genomic Med.* 2014;2(1):7–29. doi:10.1002/mgg3.22

154. van Eerde AM, Duran K, van Riel E, et al. Genes in the ureteric budding pathway: association study on vesico-ureteral reflux patients. *PLoS One.* 2012;7(4):e31327. doi:10.1371/journal.pone.0031327

155. Ninoa F, Ilari M, Noviello C, et al. Genetics of vesicoureteral reflux. *Curr Genomics.* 2016;17(1):70–79. doi:10.2174/1389202916666151014223507

156. Valério FC, Lemos RD, de C Reis AL, Pimenta LP, Vieira ÉL, Silva ACE. Biomarkers in vesicoureteral reflux: an overview. *Biomark Med.* 2020;14(8):683–696. doi:10.2217/bmm-2019-0378

157. Ludwig M, Ching B, Reutter H, Boyadjiev SA. Bladder exstrophy-epispadias complex. *Birth Defects Res A Clin Mol Teratol.* 2009;85(6):509–522. doi:10.1002/bdra.20557

158. Reutter H, Qi L, Gearhart JP, et al. Concordance analyses of twins with bladder exstrophy-epispadias complex suggest genetic etiology. *Am J Med Genet A.* 2007;143A(22):2751–2756. doi:10.1002/ajmg.a.31975

159. Reutter H, Boyadjiev SA, Gambhir L, et al. Phenotype severity in the bladder exstrophy-epispadias complex: analysis of genetic and nongenetic contributing factors in 441 families from North America and Europe. *J Pediatr.* 2011;159(5):825–831.e1. doi:10.1016/j.jpeds.2011.04.042

160. Shapiro E, Lepor H, Jeffs RD. The inheritance of the exstrophy-epispadias complex. *J Urol.* 1984;132(2):308–310. doi:10.1016/s0022-5347(17)49605-4

161. Baranowska Körberg I, Hofmeister W, Markljung E, et al. WNT3 involvement in human bladder exstrophy and cloaca development in zebrafish. *Hum Mol Genet.* 2015;24(18):5069–5078. doi:10.1093/hmg/ddv225

162. Lundin J, Söderhäll C, Lundén L, et al. 22q11.2 microduplication in two patients with bladder exstrophy and hearing impairment. *Eur J Med Genet.* 2010;53(2):61–65. doi:10.1016/j.ejmg.2009.11.004.

163. Draaken M, Baudisch F, Timmermann B, et al. Classic bladder exstrophy: frequent 22q11.21 duplications and definition of a 414 kb phenocritical region. *Birth Defects Res A Clin Mol Teratol.* 2014;100(6):512–517. doi:10.1002/bdra.23249

164. Draaken M, Reutter H, Schramm C, et al. Microduplications at 22q11.21 are associated with non-syndromic classic bladder exstrophy. *Eur J Med Genet.* 2010;53(2):55–60. doi:10.1016/j.ejmg.2009.12.005

165. Draaken M, Knapp M, Pennimpede T, et al. Genome-wide association study and meta-analysis identify ISL1 as genome-wide significant susceptibility gene for bladder exstrophy. *PLoS Genet.* 2015;11(3):e1005024.

166. Schnack TH, Zdravkovic S, Myrup C, et al. Familial aggregation of hypospadias: a cohort study. *Am J Epidemiol.* 2008;167(3):251–256. doi:10.1093/aje/kwm317

167. Kalfa N, Philibert P, Sultan C. Is hypospadias a genetic, endocrine or environmental disease, or still an unexplained malformation? *Int J Androl.* 2009;32(3):187–197. doi:10.1111/j.1365-2605.2008.00899

168. Geller F, Feenstra B, Carstensen L, et al. Genome-wide association analyses identify variants in developmental genes associated with hypospadias. *Nat Genet.* 2014;46(9):957–963. doi:10.1038/ng.3063

169. Brownlee E, Wragg R, Robb A, Chandran H, Knight M, McCarthy L. Current epidemiology and antenatal presentation of posterior urethral valves: outcome of BAPS CASS National

Audit. *J Pediatr Surg.* 2019;54(2):318–321. doi:10.1016/j.jpedsurg.2018.10.091

170. Richter F, Morton SU, Kim SW, et al. Genomic analyses implicate noncoding de novo variants in congenital heart disease. *Nat Genet.* 2020;52(8):769–777. doi:10.1038/s41588-020-0652-z

171. Cummings BB, Karczewski KJ, Kosmicki JA, et al. Transcript expression-aware annotation improves rare variant interpretation. *Nature.* 2020;581(7809):452–458. doi:10.1038/s41586-020-2329-2

172. Mohammadi P, Castel SE, Cummings BB, et al. Genetic regulatory variation in populations informs transcriptome analysis in rare disease. *Science.* 2019;366(6463):351–356. doi:10.1126/science.aay0256

173. Logsdon GA, Vollger MR, Eichler EE. Long-read human genome sequencing and its applications. *Nat Rev Genet.* 2020;21(10):597–614. doi:10.1038/s41576-020-0236-x

174. Chen K, Didsbury M, van Zwieten A, et al. Neurocognitive and educational outcomes in children and adolescents with CKD. *Clin J Am Soc Nephrol.* 2018;13(3):387–397. doi:10.2215/CJN.09650917

175. Verbitsky M, Kogon AJ, Matheson M, et al. Genomic disorders and neurocognitive impairment in pediatric CKD. *J Am Soc Nephrol.* 2017;28(8):2303–2309. doi:10.1681/ASN.2016101108

176. Lipkin PH, Macias MM. Promoting optimal development: identifying infants and young children with developmental disorders through developmental surveillance and screening. *Pediatrics.* 2020;145(1):e20193449. doi:10.1542/peds.2019-3449

177. Malinowski J, Miller DT, Demmer L, et al. Systematic evidence-based review: outcomes from exome and genome sequencing for pediatric patients with congenital anomalies or intellectual disability. *Genet Med.* 2020;22(6):986–1004. doi:10.1038/s41436-020-0771-z

178. Dimmock D, Caylor S, Waldman B, et al. Project Baby Bear: rapid precision care incorporating rWGS in 5 California children's hospitals demonstrates improved clinical outcomes and reduced costs of care. *Am J Hum Genet.* 2021;108(7):1231–1238. doi:10.1016/j.ajhg.2021.05.008

179. Dimmock DP, Clark MM, Gaughran M, et al. An RCT of rapid genomic sequencing among seriously ill infants results in high clinical utility, changes in management, and low perceived harm. *Am J Hum Genet.* 2020;107(5):942–952. doi:10.1016/j.ajhg.2020.10.003

180. Krantz ID, Medne L, Weatherly JM, et al. Effect of whole-genome sequencing on the clinical management of acutely ill infants with suspected genetic disease: a randomized clinical trial. *JAMA Pediatr.* 2021;175(12):1218–1226. doi:10.1001/jamapediatrics.2021.3496

181. Manickam K, McClain MR, Demmer LA, et al. Exome and genome sequencing for pediatric patients with congenital anomalies or intellectual disability: an evidence-based clinical guideline of the American College of Medical Genetics and Genomics (ACMG). *Genet Med.* 2021;23(11):2029–2037. doi:10.1038/s41436-021-01242-6

182. Feldenberg R, Beck A. Congenital diseases of the kidneys: prognosis and treatments. *Neoreviews.* 2017;18(6):e345–e356. doi:10.1542/neo.18-6-e345

183. Tremblay I, Grondin S, Laberge A-M, et al. Diagnostic and therapeutic misconception: parental expectations and perspectives regarding genetic testing for developmental disorders. *J Autism Dev Disord.* 2019;49(1):363–375. doi:10.1007/s10803-018-3768-6

184. Cakici JA, Dimmock DP, Caylor SA, et al. A prospective study of parental perceptions of rapid whole-genome and -exome sequencing among seriously ill infants. *Am J Hum Genet.* 2020;107(5):953–962. doi:10.1016/j.ajhg.2020.10.004

185. Li X, Nusbaum R, Smith-Hicks C, Jamal L, Dixon S, Mahida S. Caregivers' perception of and experience with variants of uncertain significance from whole exome sequencing for children with undiagnosed conditions. *J Genet Couns.* 2019;28(2):304–312. doi:10.1002/jgc4.1093.

186. Elliott AM, Friedman JM. The importance of genetic counselling in genome-wide sequencing. *Nat Rev Genet.* 2018;19(12):735–736. doi:10.1038/s41576-018-0057-3

187. Ha VTD, Frizzo-Barker J, Chow-White P. Adopting clinical genomics: a systematic review of genomic literacy among physicians in cancer care. *BMC Med Genomics.* 2018;11(1):18. doi:10.1186/s12920-018-0337-y

188. Kiryluk K, Goldstein DB, Rowe JW, Gharavi AG, Wapner R, Chung WK. Precision Medicine in internal medicine. *Ann Intern Med.* 2019;170(9):635–642. doi:10.7326/M18-0425

189. Goldman L, Goldman JS. Precision medicine for clinicians: the future begins now. *Ann Intern Med.* 2019;170(9):660–661

190. Zimani AN, Peterlin B, Kovanda A. Increasing genomic literacy through national genomic projects. *Front Genet.* 2021;12:693253. doi:10.3389/fgene.2021.693253

191. Milo Rasouly H, Cuneo N, Marasa M, et al. GeneLiFT: a novel test to facilitate rapid screening of genetic literacy in a diverse population undergoing genetic testing. *J Genet Couns.* 2020;30(3):742–754. doi:10.1002/jgc4.1364

192. Giuse NB, Kusnoor SV, Koonce TY, et al. Guiding oncology patients through the maze of precision medicine. *J Health Commun.* 2016;21(suppl 1):5–17. doi:10.1080/10810730.2015.1131772

193. Canedo JR, Miller ST, Myers HF, Sanderson M. Racial and ethnic differences in knowledge and attitudes about genetic testing in the US: systematic review. *J Genet Couns.* 2019;28(3):587–601. doi:10.1002/jgc4.1078

194. Hamilton JG, Shuk E, Arniella G, et al. Genetic testing awareness and attitudes among Latinos: exploring shared perceptions and gender-based differences. *Public Health Genomics.* 2016;19(1):34–46. doi:10.1159/000441552

195. Reuter CM, Kohler JN, Bonner D, et al. Yield of whole exome sequencing in undiagnosed patients facing insurance coverage barriers to genetic testing. *J Genet Couns.* 2019;28(6):1107–1118. doi:10.1002/jgc4.1161

196. Iglesias A, Anyane-Yeboa K, Wynn J, et al. The usefulness of whole-exome sequencing in routine clinical practice. *Genet Med.* 2014;16(12):922–931. doi:10.1038/gim.2014.58

197. Jensen TS, Chin J, Evans MA, et al. *Next Generation Sequencing (NGS) for Medicare Beneficiaries with Advanced Cancer.* Centers for Medicare & Medicaid Services; Published 2020. Available at: https://www.cms.gov/medicare-coverage-database/view/ncacal-decision-memo.aspx?proposed=N&NCAId=296

198. Manolio TA, Abramowicz M, Al-Mulla F, et al. Global implementation of genomic medicine: we are not alone. *Sci Transl Med.* 2015;7(290):290ps13. doi:10.1126/scitranslmed.aab0194

199. Abacan MA, Alsubaie L, Barlow-Stewart K, et al. The global state of the genetic counseling profession. *Eur J Hum Genet.* 2019;27(2):183–197. doi:10.1038/s41431-018-0252-x

200. Sirisena ND, Dissanayake VHW. Strategies for genomic medicine education in low- and middle-income countries. *Front Genet.* 2019;10:944. doi:10.3389/fgene.2019.00944

201. Hillyer GC, Schmitt KM, Reyes A, et al. Community education to enhance the more equitable use of precision medicine in

Northern Manhattan. *J Genet Couns*. 2020;29(2):247–258. doi:10.1002/jgc4.1244

202. Splinter K, Adams DR, Bacino CA, et al. Effect of genetic diagnosis on patients with previously undiagnosed disease. *N Engl J Med*. 2018;379(22):2131–2139. doi:10.1056/NEJMoa1714458

203. Richards S, Aziz N, Bale S, et al. Standards and guidelines for the interpretation of sequence variants: a joint consensus recommendation of the American College of Medical Genetics and Genomics and the Association for Molecular Pathology. *Genet Med*. 2015;17(5):405–424. doi:10.1038/gim.2015.30

204. Popejoy AB, Fullerton SM. Genomics is failing on diversity. *Nature*. 2016;538(7624):161–164. doi:10.1038/538161a

205. Denny JC, Rutter J, Goldstein DB, et al. The "All of Us" research program. *N Engl J Med*. 2019;381(7):668–676. doi:10.1056/NEJMsr1809937

206. Nestor JG, Groopman EE, Gharavi AG. Towards precision nephrology: the opportunities and challenges of genomic medicine. *J Nephrol*. 2018;31(1):47–60. doi:10.1007/s40620-017-0448-0

207. Bell EF, Hintz SR, Hansen NI, et al. Mortality, in-hospital morbidity, care practices, and 2-year outcomes for extremely preterm infants in the US, 2013-2018. *JAMA*. 2022;327(3):248–263. doi:10.1001/jama.2021.23580

208. Horbar JD, Carpenter JH, Badger GJ, et al. Mortality and neonatal morbidity among infants 501 to 1500 grams from 2000 to 2009. *Pediatrics*. 2012;129(6):1019–1026. doi:10.1542/peds.2011-3028

209. Petrikin JE, Cakici JA, Clark MM, et al. The NSIGHT1-randomized controlled trial: rapid whole-genome sequencing for accelerated etiologic diagnosis in critically ill infants. *NPJ Genom Med*. 2018;3(1):1–11. doi:10.1038/s41525-018-0045-8

210. Saunders CJ, Miller NA, Soden SE, et al. Rapid whole-genome sequencing for genetic disease diagnosis in neonatal intensive care units. *Sci Transl Med*. 2012;4(154):154ra135. doi:10.1126/scitranslmed.3004041

211. Mestek-Boukhibar L, Clement E, Jones WD, et al. Rapid paediatric sequencing (RaPS): comprehensive real-life workflow for rapid diagnosis of critically ill children. *J Med Genet*. 2018;55(11):721–728. doi:10.1136/jmedgenet-2018-105396

212. French CE, Delon I, Dolling H, et al. Whole genome sequencing reveals that genetic conditions are frequent in intensively ill children. *Intensive Care Med*. 2019;45(5):627–636. doi:10.1007/s00134-019-05552-x

213. Powis Z, Farwell Hagman KD, Speare V, et al. Exome sequencing in neonates: diagnostic rates, characteristics, and time to diagnosis. *Genet Med*. 2018;20(11):1468–1471. doi:10.1038/gim.2018.11

214. Wojcik MH, Schwartz TS, Yamin I, et al. Genetic disorders and mortality in infancy and early childhood: delayed diagnoses and missed opportunities. *Genet Med*. 2018;20(11):1396–1404. doi:10.1038/gim.2018.17

215. Bertoli-Avella AM, Beetz C, Ameziane N, et al. Successful application of genome sequencing in a diagnostic setting: 1007 index cases from a clinically heterogeneous cohort. *Eur J Hum Genet*. 2021;29(1):141–153. doi:10.1038/s41431-020-00713-9

216. Hausman-Kedem M, Malinger G, Modai S, et al. Monogenic causes of apparently idiopathic perinatal intracranial hemorrhage. *Ann Neurol*. 2021;89(4):813–822. doi:10.1002/ana.26033

217. Elliott AM, du Souich C, Lehman A, et al. RAPIDOMICS: rapid genome-wide sequencing in a neonatal intensive care unit—successes and challenges. *Eur J Pediatr*. 2019;178(8):1207–1218. doi:10.1007/s00431-019-03399-4

218. Stark Z, Tan TY, Chong B, et al. A prospective evaluation of whole-exome sequencing as a first-tier molecular test in infants with suspected monogenic disorders. *Genet Med*. 2016;18(11):1090–1096. doi:10.1038/gim.2016.1

219. Farnaes L, Hildreth A, Sweeney NM, et al. Rapid whole-genome sequencing decreases infant morbidity and cost of hospitalization. *NPJ Genom Med*. 2018;3:10. doi:10.1038/s41525-018-0049-4

220. Meng L, Pammi M, Saronwala A, et al. Use of exome sequencing for infants in intensive care units: ascertainment of severe single-gene disorders and effect on medical management. *JAMA Pediatr*. 2017;171(12):e173438. doi:10.1001/jamapediatrics.2017.3438

221. van Diemen CC, Kerstjens-Frederikse WS, Bergman KA, et al. Rapid targeted genomics in critically ill newborns. *Pediatrics*. 2017;140(4):e20162854. doi:10.1542/peds.2016-2854

222. Willig LK, Petrikin JE, Smith LD, et al. Whole-genome sequencing for identification of Mendelian disorders in critically ill infants: a retrospective analysis of diagnostic and clinical findings. *Lancet Respir Med*. 2015;3(5):377–387. doi:10.1016/S2213-2600(15)00139-3

223. Zhu X, Petrovski S, Xie P, et al. Whole-exome sequencing in undiagnosed genetic diseases: interpreting 119 trios. *Genet Med*. 2015;17(10):774–781. doi:10.1038/gim.2014.191

224. Ceyhan-Birsoy O, Murry JB, Machini K, et al. Interpretation of genomic sequencing results in healthy and ill newborns: results from the BabySeq Project. *Am J Hum Genet*. 2019;104(1):76–93. doi:10.1016/j.ajhg.2018.11.016

Chapter 9

Evidence-Based Approach to Diuretic Therapy in the Neonate

Jeffrey L. Segar, MD

Chapter Outline

Introduction

Diuretics are commonly used in the neonatal population to treat infants with bronchopulmonary dysplasia (BPD), cardiac disease associated with congestive heart failure, and acute kidney injury (AKI). The relatively high frequency of diuretic use has been documented by several large retrospective cohorts. Laughon et al. utilized the Pediatrix Medical Group data warehouse (1997–2011) to identify that 37% of almost 40,000 infants <32 weeks' gestation and <1500 g birth weight were exposed to at least one diuretic, with 93% of these infants receiving at least a single dose of furosemide.[1] Using this same database, Clark et al. reported that furosemide was the seventh most commonly reported medication in the neonatal intensive care unit (NICU), with over 8% of all NICU patients being exposed to the agent.[2] This widespread use of diuretics occurs despite the lack of evidence demonstrating a beneficial effect of long-term diuretic therapy on clinical outcomes in infants with BPD and other medical conditions. A survey of US neonatologists

involving hypothetical clinical scenarios suggests diuretic therapy for very low birth weight infants in the first 28 days of life is commonly used, despite limited evidence of benefit from randomized trials.[3] A majority of respondents expected sustained improvements in pulmonary mechanics, decreased days on mechanical ventilation, and decreased length of stay, despite the lack of evidence in current literature. Finally, although the list of potential complications from diuretic therapy is extensive, including electrolyte abnormalities, bone demineralization, and growth failure, these appear to have limited influence on the decision-making process. This disparity underscores the reasons for both furosemide and hydrochlorothiazide being included on the 2020–2021 Best Pharmaceuticals for Children Act (BPCA) Priority list of needs in pediatric therapeutics.[4]

A rational, patient-centered approach to diuretic therapy in neonates requires a basic understanding of developmental renal physiology and function, knowledge of the mechanisms of action of diuretics, evidence of their efficacy relative to specific disease states, and familiarity with the potential adverse effects. This chapter seeks to fulfill these needs of the clinician with a particular focus on the use of diuretics in neonates with lung disease, congenital heart disease, and AKI.

Developmental Renal Physiology and Function

During the last trimester of gestation, the fetal kidneys receive only 2%–4% of the combined ventricular blood output.[5] Following birth there is a decrease in renal vascular resistance associated with a rise in arterial pressure, both contributing to an increase in renal blood flow during the weeks following birth such that the newborn kidney receives 8%–10% of cardiac output at the end of the first week of life and 15%–18% by a few months of age. In comparison, 25% of cardiac output is distributed to the kidneys in the normal adult.[6] Accompanying postnatal changes in blood flow are marked increases in the glomerular filtration rate (GFR) and sodium reabsorption. In a longitudinal study of preterm infants whose gestational ages at birth ranged from 27 to 31 weeks, Vieux et al. identified that GFR, as measured by creatinine clearance, increased from 18.5 ± 12.6 (day 7) to 26.2 ± 19.6 mL/min per 1.73 m² (day 28).[7] GFR was approximately two times higher in 31-week gestation infants compared with 27-week gestation infants throughout this period. It is estimated that GFR increases at least 50% during the first day of life in the term infant and doubles by 2 weeks of age.[8] Studies in animal models suggest anatomical and neurohumoral factors, including the renin-angiotensin system, nitric oxide, and prostaglandins, contribute to these developmental changes that have important implications regarding the pharmacokinetics of diuretics in neonates.

Sodium is the principal cation in the extracellular water compartment and is instrumental in maintaining the size of the extracellular space, including intravascular volume. Because preservation of extracellular and intravascular volume is essential for life, the mature kidney displays redundant sodium transport systems that allow for a high degree of renal tubular sodium reabsorption. In contrast, the developing kidney exhibits obligate urine sodium loss because of immaturity of renal tubular sodium transport. In utero, urinary fractional excretion of sodium (FENa) is remarkably high, averaging 10%–15%.[9] Urine sodium losses remain high in preterm infants 22–32 weeks' gestation (FENa 5%–10% during first few days of life) and slowly decrease with advancing postnatal age, typically achieving an FENa of 0.5%–1% by 36 weeks postmenstrual age.[10,11] In full-term infants, FENa decreases to 2%–4% in the first few hours after birth and to lower values in the subsequent 48 hours. Changes in renal sodium excretion appear to be related to changes in renal blood flow distribution, proximal tubule length, expression and activity of sodium-potassium ATPase and luminal membrane sodium-hydrogen exchanger, and response to hormones.[12]

Sodium Reabsorption in the Kidney

The majority of sodium filtered by the glomerulus is reabsorbed along the renal tubule by a variety of ion pumps and transport proteins.[13] The primary site of sodium reabsorption is within the proximal tubule (50%–70% of total renal sodium reabsorption), with lesser amounts reabsorbed in the loop of Henle (25%–30%), the distal tubule (5%), and the collecting duct (3%). The basolateral sodium-potassium ATPase (Na^+-K^+-ATPase) provides the electrochemical driving force for sodium reabsorption along the nephron tubule, decreasing intracellular sodium concentration and generating a negative cellular potential difference. With the proximal tubule, sodium is reabsorbed along with organic solutes, via the Na-H exchanger in the apical membrane, and passively across tight junctions. Within the thick ascending loop of Henle, the Na^+-K^+-$2Cl^-$ cotransporter in the apical membrane is primarily responsible for sodium reabsorption. This is the transporter that is inhibited by loop diuretics, such as furosemide. Sodium transport in the distal convoluted tubule occurs via the Na-Cl transporter (NCC), which is inhibited by thiazide diuretics, while the collecting tubule primarily utilizes the epithelial sodium channel (ENaC) on principal cells and a Na^+-dependent Cl^-/HCO_3 exchanger on intercalated cells. Different classes of diuretics, described later, target these different, apically located transporters to block sodium, chloride, and ultimately water reabsorption in the kidney, leading to various degrees of natriuresis, chloruresis, and diuresis.

Diuretic Classes Based Upon Mechanisms of Action

Diuretics are designed to reduce sodium and chloride reabsorption within the renal tubules and in doing so reduce the luminal-to-cellular osmotic gradient, which in turn limits water reabsorption and increases urine production (i.e., water loss). Diuretics are typically classified by their sites and mechanisms of action. The two most common types of diuretics used in the neonatal population, loop diuretics (acting in the thick ascending limb) and thiazide diuretics (acting in the distal convoluted tubule), are described herein. Potassium-sparing diuretics, which represent a third class of diuretics and act in the aldosterone-sensitive distal nephron, are less commonly used and then typically in combination with thiazides. Diuretics with limited use or pharmacologic/pharmacokinetic data in the neonatal population will only briefly be mentioned.

LOOP DIURETICS

The loop diuretics furosemide and bumetanide exert their principal action by inhibiting the Na^+-K^+-$2Cl^-$ symport in the thick ascending loop of Henle and are characterized by a prompt onset of action and short duration of diuresis. Because this portion of the renal tubule has a high capacity to reabsorb sodium (approximately 25% of all filtered sodium), loop diuretics are the most potent natriuretic agents. Loop diuretics are highly protein bound and not readily filtered at the glomerulus; rather, they require delivery into the proximal tubular lumen via organic acid transporters (OAT1 and OAT3) to be functional. They act in the thick ascending loop of Henle to block the Na^+-K^+-$2Cl^-$ transporter, thereby inhibiting sodium, chloride, and potassium reabsorption. The pharmacokinetics of furosemide differ greatly between preterm and term infants and demonstrate extensive interindividual variability.[14] Compared with adults, in which half-life of furosemide is 1.3 ± 0.8 hours, the half-life in preterm infants (on average 30 weeks' gestation, postmenstrual age of 1–4 weeks) is 15- to 20-fold longer, and in term infants approximately 6- to 10-fold longer. These differences in half-life likely relate to differences in renal blood flow, the low rate of tubular secretion, and reduced metabolic elimination.[15]

Repeated administration of loop diuretics produces pharmacologic tolerance resulting in a significant reduction in its diuretic and natriuretic efficacy and rebound sodium retention.[16,17] The mechanisms responsible for this "breaking phenomenon" remain unclear, though likely result in part from a decrease in extracellular fluid volume, leading to activation of the renin-angiotensin-aldosterone system and compensatory increases in water and sodium absorption in the proximal convoluted and distal renal tubule.[18] In addition, decreased sodium reabsorption in the thick ascending loop of Henle leads to increased sodium delivery to the distal and collecting tubules, further contributing to a compensatory increase in sodium reabsorption. Therefore, blockade of sodium reabsorption within these different nephron segments using thiazide or thiazide-like diuretics (described later) offers the opportunity to overcome diuretic resistance. In preterm infants with chronic lung disease, coadministration of metolazone, a thiazide-like diuretic, with furosemide enhances diuresis, natriuresis, and chloruresis and overcomes the development of tolerance to furosemide.[19] Similar findings using combined diuretic therapies have been reported in pediatric patients with chronic renal failure and furosemide-resistant edema.[20,21]

Appropriate dosing of furosemide is dependent upon gestational and postnatal age of the infant. Because of the prolonged half-life, consideration should be given to dosing preterm infants (<31 weeks' postmenstrual age) no more often than every 24 hours (1 mg/kg IV). Older infants may receive furosemide every 12 hours.[14] Because the bioavailability of orally administered furosemide is low and relatively variable, most clinicians consider a parenteral dose of 1 mg/kg to be equivalent to an enteral dose of 2 mg/kg.[22]

THIAZIDE DIURETICS

Thiazide diuretics are sulfonamide derivatives that differ from loop diuretics with respect to mechanism and sites of action, efficacy, and side effects. Like loop diuretics, thiazide diuretics require active transport into the lumen of the proximal tubules via organic acid transporters where they inhibit the potassium-independent Na^+-Cl^- symporter in the distal convoluted tubule. Thiazide-like diuretics (i.e., metolazone) have different chemical structures than thiazide agents, though have similar action. Because less sodium is typically reabsorbed in this region of the tubule compared with the ascending loop of Henle, thiazides display only moderate potency as diuretics. Increased activation of the Na^+-K^+-ATPase in the collecting duct resulting from stimulation of the renin-angiotensin-aldosterone system and increased sodium delivery results in increased urine potassium secretion.[23] As opposed to loop diuretics, thiazides do not increase urinary calcium or magnesium excretion and may increase distal tubule calcium reabsorption. This hypocalciuric effect is lost when sodium supplementation is provided as increased luminal sodium impairs calcium reuptake.[24]

There has been little to no study of thiazide pharmacokinetics in the neonate. Dosing recommendations for infants <6 months of age provided by various sources appear to be extrapolated from adult and animal studies as well as clinical experience. An average, the oral dose of hydrochlorothiazide is typically 2–3 mg/kg per day divided every 12 hours, with the equivalent oral dose of chlorothiazide being 20–40 mg/kg per day divided every 12 hours.[25]

SPIRONOLACTONE

The synthetic steroid spironolactone acts as a competitive aldosterone receptor antagonist. Upon binding to the mineralocorticoid receptor, aldosterone upregulates the Na^+-K^+-ATPase in the distal tubule and collecting duct to increase reabsorption of sodium in exchange for potassium. By inhibiting aldosterone, spironolactone attenuates sodium reabsorption, thereby sparing potassium excretion. Because little filtered sodium load reaches the distal tubule, spironolactone is a weak diuretic and is primarily prescribed in the neonatal population for its reported potassium-sparing effects in conjunction with a thiazide diuretic. However, in comparing outcomes of infants treated with the combination of chlorothiazide and spironolactone or chlorothiazide alone, Hoffman et al. found no difference in the need for electrolyte supplementation.[26] Spironolactone also exerts antiandrogen activity by competitive binding to the androgen receptor and inhibition of formation of the receptor complex, although it is unknown whether these effects occur at the doses commonly prescribed to infants.[27]

Clinical Uses/Indications for Loop and Thiazide Diuretics

RESPIRATORY DISTRESS SYNDROME

The use of diuretics in treating respiratory distress syndrome (RDS) and lessening the need for mechanical

ventilator support has been evaluated in a limited number of trials. Rationale for these trials were derived from observations that RDS is associated with fluid in the alveolar and interstitial spaces impairing gas exchange and lowering lung compliance and that in the presurfactant era, spontaneous diuresis often preceded improvement in infants with RDS.[28,29] In preterm infants with RDS, a single dose of furosemide resulted in acute improvements in lung compliance and alveolar-arterial oxygen gradient prior to any significant diuresis, both findings suggesting a direct effect of furosemide on lung fluid dynamics.[30] However, further studies have failed to identify a clinically beneficial effect of diuretics for RDS. A 2011 Cochrane Review, which included seven studies, concluded there are no data to support the routine administration of furosemide in infants with RDS.[31] Six studies involving a total of only 124 patients were included in the analysis of comparing mortality of infants receiving furosemide compared with placebo, no diuretic, or as needed diuretic administration. Diuretic use showed a trend toward increased mortality, with a relative risk of 1.35 (95% confidence interval [CI] 0.71–2.56) and no effect on the incidence of BPD or other long-term outcomes. In summary, there are no data to support the routine administration of furosemide in preterm infants with RDS.

BRONCHOPULMONARY DYSPLASIA

Furosemide is the most widely prescribed medication for the management of BPD.[32] This high rate of use has occurred despite few studies having prospectively examined the short- and long-term effects of furosemide in these infants and the absence of data supporting its use. In 11-week-old infants with stage 3 or 4 BPD, furosemide (1 mg/kg IV) improved airway resistance, airway conductance, and pulmonary compliance within 1 hour of administration, though no significant effect of furosemide on subsequent measurements between 1 and 24 hours after administration was identified.[33] Engelhardt et al. found that administration of furosemide over a 6- to 10-day period to spontaneously breathing infants with BPD improved mechanical lung properties but had limited effect on gas exchange.[34] A 2011 Cochrane Review of loop diuretics for preterm infants with (or developing) chronic lung disease found only six studies met criteria for inclusion in the analysis.[35] The authors concluded that because of "lack of data from randomized trials concerning effects on important clinical outcomes, routine or sustained use of systemic loop diuretics in infants with (or developing) CLD cannot be recommended based on current evidence."

Thiazide diuretics have also been studied for neonatal lung disease and are commonly used in infants with BPD. In a double-blinded crossover design trial allocating nonventilated infants with BPD to either diuretics or placebo for 1 week, Kao et al. found the combination of chlorothiazide (20 mg/kg per dose and spironolactone 1.5 mg/kg per dose, both given twice a day) resulted in significant decreases in airway resistance and dynamic compliance compared with placebo.[36] In a separate study of 43 infants with oxygen-dependent lung disease randomized to either chlorothiazide and spironolactone or placebo until no longer requiring supplemental oxygen diuretics improved lung function, but did not decrease the total number of days requiring supplemental oxygen.[37] In a small randomized trial ($n = 34$), Albersheim et al. found hydrochlorothiazide and spironolactone, compared with placebo, had no effect on the number of hospital or ventilator days in infants requiring $\geq 30\%$ FiO_2 and greater than 30 days of age, although survival to discharge was significantly increased (84%) in the treatment compared with placebo (47%).[38] A 2011 Cochrane Review found six studies in which preterm infants with or developing chronic lung disease and at least 5 days of age were randomly allocated to receive a thiazide-like diuretic though most studies failed to assess important clinical outcomes.[39] Because of the paucity of randomized controlled trials and numbers of patients studied, the authors concluded there is no strong evidence of benefit from the routine use of distal diuretics in preterm infants with chronic lung disease. More recently, Tan et al. published their single-center experience with administering hydrochlorothiazide and spironolactone to infants <28 weeks' gestation with evolving or established BPD.[40] No improvements in mean airway pressure or oxygen requirement were present 1 week after initiating diuretics. Additionally, 84% developed hyponatremia, and weight gain significantly decreased from 18 mg/kg per day to 10 mg/kg per day.

Several large, retrospective analyses have attempted to address the utility of diuretics in improving clinical outcomes of infants with chronic lung disease. An observational study from England involving over 9000 infants <29 weeks' gestation found that postnatal diuretic exposure, defined as receiving diuretics for ≥ 7 days, was associated with *increased* probability of being discharged home on supplemental oxygen.[41] Unfortunately, all diuretic types were combined in this study, and no data regarding dosage or timing of diuretic exposure were provided. Bamat et al. described wide variation (more than sixfold) among 43 centers in furosemide usage in infants ($n = 3252$) with severe BPD.[42] Mortality and postmenstrual age at discharge did not differ between low-use and high-use centers. A lack of efficacy was also reported by Blaisdell et al., who found the probability of decreasing respiratory support requirements did not improve in infants exposed to diuretics compared with unexposed infants, but significantly *increased* in the 1–7 days after diuretics were started.[43] In contrast, in a cohort of almost 40,000 infants born at 23–29 weeks' gestation, half of whom received furosemide, greater furosemide exposure between postnatal day 7 and 36 weeks' postmenstrual age was associated with decreased risk of BPD or a combined outcome of BPD and death.[44]

What is most evident from review of published literature is that data on relevant long-term clinical outcomes of diuretic use in infants with chronic lung disease are lacking. Although a role for diuretics in the management of selected infants with BPD likely exits, routine use of these medications in this population cannot be recommended based upon current literature. Prospective studies are urgently needed to assess whether diuretic administration to infants with BPD improves mortality, duration of oxygen dependency, duration of ventilator-dependency, length of hospital stay and neurodevelopmental outcomes.

PATENT DUCTUS ARTERIOSUS

The renal side effects of nonsteroidal antiinflammatory drugs (NSAIDs) used for pharmacologic closure of patent ductus arteriosus (PDA) therapy are well known, with an increase in renal vascular resistance and decrease in renal blood flow related to inhibition of the prostaglandin system. Because furosemide may increase renal blood flow through the stimulation of renal prostaglandin E2 production, it has been proposed that administration of furosemide during NSAID therapy could ameliorate drug-related renal toxicity.[45] A

2001 Cochrane Review found insufficient evidence to support the administration of furosemide to premature infants treated with indomethacin for PDA.[46] This metaanalysis, involving 70 patients enrolled in three trials, failed to show any reduction in toxicity of indomethacin therapy in PDA or increase in treatment failure (relative risk = 1.25; 95% CI 0.62–2.52). In subsequent studies the incidence of renal dysfunction was significantly *increased* by furosemide exposure.[47,48] Thus, the use of furosemide to decrease the renal side effects of NSAIDs cannot be supported.

Concern about the potential for furosemide to induce prostaglandin-regulated dilation of the ductus arteriosus in the preterm infant also exists. In neonatal rats, furosemide delays ductal closure and dilates the constricted ductus arteriosus in a dose-dependent manner.[49] Furosemide increased the incidence of PDA compared with chlorothiazide in premature infants prescribed diuretics for treatment of RDS.[50] In contrast, analysis of a large data set found furosemide exposure was not associated with increased odds of PDA treatment in very low birth weight infants.[51]

CONGENITAL HEART DISEASE/HEART FAILURE

Neonatal heart failure may result from congenital heart diseases associated with a left-to-right shunt and systemic processes (inflammatory, metabolic, idiopathic) that result in cardiomyopathy. In adults, diuretics play a key role in the management of patients with symptomatic heart failure associated with fluid overload. The goal of diuretic therapy is to achieve short-term negative sodium and water balance while chronically reducing extracellular fluid volume. Though the underlying pathophysiology and clinical experience support the use, limited controlled data in adults exist to provide evidence-based approaches. The most recent Cochrane Review on the subject found only seven placebo-controlled trials totally only several hundred patients.[52] These studies identified that diuretic use was associated with decreased mortality, decreased admission, and improved exercise capacity compared with placebo in adults. Evidence for the use of diuretics within pediatric populations is even more limited. In 1978, Engle et al. reported their observations following furosemide administration to 62 pediatric patients with heart disease and edema, 28 of whom were 1 day to 3 months of age.[53] Within this population,

all of whom were also receiving digoxin, a single dose of furosemide significantly increased urine output and decreased tachypnea in about two-thirds of patients. Based upon studies in adults and empiric/observational data such as that provided by Engle, the Canadian Cardiovascular Society recommended routine use of diuretics in the emergency setting in children with heart failure.[54] The guidelines do not comment specifically on the use of diuretics for chronic heart failure, focusing instead on angiotensin-converting enzyme inhibition. The clinical experience of providers suggests that signs consistent with neonatal heart failure, including cyanosis, tachypnea, tachycardia, diaphoresis, and feeding difficulty, are often alleviated by chronic diuretic therapy. However, whether chronic diuretic therapy, other pharmacologic agents, or combined therapy provides optimal medical management in this population has not been studied.

Loop diuretics are commonly prescribed to newborns following cardiac surgery. Because of concern for acute fluctuations in intravascular volume associated with bolus administration of loop diuretics, some clinicians choose to use continuous intravenous administration. Continuous furosemide infusion for 72 hours (loading bolus [1–2 mg/kg] followed by a continuous infusion at 0.2 mg/kg per hour) in hemodynamically unstable infants after cardiac surgery appeared to be a safe and effective treatment for volume overload.[55] In cardiac postoperative patients less than 6 months of age, urinary output per dose of drug was significantly greater in a group receiving continuous (0.1 mg/kg per hour) furosemide compared with intermittent dosing (1 mg/kg IV every 4 hours), and the need for fluid replacement was decreased.[56] In contrast, using an adjustable dosing of furosemide based upon clinical parameters, Klinge et al. found urine production was greater (per milligram of drug) in the intermittent compared with continuous group and required a significantly lower total daily dose of the drug.[57] Continuous furosemide administration has also been utilized for infants treated with extracorporeal membrane oxygenation. Although furosemide infusion appears to be effective in promoting urine output and reducing volume overload, optimal infusion rates likely vary widely depending upon patient characteristics and adsorption of furosemide onto extracorporeal membrane oxygenation circuit components.[14]

ACUTE KIDNEY INJURY

At the organ level, furosemide offers the potential to ameliorate injury by increasing renal blood flow through the stimulation of prostaglandin production, clearing of tubular debris by maintaining luminal salt and water and thus urine flow, and decreasing renal oxygen consumption.[58,59] This latter concept is based on the understanding that renal oxygen consumption is proportional to renal tubular sodium reabsorption, with up to 80% of renal oxygen consumption related to the activity of the Na-H antiporter.[60] Although experimental evidence suggest renal workload may be reduced by diuretics, there is contradictory clinical evidence to support its use to prevent or decrease the severity of AKI. A metaanalysis of furosemide to prevent or treat acute renal failure in adults found no significant clinical benefit, although the risk for ototoxicity may have been increased.[61] A recent retrospective analysis of 456 patients admitted to a pediatric intensive care unit, of whom 43.4% received furosemide in the first week of admission, reported mortality was twice that in the furosemide-treated group, even after adjusting for severity of illness.[62] In contrast, analysis of a large adult intensive care database reported that in patients with AKI furosemide administration was associated with reduced in-hospital and 90-day mortality (hazard ratio 0.67; 95% CI 0.61–0.74; $P < .001$; hazard ratio 0.69; 95% CI 0.64–0.75; $P < .001$, respectively).[63] Despite an absence of data supporting the clinical use of furosemide in the setting of neonatal AKI, furosemide is commonly used for the management of oliguria and fluid overload. A recent review of a large clinical database from 46 US children's hospitals found that 76% of preterm infants (<37 weeks' gestational age at birth) diagnosed with AKI were administered diuretics (99% receiving furosemide).[64] Notably, in neonates with AKI, treatment with diuretics was significantly associated with *increased* mortality, need for mechanical ventilation, and length of stay. As in other NICU patient populations, additional evaluation of the use of furosemide in AKI, including indications for, dosing, and duration of use, is required. For subpopulations of infants with AKI, such as those with significant fluid overload or hyperkalemia or those for whom no kidney supportive therapy options exist, prudent use of diuretics may be appropriate.[65] Because AKI is associated with reduced renal blood flow and there is a need for proximal renal tubular excretion for the drug to be active, consideration should be given to using larger than traditional doses (i.e., 2–5 mg/kg IV). However, in the absence of the desired clinical response and with knowledge of potential side effects, there is little justification for continued dosing.

Adverse Effects of Furosemide

The prescription of diuretics necessitates careful attention to fluid and electrolyte homeostasis, particularly when first initiating therapy. Because of the effects on charge across the apical membrane, passive reabsorption of potassium, calcium, and magnesium is inhibited. Therefore, in addition to hyponatremia and hypochloremic metabolic alkalosis, patients receiving furosemide should be monitored for hypokalemia, hypomagnesemia, and hypocalcemia. A retrospective cohort study of NICU patients identified that 92% of those infants exposed to diuretics experienced derangements of at least one serum electrolyte and/or required electrolyte supplementation.[66]

Because significant amounts of divalent cations such as Ca^{2+} are reabsorbed in the loop of Henle by mechanisms that depend upon the transport of sodium chloride, administration of furosemide may result in hypercalciuria, bone demineralization, and renal calcifications.[67,68] Exposure to furosemide above 10 mg/kg body weight cumulative dose has recently been shown by multivariate analysis to be the strongest independent risk factor for nephrocalcinosis (odds ratio 48.1, 95% CI 4.0–58.5, $P < .01$).[69] In infants with BPD, diuretic use of any type longer than 2 weeks in duration was associated with significantly increased risk of metabolic bone disease (odds ratio 5.45, 95% CI 1.25–23.84).[70]

Although uncommon, ototoxicity remains a risk in neonates with impaired drug clearance and concomitant administration of other ototoxic drugs or agents that impair furosemide clearance. In a study of survivors of the Canadian arm of the Neonatal Inhaled Nitric Oxide Study, cumulative dosage and duration of loop diuretic use were linked to sensorineural hearing loss.[71]

Administration of furosemide may directly or via induced sodium and water loss activate several neurohumoral systems that counteract diuretic effects on body fluid and electrolyte balance and impact cardiopulmonary hemodynamics. Those mechanisms triggered may include the renin-angiotensin-aldosterone system, sympathetic nervous system, prostaglandins, and vasopressin.[72] Animal and human studies suggest that short courses and even single doses of furosemide increase plasma renin activity, angiotensin II, and aldosterone. In neonates, a single dose of furosemide significantly increased plasma renin activity and aldosterone as well as urinary aldosterone excretion.[73,74]

Activation of the renin-angiotensin signaling system promotes pulmonary artery smooth muscle proliferation, migration, fibrosis, oxidant stress inflammation, vasoconstriction, and impaired endothelial function.[75] Aldosterone, via mineralocorticoid receptors located on pulmonary artery endothelial and smooth muscle cells, regulates genes involved in oxidative stress, smooth muscle proliferation, and hypertrophy as well as extracellular matrix formation and fibrosis.[76] Activation of these systems may be particularly deleterious to infants with moderate to severe BPD, in whom the reported incidence of pulmonary hypertension has been reported between 17% and 40%.[77] Given the frequency that diuretics are administered to infants with BPD at high risk for the development of BPD-associated pulmonary hypertension, a deeper understanding of neurohumoral consequences of diuretics is needed.

The potential impact of chronic diuretic therapy on somatic growth should not be overlooked. Data from animal studies and in human infants demonstrate sodium depletion negatively impacts energy efficiency, weight, and linear growth.[78–80] Studies in infants with excessive sodium losses from intestinal ostomies and cystic fibrosis suggest that sodium replacement promotes growth independent of sodium intake.[81,82] Chronic diuretic therapy, as often occurs in infants with BPD or congenital heart disease, may result in a state of total body sodium depletion that may go unrecognized, as serum sodium values are not reflective of total body sodium stores.

Novel Diuretics, Uses, and Strategies

In addition to it use in fluid overload states, thiazide diuretics have additionally found use in the treatment of diabetes insipidus (DI).[83] DI results from the impaired synthesis and secretion of vasopressin (central DI) or an unresponsiveness of the kidneys to the hormone (nephrogenic DI) and is characterized by the excretion of large amounts of dilute urine. Though mechanisms continue to be debated, thiazides exert a paradoxical antidiuretic effect in these patients and have been a key agent in the treatment of DI. Mannitol is an osmotic diuretic, filtered by the glomerulus and not reabsorbed, thus increasing osmolality of tubular fluid with a resultant decrease in water reabsorption. Carbonic anhydrase inhibitors, such as acetazolamide, block bicarbonate absorption by inhibiting the reaction $CO_2 + H_2O \leftrightharpoons H_2CO_3 \leftrightharpoons H^+ + HCO_3^-$, leading to decreased sodium reuptake and a mild diuresis. Although previously suggested as a therapy for posthemorrhagic hydrocephalus due to its effects on decreasing cerebral spinal fluid production, randomized trials demonstrated a lack of efficacy in decreasing the rate of shunt placement and an association with increased neurologic morbidity.[84] Use of the agent may also lead to a hyperchloremic metabolic acidosis. Amiloride is a weak diuretic that acts by inhibiting the ENaC channel in collecting ducts of the kidney, promoting sodium and water loss while sparing potassium. Aside from its potential use in patients with Liddle syndrome or hypoaldosteronism, amiloride has little role in the neonatal population.[85,86]

Though not typically considered a diuretic, methylxanthines (aminophylline, theophylline, caffeine), which function as nonselective adenosine receptor antagonists, appear to promote diuresis when used in states of hypoxemic kidney injury. Specifically, aminophylline or theophylline, administered as a single dose soon after birth, decreases the incidence of AKI (defined by oliguria) in infants with hypoxic-ischemic encephalopathy.[87] In infants with encephalopathy and early evidence of renal dysfunction, aminophylline administration at 25 ± 14 hours after birth increased urine output compared with control infants.[88]

The limited evidence of therapeutic efficacy coupled with known adverse effects of current diuretic agents should promote investigation of additional pharmacologic agents to induce diuresis and/or natriuresis. Tolvaptan, a vasopressin type 2 receptor antagonist, inhibits free water absorption within the kidney collecting tubules, resulting in diuresis without concomitant natriuresis. Although clinical efficacy has been demonstrated in adult populations, there is limited experience with the drug in neonates. Successful use of tolvaptan has been reported in infants with autosomal dominant polycystic kidney disease, syndrome of inappropriate ADH secretion, and volume overload after cardiac surgery.[89–91] Carperitide, a synthetic α-human atrial natriuretic peptide, induces natriuresis and vasodilation while inhibiting the renin-angiotensin system. Carperitide's use has primarily been limited to adults with acute, decompensated heart failure. Nesiritide, a β-type human natriuretic peptide, elicited improvement in diuresis in a small population of infants and children with congestive heart failure already receiving inotropic and diuretic therapy.[92] Presently, however, there appears to be little role for recombinant natriuretic peptides in the neonatal population.

Summary

Although data on the benefits of diuretic therapy in neonates with chronic medical conditions are lacking, most practitioners can identify infants who clinically benefited for variable lengths of time after the initiation of diuretic therapy. Practitioners should develop a rational and individualized approach to diuretic therapy, acknowledging potential side effects and assessing the risk-benefit balance. Use of diuretics in infants with BPD may be considered for those displaying deterioration in pulmonary status or infants whose progress of resolution of lung injury has ceased. If the decision to initiate diuretic therapy is made, the clinician should decide a priori the duration of the initial course of diuretics and the extent of expected improvement in lung function (i.e., goal of therapy). In the absence of clinical improvement, justification for continuation of diuretic therapy is limited. A similar, thoughtful approach should also be taken for infants with other fluid overload states. Diuretic dosing regimens need to consider the developmental state of the kidney, accounting for postnatal changes in renal blood flow and nephrogenesis.

REFERENCES

1. Laughon MM, Chantala K, Aliaga S, et al. Diuretic exposure in premature infants from 1997 to 2011. *Am J Perinatol.* 2015; 32:49–56.
2. Clark RH, Bloom BT, Spitzer AR, et al. Reported medication use in the neonatal intensive care unit: data from a large national data set. *Pediatrics.* 2006;117:1979–1987.
3. Hagadorn JI, Sanders MR, Staves C, et al. Diuretics for very low birth weight infants in the first 28 days: a survey of the US neonatologists. *J Perinatol.* 2011;31:677–681.
4. *Best Pharmaceuticals for Children Act (BPCA) Priority List of Needs in Pediatric Therapeutics.* Available at: https://www.nichd.nih.gov/sites/default/files/inline-files/2020PriorityListFeb20.pdf. Accessed January 15, 2022.
5. Robillard JE, Nakamura KT, Matherne GP, et al. Renal hemodynamics and functional adjustments to postnatal life. *Semin Perinatol.* 1988;12:143–150.
6. Solhaug MJ, Jose PA. Postnatal maturation of renal blood flow. In: Polin RA, Fox WW, Abman SH, eds. *Fetal and Neonatal Physiology.* 3rd ed. WB Saunders; 2004:1242–1249.
7. Vieux R, Hascoet JM, Merdariu D, et al. Glomerular filtration rate reference values in very preterm infants. *Pediatrics.* 2010;125:e1186–e1192.
8. Guignard JP. Postnatal development of glomerular filtration rate in neonates. In: Polin RA, Fox WW, Abman SH, eds. *Fetal and Neonatal Physiology.* 3rd ed. WB Saunders; 2004:1256–1266.
9. Chevalier RL. The moth and the aspen tree: sodium in early postnatal development. *Kidney Int.* 2001;59:1617–1625.
10. Segar JL, Grobe CC, Grobe JL. Maturational changes in sodium metabolism in periviable infants. *Pediatr Nephrol.* 2021;36: 3693–3698.
11. Bueva A, Guignard JP. Renal function in preterm neonates. *Pediatr Res.* 1994;36:572–577.
12. Segar JL. Renal adaptive changes and sodium handling in the fetal-to-newborn transition. *Semin Fetal Neonatal Med.* 2017; 22:76–82.
13. Baum M. Renal transport of sodium during development. In: Polin RA, Abman SH, Rowitch DH, Benitz WE, Fox WW, eds. *Fetal and Neonatal Physiology.* 5th ed. Elsevier; 2017: 1002–1010.
14. Pacifici GM. Clinical pharmacology of furosemide in neonates: a review. *Pharmaceuticals (Basel).* 2013;6:1094–1129.
15. Aranda JV, Perez J, Sitar DS, et al. Pharmacokinetic disposition and protein binding of furosemide in newborn infants. *J Pediatr.* 1978;93:507–511.
16. Mirochnick MH, Miceli JJ, Kramer PA, et al. Renal response to furosemide in very low birth weight infants during chronic administration. *Dev Pharmacol Ther.* 1990;15:1–7.
17. Chemtob S, Doray JL, Laudignon N, et al. Alternating sequential dosing with furosemide and ethacrynic acid in drug tolerance in the newborn. *Am J Dis Child.* 1989;143:850–854.
18. Ellison DH. Diuretic resistance: physiology and therapeutics. *Semin Nephrol.* 1999;19:581–597.
19. Segar JL, Robillard JE, Johnson KJ, et al. Addition of metolazone to overcome tolerance to furosemide in infants with bronchopulmonary dysplasia. *J Pediatr.* 1992;120:966–973.
20. Arnold WC. Efficacy of metolazone and furosemide in children with furosemide-resistant edema. *Pediatrics.* 1984;74:872–875.
21. Garin EH. A comparison of combinations of diuretics in nephrotic edema. *Am J Dis Child.* 1987;141:769–771.
22. Peterson RG, Simmons MA, Rumack BH, et al. Pharmacology of furosemide in the premature newborn infant. *J Pediatr.* 1980;97:139–143.
23. Martinez-Maldonado M, Cordova HR. Cellular and molecular aspects of the renal effects of diuretic agents. *Kidney Int.* 1990;38:632–641.
24. Campfield T, Braden G, Flynn-Valone P, et al. Effect of diuretics on urinary oxalate, calcium, and sodium excretion in very low birth weight infants. *Pediatrics.* 1997;99:814–818.

25. Guignard JP, Iacobelli S. Use of diuretics in the neonatal period. *Pediatr Nephrol.* 2021;36:2687–2695.
26. Hoffman DJ, Gerdes JS, Abbasi S. Pulmonary function and electrolyte balance following spironolactone treatment in preterm infants with chronic lung disease: a double-blind, placebo-controlled, randomized trial. *J Perinatol.* 2000;20:41–45.
27. Dorrington-Ward P, McCartney AC, Holland S, et al. The effect of spironolactone on hirsutism and female androgen metabolism. *Clin Endocrinol (Oxf).* 1985;23:161–167.
28. Heaf DP, Belik J, Spitzer AR, et al. Changes in pulmonary function during the diuretic phase of respiratory distress syndrome. *J Pediatr.* 1982;10:103–107.
29. Bland RD, McMillan DD, Bressack MA. Decreased pulmonary transvascular fluid filtration in awake newborn lambs after intravenous furosemide. *J Clin Invest.* 1978;62:601–609.
30. Najak ZD, Harris EM, Lazzara A Jr, et al. Pulmonary effects of furosemide in preterm infants with lung disease. *J Pediatr.* 1983;102:758–763.
31. Stewart A, Brion LP, Soll R. Diuretics for respiratory distress syndrome in preterm infants. *Cochrane Database Syst Rev.* 2011;(12):CD001454.
32. Bamat NA, Kirpalani H, Feudtner C, et al. Medication use in infants with severe bronchopulmonary dysplasia admitted to United States children's hospitals. *J Perinatol.* 2019;39:1291–1299.
33. Kao LC, Warburton D, Sargent CW, et al. Furosemide acutely decreases airways resistance in chronic bronchopulmonary dysplasia. *J Pediatr.* 1983;103:624–629.
34. Engelhardt B, Elliott S, Hazinski TA. Short- and long-term effects of furosemide on lung function in infants with bronchopulmonary dysplasia. *J Pediatr.* 1986;109:1034–1039.
35. Stewart A, Brion LP. Intravenous or enteral loop diuretics for preterm infants with (or developing) chronic lung disease. *Cochrane Database Syst Rev.* 2011;(9):CD001453.
36. Kao LC, Warburton D, Cheng MH, et al. Effect of oral diuretics on pulmonary mechanics in infants with chronic bronchopulmonary dysplasia: results of a double-blind crossover sequential trial. *Pediatrics.* 1984;74:37–44.
37. Kao LC, Durand DJ, McCrea RC, et al. Randomized trial of long-term diuretic therapy for infants with oxygen-dependent bronchopulmonary dysplasia. *J Pediatr.* 1994;124:772–781.
38. Albersheim SG, Solimano AJ, Sharma AK, et al. Randomized, double-blind, controlled trial of long-term diuretic therapy for bronchopulmonary dysplasia. *J Pediatr.* 1989;115:615–620.
39. Stewart A, Brion LP, Ambrosio-Perez I. Diuretics acting on the distal renal tubule for preterm infants with (or developing) chronic lung disease. *Cochrane Database Syst Rev.* 2011;9:CD001817.
40. Tan C, Sehgal K, Sehgal K, et al. Diuretic use in infants with developing or established chronic lung disease: a practice looking for evidence. *J Paediatr Child Health.* 2020;56:1189–1193.
41. Williams EE, Gunawardana S, Donaldson NK, et al. Postnatal diuretics, weight gain and home oxygen requirement in extremely preterm infants. *J Perinat Med.* 2021;50:100–107.
42. Bamat NA, Nelin TD, Eichenwald EC, et al. Loop diuretics in severe bronchopulmonary dysplasia: cumulative use and associations with mortality and age at discharge. *J Pediatr.* 2021;231:43–49.e3.
43. Blaisdell CJ, Troendle J, Zajicek A, et al. Acute responses to diuretic therapy in extremely low gestational age newborns: results from the Prematurity and Respiratory Outcomes Program Cohort Study. *J Pediatr.* 2018;197:42–47.
44. Greenberg RG, Gayam S, Savage D, et al. Best Pharmaceuticals for Children Act—Pediatric Trials Network Steering Committee. Furosemide exposure and prevention of bronchopulmonary dysplasia in premature infants. *J Pediatr.* 2019;208:134–140.e2.
45. Patak RV, Fadem SZ, Rosenblatt SG, et al. Diuretic-induced changes in renal blood flow and prostaglandin E excretion in the dog. *Am J Physiol.* 1979;236:F494–F500.
46. Brion LP, Campbell DE. Furosemide for symptomatic patent ductus arteriosus in indomethacin-treated infants. *Cochrane Database Syst Rev.* 2001;(3):CD001148.
47. Lee BS, Byun SY, Chung ML, et al. Effect of furosemide on ductal closure and renal function in indomethacin-treated preterm infants during the early neonatal period. *Neonatology.* 2010;98:191–199.
48. Andriessen P, Struis NC, Niemarkt H, et al. Furosemide in preterm infants treated with indomethacin for patent ductus arteriosus. *Acta Paediatr.* 2009;98:797–803.
49. Toyoshima K, Momma K, Nakanishi T. In vivo dilatation of the ductus arteriosus induced by furosemide in the rat. *Pediatr Res.* 2010;6:173–176.
50. Green TP, Thompson TR, Johnson DE, et al. Furosemide promotes patent ductus arteriosus in premature infants with the respiratory-distress syndrome. *N Engl J Med.* 1983;308:743–748.
51. Thompson EJ, Greenberg RG, Kumar K, et al. Association between furosemide exposure and patent ductus arteriosus in hospitalized infants of very low birth weight. *J Pediatr.* 2018;199:231–236.
52. Faris RF, Flather M, Purcell H, et al. Diuretics for heart failure. *Cochrane Database Syst Rev.* 2011;(2):CD003838.
53. Engle MA, Lewy JE, Lewy PR, et al. The use of furosemide in the treatment of edema in infants and children. *Pediatrics.* 1978;62:811–818.
54. Kantor PF, Lougheed J, Dancea A, et al. Presentation, diagnosis, and medical management of heart failure in children: Canadian Cardiovascular Society guidelines. *Can J Cardiol.* 2013;29:1535–1552.
55. van der Vorst MM, Kist-van Holthe JE, den Hartigh J, et al. Absence of tolerance and toxicity to high-dose continuous intravenous furosemide in haemodynamically unstable infants after cardiac surgery. *Br J Clin Pharmacol.* 2007;64:796–803.
56. Luciani GB, Nichani S, Chang AC, et al. Continuous versus intermittent furosemide infusion in critically ill infants after open heart operations. *Ann Thorac Surg.* 1997;64:1133–1139.
57. Klinge JM, Scharf J, Hofbeck M, et al. Intermittent administration of furosemide versus continuous infusion in the postoperative management of children following open heart surgery. *Intensive Care Med.* 1997;23:693–697.
58. Moghal NE, Shenoy M. Furosemide and acute kidney injury in neonates. *Arch Dis Child Fetal Neonatal Ed.* 2008;93:F313–F316.
59. Iguchi N, Lankadeva YR, Mori TA, et al. Furosemide reverses medullary tissue hypoxia in ovine septic acute kidney injury. *Am J Physiol Regul Integr Comp Physiol.* 2019;317:R232–R239.
60. Ricksten SE, Bragadottir G, Redfors B. Renal oxygenation in clinical acute kidney injury. *Crit Care.* 2013;17(2):221.
61. Ho KM, Sheridan DJ. Meta-analysis of frusemide to prevent or treat acute renal failure. *BMJ.* 2006;333(7565):420.
62. Dai X, Chen J, Li W, et al. Association between furosemide exposure and clinical outcomes in a retrospective cohort of critically ill children. *Front Pediatr.* 202;8:589124.

63. Zhao GJ, Xu C, Ying JC, et al. Association between furosemide administration and outcomes in critically ill patients with acute kidney injury. *Crit Care*. 2020;24:75.

64. Mohamed TH, Klamer B, Mahan JD, et al. Diuretic therapy and acute kidney injury in preterm neonates and infants. *Pediatr Nephrol*. 2020;36:3981–3991.

65. Segar J, Jetton JG. Diuretic use, acute kidney injury, and premature infants: the call for evidence-based guidelines. *Pediatr Nephrol*. 2020;36:3807–3811.

66. Dartois LL, Levek C, Grover TR, et al. Diuretic use and subsequent electrolyte supplementation in a level IV neonatal intensive care unit. *J Pediatr Pharmacol Ther*. 2020;25:124–130.

67. Chang HY, Hsu CH, Tsai JD, et al. Renal calcification in very low birth weight infants. *Pediatr Neonatol*. 2011;52:145–149.

68. Atkinson SA, Shah JK, McGee C, et al. Mineral excretion in premature infants receiving various diuretic therapies. *J Pediatr*. 1988;113:540–545.

69. Gimpel C, Krause A, Franck P, et al. Exposure to furosemide as the strongest risk factor for nephrocalcinosis in preterm infants. *Pediatr Int*. 2010;52:51–56.

70. Chen W, Zhang Z, Dai S, et al. Risk factors for metabolic bone disease among preterm infants less than 32 weeks gestation with bronchopulmonary dysplasia. *BMC Pediatr*. 2021;21(1):235.

71. Robertson CM, Tyebkhan JM, Peliowski A, et al. Ototoxic drugs and sensorineural hearing loss following severe neonatal respiratory failure. *Acta Paediatr*. 2006;95:214–223.

72. Huang X, Dorhout Mees E, Vos P, et al. Everything we always wanted to know about furosemide but were afraid to ask. *Am J Physiol Renal Physiol*. 2016;310:F958–F971.

73. Sulyok E, Varga F, Nemeth M, et al. Furosemide-induced alterations in the electrolyte status, the function of renin-angiotensin-aldosterone system, and the urinary excretion of prostaglandins in newborn infants. *Pediatr Res*. 1980;14:765–768.

74. Costa S, Gallini F, De Carolis MP, et al. Urinary aldosterone excretion and renal function in extremely-low-birth-weight infants following acute furosemide therapy. *Neonatology*. 2009;96:171–174.

75. Maron BA, Leopold JA. The role of the renin-angiotensin-aldosterone system in the pathobiology of pulmonary arterial hypertension (2013 Grover Conference series). *Pulm Circ*. 2014;4:200–210.

76. DuPont JJ, Jaffe IZ. 30 Years of the mineralocorticoid receptor: the role of the mineralocorticoid receptor in the vasculature. *J Endocrinol*. 2017;234:T67–T82.

77. Mirza H, Ziegler J, Ford S, et al. Pulmonary hypertension in preterm infants: prevalence and association with bronchopulmonary dysplasia. *J Pediatr*. 2014;165:909–914.e1.

78. Wassner SJ. Altered growth and protein turnover in rats fed sodium-deficient diets. *Pediatr Res*. 1989;26:608–613.

79. Fine BP, Ty A, Lestrange N, et al. Sodium deprivation growth failure in the rat: alterations in tissue composition and fluid spaces. *J Nutr*. 1987;117:1623–1628.

80. Segar JL, Grobe CC, Balapattabi K, et al. Dissociable effects of dietary sodium in early life upon somatic growth, fluid homeostasis, and spatial memory in mice of both sexes. *Am J Physiol Regul Integr Comp Physiol*. 2021;320:R438–R451.

81. Mansour F, Petersen D, De Coppi P, et al. Effect of sodium deficiency on growth of surgical infants: a retrospective observational study. *Pediatr Surg Int*. 2014;30:1279–1284.

82. Coates AJ, Crofton PM, Marshall T. Evaluation of salt supplementation in CF infants. *J Cyst Fibros*. 2009;8:382–385.

83. Pogacar PR, Mahnke S, Rivkees SA. Management of central diabetes insipidus in infancy with low renal solute load formula and chlorothiazide. *Curr Opin Pediatr*. 2000;12:405–411.

84. Kennedy CR, Ayers S, Campbell MJ, et al. Randomized, controlled trial of acetazolamide and furosemide in posthemorrhagic ventricular dilation in infancy: follow-up at 1 year. *Pediatrics*. 2001;108:597–607.

85. Assadi FK, Kimura RE, Subramanian U, et al. Liddle syndrome in a newborn infant. *Pediatr Nephrol*. 2002;17:609–611.

86. Griffing GT, Cole AG, Aurecchia SA, et al. Amiloride in primary hyperaldosteronism. *Clin Pharmacol Ther*. 1982;31:56–61.

87. Bhatt GC, Gogia P, Bitzan M, et al. Theophylline and aminophylline for prevention of acute kidney injury in neonates and children: a systematic review. *Arch Dis Child*. 2019;104: 670–679.

88. Chock VY, Cho SH, Frymoyer A. Aminophylline for renal protection in neonatal hypoxic-ischemic encephalopathy in the era of therapeutic hypothermia. *Pediatr Res*. 2021;89: 974–980.

89. Kerling A, Toka O, Rüffer A, et al. First experience with Tolvaptan for the treatment of neonates and infants with capillary leak syndrome after cardiac surgery. *BMC Pediatr*. 2019;19:57.

90. Gilbert RD, Evans H, Olalekan K, et al. Tolvaptan treatment for severe neonatal autosomal-dominant polycystic kidney disease. *Pediatr Nephrol*. 2017;32:893–896.

91. Marx-Berger D, Milford DV, Bandhakavi M, et al. Tolvaptan is successful in treating inappropriate antidiuretic hormone secretion in infants. *Acta Paediatr*. 2016;105:e334–e337.

92. Mahle WT, Cuadrado AR, Kirshbom PM, et al. Nesiritide in infants and children with congestive heart failure. *Pediatr Crit Care Med*. 2005;6:543–546.

Chapter 10

Effect of Preterm Birth on Renal Outcomes

Marissa J. DeFreitas, MD, and Carolyn L. Abitbol, MD

Chapter Outline

Introduction

Preterm birth is estimated to impact 15 million births worldwide annually.[1] Due to advancements in the treatment of preterm infants, survival of these infants has improved, albeit with increased morbidity due to the development of chronic diseases, especially in those born extremely preterm.[2,3] The renal consequences of preterm birth are relevant in the short term, during the neonatal intensive care unit (NICU) course, as well as in the long term over the life span.[4,5] Preterm birth has been repeatedly shown in large epidemiologic studies to be associated with an increased risk of chronic kidney disease (CKD) and hypertension in adulthood as part of the developmental origins of cardiovascular and renal disease model.[6–8] This phenomenon was initially described by Barker several decades ago after his observation that individuals in specific regions during periods of famine or high infant mortality rates were born of lower birth weight and developed cardiovascular disease and metabolic syndrome in late adulthood disproportionately to those not exposed in utero to harsh environmental stressors.[9,10] This paradigm has now spawned both clinical and experimental studies

looking at various exposures from the womb, including preterm birth and low birth weight (LBW), and the impact on how adaptive responses in utero to various stressors becomes maladaptive in early life and can lead to various chronic disease phenotypes, coined the "thrifty phenotype." In this chapter, we will highlight the unique impact of preterm birth on the developing kidney as well as summarize important tools available to monitor renal health after preterm birth.

Nephrogenesis Interrupted by Preterm Birth and Physiologic Adaptations

Nephrogenesis in humans, as opposed to other species, is ongoing through 36 weeks' gestation, with most of the nephron development occurring in the second and third trimesters.[11,12] Thus preterm infants are born with an incomplete complement of nephrons—oligonephronia—which is proportional to the degree of prematurity.[5,12] Autopsy studies of infants born preterm have shown that more advanced nephrogenesis correlated with gestational age (GA), that preterm infants had a lower radial glomerular count than term infants[13] and that preterm infants had

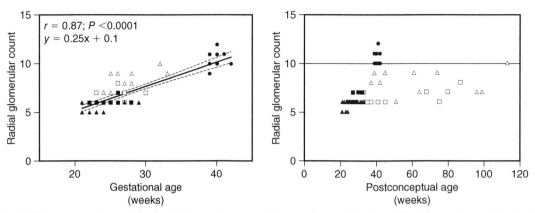

Fig. 10.1. *(Left)* Linear regression analysis of radial glomerular counts with increasing gestational age. *(Right)* Regression analysis of radial glomerular counts with lack of correlation with increasing postconceptual age. The line at "10" shows the minimum normal glomerular generation by 36 weeks' gestation. *Closed triangles*, group 1A = survived < 40 days with renal failure; *closed squares*, group 1B = survived < 40 days without renal failure; open squares, group 2A = survived ≥ 40 days with renal failure; *open triangles*, group 2B = survived ≥ 40 days without renal failure; and *closed circles*, group 3, full-term controls.[12]

a greater percentage of morphologically abnormal glomeruli and evidence of renal hyperfiltration[14] (Fig. 10.1). In fact, the number of nephrons has been shown to increase by 25,743 for each additional 100 g of birth weight.[15] Additionally, among all humans, there is a wide normal distribution in congenital nephron endowment, with a 10-fold variance in nephron numbers ranging from approximately 200,000 to over 2 million per kidney, which is likely reflective of evolutionary developmental plasticity and epigenetic processes that alter phenotype in response to environmental stimuli.[16–18] Similarly, infants born preterm have a high interindividual variability in radial glomerular counts and glomerular morphology, which implies that some infants born preterm have more resilience in nephron mass and function at birth than others.[19]

In addition, postnatal nephrogenesis in preterm infants has been noted to occur aberrantly in the first 40 days of life. Unsurprisingly, even outside this initial period, postnatal nephrogenesis is negatively impacted by the presence of acute kidney injury (AKI) (Fig. 10.2).[13] Various extrauterine stressors encountered frequently by the preterm neonate including nephrotoxin exposures, hemodynamic instability, sepsis, and oxidative stress from hyper- and hypoxic insults are cumulatively detrimental during the limited 4- to 6-week period of ongoing nephron formation after birth.[20] Once nephrogenesis ceases, only tubular and interstitial tissue expansion and vascular growth continue to occur.[21]

At the time of birth, the kidneys undergo a significant hemodynamic transition from the fetal to extrauterine environment that is heralded by an abrupt increase in renal perfusion pressure mediated by a larger proportion of the cardiac output (3% fetal → 20% postnatal) directed toward the kidneys.[22] This transition characterizes the increase in glomerular filtration rate (GFR) seen during the switch from fetal to extrauterine life given that the mean arterial pressure increases while the renal vascular resistance decreases allowing for improved renal blood flow.[23] This phenomenon is further orchestrated by several intrarenal vasoconstrictive (i.e., renin-angiotensin-aldosterone system [RAAS], endothelin) and vasodilator (i.e., atrial natriuretic peptide, bradykinin, prostaglandins, nitric oxide) forces that are essential in maintaining an appropriate balance in renal perfusion and avoiding vasomotor nephropathy.[24] There is also a gradual decrease in filtration fraction (filtration fraction = GFR/renal plasma flow), which is the proportion of the plasma reaching the kidneys that ultimately passes into the renal tubules, from 50% after birth to a mature level of 20% once renal vascular resistance decreases and tubular expansion occurs. However, in preterm infants the filtration fraction is higher and takes longer to mature.[22] The urinary flow rate is positively correlated with increasing GFR during the first few days of life in both term and preterm infants. Of note, the rate of increase of GFR is less in preterm than in term infants and continues to be discrepant

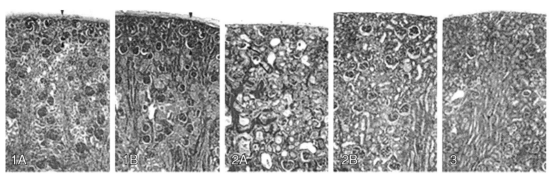

Fig. 10.2 Renal autopsy tissue from extremely preterm infants with (group A) and without (group B) renal failure with short (group 1: <40 days) and long-term survival (group 2: ≥40 days). Preterm infants with short survival (1A and 1B) show "S-shaped bodies" from early glomeruli and immature tubular structures in the glomerulogenic zone. New glomerular formation has disappeared in longer-term preterm survivors and term infants (2A, 2B, and 3). Long-term preterm infants with acute kidney injury (*AKI*) (2A) showed cystic dilatation of Bowman capsule (*arrows*) and some cystically dilated tubules and smaller glomerular tuft areas than those without AKI (2B). Glomerulomegaly is present (2B) indicating hyperfiltration. Group 1A = survived < 40 days with renal failure, group 1B = survived < 40 days without renal failure, group 2A = survived ≥ 40 days with renal failure, group 2B = survived ≥ 40 days without renal failure, and group 3, full term controls. (Adapted from Rodríguez MM, Gómez AH, Abitbol CL, Chandar JJ, Duara S, Zilleruelo GE. Histomorphometric analysis of postnatal glomerulogenesis in extremely preterm infants. *Pediatr Dev Pathol.* 2004;7(1):17–25.)

during the early childhood years.[12,22,25] Significant debate still exists as to how to best calculate GFR and define AKI in the neonatal period given the limitations of current biomarkers.[5,26,27] At birth, immature renal tubules result in a limited urinary concentrating ability and increased fractional excretion of sodium, which gradually matures with time.[25]

One important consequence of having a congenital nephron deficit and hence reduced glomerular filtration surface area is the development of hyperfiltration known as the Brenner hypothesis.[23] This phenomenon describes the adaptation to a reduction in the number of nephrons by increasing the single nephron GFR. Although this compensation helps to maintain GFR initially, over time the rise in intraglomerular pressure related in part to activation of the RAAS leads to albuminuria, glomerulosclerosis, and clinically significant CKD (Fig. 10.3).[28,29]

Developmental Programming of Kidney and Cardiovascular Disease

Prematurity alone does not adequately capture the risk for abnormal nephrogenesis and long-term kidney disease. Often the causes for preterm delivery and their impacts on the fetus are also independent risk factors for renal health. For example, there is significant overlap with growth restriction on those infants born prematurity.[30] In fact, preterm birth accounts for approximately

80% of LBW individuals weighing <2500 g at birth.[20] Hence, although prematurity is independently associated with a reduced nephron number, preterm infants are often born LBW or small for gestational age, or following maternal disorders such as diabetes and preeclampsia, which are also uniquely associated with reduced nephron number and developmental programming of kidney and cardiovascular disease in later life.[31] Teasing apart the individual contribution of each of these often-overlapping factors on reduction of nephron number can be difficult. In fact, large population-based epidemiologic studies have shown that it is the combination of growth restriction (LBW/small for gestational age) and preterm birth that are most associated with the development of CKD, end-stage kidney disease, and hypertension in adult life.[8,32]

Animal studies largely in rodents have used maternal exposures such as low-protein diet, diabetes, or prenatal steroids to induce growth restriction and low nephron number in offspring to monitor for future development of hypertension and kidney disease. Stelloh et al. examined the effect of preterm birth on the kidneys of mice delivered 2 days before the end of gestation and found in adulthood that the mice developed CKD, elevated blood pressure, and albuminuria.[33] In addition, recently it was shown in a similar preterm mouse model that early cessation of nephrogenesis occurred, resulting in lower glomerular density with premature differentiation of nephron progenitor

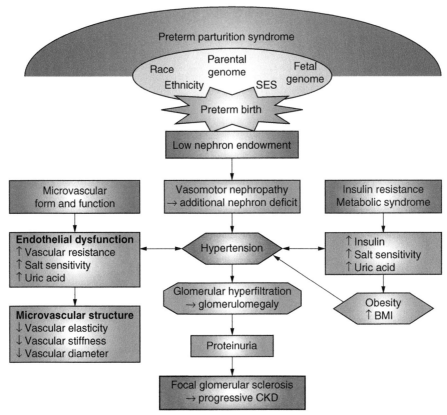

Fig. 10.3 A multidimensional scheme showing the effects that preterm birth can have on the risks of cardiovascular and renal disease in later life.[19] *BMI*, body mass index; *CKD*, chronic kidney disease; *SES*, socioeconomic status.

cells.[34] Further work in preterm animal models and translational studies can help to direct therapeutic development aimed at reprogramming the differential impact of growth restriction versus prematurity related nephron deficit.

Oligonephronia: Kidney Size as a Surrogate Marker for Nephron Mass

In clinical practice, a limited tool set exists to identify which preterm and other vulnerable neonatal populations have evidence of oligonephropathy and should be monitored closely in the NICU and beyond. One longstanding, validated, and noninvasive tool is renal ultrasonography to measure kidney size as a surrogate for nephron mass. The kidney is an ellipsoid-shaped organ that can be measured using a variety of parameters, including length, volume (equation for ellipsoid = Length × Width × Anteroposterior diameter × 0.523),

parenchymal thickness/area, or cortical thickness/volume.[35] These values can be expressed per kidney or as a sum of both kidneys expressed as total kidney volume (TKV) or parenchymal area. Brennan et al. recently compared the renal parenchymal thickness of preterm infants born <32 weeks without growth restriction to GA-matched intrauterine controls and found that at 32 weeks' postmenstrual age[36] the preterm infants had a significantly thinner parenchyma than GA-matched fetuses, suggesting a nephron deficit. However, this discrepancy resolved by 37 weeks' postmenstrual age, suggesting evidence of early compensatory hyperfiltration.[37]

In addition, kidney area and volume measures have each been indexed to a variety of body anthropometric parameters (i.e., body weight, height, body surface area [BSA]). This effort is to normalize kidney size to body habitus, as they are known to be tightly correlated.[38] There is a normal Gaussian distribution of TKV individualized to BSA (TKV/m^2 = mL/m^2) when

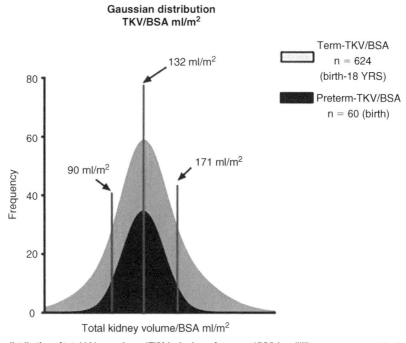

Fig. 10.4. The Gaussian distribution of total kidney volume (*TKV*) by body surface area (*BSA*) in milliliters per square meter (mL/m²). The predominant distribution is derived from the data of 624 health German individuals from <1 month to 18 years of age.[36] The mean and 90% confidence intervals define the normal distribution of kidney mass and by inference, "nephron endowment" since kidney volume correlates closely with kidney weight. An individual whose TKV/m² falls below the 10th percentile (<90 mL/m²) should be observed closely for the development of chronic kidney disease due to nephropenia. The darker curve within the larger German cohort is data from our cohort of 60 preterm infants.[5] This demonstrates that preterm infants have a similar normal distribution of nephron endowment at birth and suggests that they have potential for normal attainment of nephron mass in the extrauterine environment. Most importantly, preterm infants should be followed sequentially for kidney growth by TKV/m² throughout childhood.

measured by noninvasive renal ultrasound from birth to adulthood.[38] A cross-sectional study of renal ultrasounds in 624 healthy German children from birth to 18 years of age showed an average TKV/m² to be 132 mL/m², with the 10th and 90th percent confidence intervals being 90 and 171 mL/m², respectively.[38] In a separate Canadian cohort of 168 full-term, healthy Caucasian infants < 3 months of age, an identical curve was generated with the mean TKV/m² = 132 ± 29 mL/m².[39] When the Gaussian distribution of TKV/m² of the normal population of 624 infants, children, and adults was superimposed on that of 60 preterm infants at birth from a diverse American cohort, they were similarly normally distributed (Fig. 10.4).[5] This suggests that not all preterm born individuals have oligonephronia but rather those whose TKV/m² falls below the 10th percentile are at higher risk and should be monitored for hypertension and progression to CKD.

It has been shown that neonatal GFR is dependent primarily on GA, TKV, and MAP.[40] In addition, TKV and TKV individualized to BSA correlates closely with kidney function across all age groups and in various disease pathologies.[41–44] TKV has been noted to be smaller in preterm and LBW infants compared with their term counterparts.[44–47] In addition, multiple gestation poses a competitive intrauterine environment, which has been linked to different TKV among twin pairs with and without twin-twin transfusion syndrome.[48] Importantly, follow-up studies of individuals born preterm have shown that TKV continues to be discrepant for some and can be a useful marker of kidney health in childhood and adolescence with correlates to kidney function, albuminuria, and elevated blood pressure.[49–55]

More advanced imaging modalities to count nephron number such as MRI are still in the experimental stages of development.[56] The use of MRI/CT scans in neonatal populations requires the use of sedation, radiation in the case of CT, and increased cost and limited availability in the case of MRI. Given their limited use for evaluation of nephron number, these are not currently used clinically. The use of 3D ultrasonography may have benefit over 2D ultrasonography to more accurately measure TKV; however, this is also not universally available and requires trained sonographers as well as cost for the appropriate probe.[35]

Early Nephron Loss and Accelerated Aging of the Kidney After Preterm Birth

The timing of nephron loss is key in relation to the risk of progression to CKD. Early nephron loss related to preterm birth during active nephrogenesis is not equivalent to nephron loss in later life. For example, unilateral nephrectomy for living kidney donation is rarely associated with hypertension and CKD in later life.[31] In fact, it has been shown in a rodent model that unilateral nephrectomy during ongoing nephrogenesis leads to more severe glomerular and tubulointerstitial damage at adult age than undergoing nephron loss after nephrogenesis is completed.[57] Investigators have also shown that nephron loss during nephrogenesis affects renal development and induces a specific upregulation of genes that might hinder tissue repair after secondary kidney injury.[58]

Part of the developmental programming model has looked at markers of early aging and cumulative oxidative stress to explain the multiorgan dysfunction seen after preterm birth.[59] The loss of nephrons with natural aging is due to atrophy and reabsorption of globally sclerotic glomeruli with hypertrophy of remaining nephrons. One proposed mechanism is that aging is a function of increasing intracellular oxidative stress associated with free-radical leakage from aging mitochondria, which stimulates an inflammatory response and organ-specific injury including the kidney.[60] Luyckx et al. showed the impact of early kidney aging in a rodent model in which stress-induced senescence marker p16 was increased in kidneys from LBW rodents at birth through 6 months of age and worsened after catch-up growth.[61] Preterm infants are in fact exposed to oxidative stress by way of variable periods of hypoxia and hyperoxia, the latter due often to prolonged supplemental oxygen needs with a reduced antioxidant capacity, which is known to result

in kidney injury that persists into adulthood.[62,63] Limited studies have investigated the use of antioxidants on ameliorating prematurity-related kidney injury due to oxidative stress.[62,63]

Multiple Hit Pathways From Prematurity to Chronic Kidney Disease: Short- and Long-Term Risk Factors

It is believed that oligonephropathy of prematurity or LBW is only the initial "hit" for programming of kidney and cardiovascular disease. Ex utero preterm infants, especially those most preterm, are exposed to multiple insults that contribute in the short term to further acquired nephron loss and predispose to developing clinically significant CKD (Fig. 10.5).[5,64] These additional hits include AKI (recently redefined by the modified Kidney Disease: Improving Global Outcomes guidelines in neonates), hypotension, hyper- and hypoxia, sepsis, and nephrotoxic drug exposures (aminoglycosides, nonsteroidal antiinflammatory drugs, etc.). CKD can ensue because of any of these insults.[65] In fact, a recent international multicenter study found that AKI among preterm was approximately 25% and that this was associated with increased length of NICU stay and increased mortality.[66] Importantly, the AWAKEN Assessment of Worldwide Acute Kidney Epidemiology in Neonates (AWAKEN) study showed other risk factors for neonatal AKI including outborn delivery; other factors were associated with a lower risk of AKI including exposure to maternal hypertensive disorders and use of methylxanthines.[67–70] Efforts to systematically reduce the incidence of medication-induced AKI in the NICU have been published and have shown that use of the electronic medical record and pharmacy supervision to flag high-risk cases with more frequent monitoring of the serum creatinine has significantly reduced the number of AKI episodes.[71] However, these quality improvement measures require time and resources that are center specific and have not been universally adopted. AKI has been shown in neonatal and pediatric populations to be associated with the development of CKD in childhood and requires long-term follow-up.[5,20,64,65,72] Hence, improved awareness of the importance and detection of AKI in the neonatal period can help to proactively surveil these vulnerable patients after NICU discharge.

Exposures

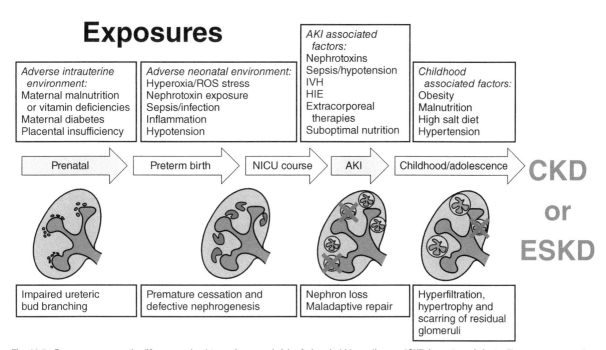

Fig. 10.5. Exposures across the life course lead to an increased risk of chronic kidney disease (*CKD*) in preterm infants. There are many unique exposures incurred by the preterm neonate that lead to an enhanced risk of acute kidney injury (*AKI*) as well as CKD. Prior to birth, a hostile intrauterine environment can affect branching and nephron development. Following preterm birth, there may be acceleration and early cessation of normal nephron development. In addition, disruption of normal nephron development may be related to nephrotoxic exposures from the neonatal intensive care unit (*NICU*) environment. Preterm neonates face high rates of AKI, which may lead to nephron loss. The low nephron endowment and nephron loss lead to risk for glomerular hyperfiltration and additional damage to residual glomeruli. After leaving the NICU, exposures including obesity, high-sodium diet, and hypertension may be additional stressors that accelerate the progression to CKD in the preterm population.[62] *IVH*, intraventricular hemorrhage; *HIE*, hypoxic ischemic encephalopathy; *ROS*, reactive oxygen species; *ESKD*, end-stage kidney disease.

In the long term, additional stressors can lead to progression of hyperfiltration and glomerulosclerosis. The most prevalent and potentially reversible of these is rapid catch-up growth and the development of obesity.[73] Growth trajectories and neonatal nutrition are known to contribute to the developmental programming of nephron endowment, insulin resistance, and cardiovascular and renal disease in later life.[74–76] Accelerated postnatal growth in preterm infants, whether small or appropriate for GA, contributes to the development of the metabolic syndrome with insulin resistance in early childhood, which is further confounded by excessive adiposity.[76,77] This, in turn, contributes to the early progression of CKD, especially in those born preterm with low nephron endowment.[73,78,79] The adverse long-term effects of perinatal exposure to excessive carbohydrate energy, low-protein diet, high-fat diet, high-fructose diet, high- and low-salt diets, as well as micronutrient deficiencies

have been documented in human and laboratory studies.[76,78] These effects are established during "developmental time slots" when the system is primed for staged development during fetal life and the perinatal period. As such, specific alterations in the nutritional environment may program for nephron endowment, blood pressure dysregulation, and endothelial and mitochondrial dysfunction. Much of these programmed effects are mediated by oxidative stress and metabolic pathways that are perpetuated throughout the lifetime of the individual. The follow-up of infants with predisposition to CKD including those with extreme preterm birth and growth restriction should include monitoring of the diet and avoidance of excess salt, hypercaloric formulas, and overweight/obesity.

Obesity-related glomerulopathy in preterm born individuals has been widely reported and is thought to be related to increased metabolic stress and hyperfiltration on a lower nephron mass leading to glomerulosclerosis,

TABLE 10.1	Reference Ranges for Kidney Risk Assessment Within the First Year of Life	
	Low Risk	**High Risk**
Blood pressure	≤50th percentile	≥90th percentile
Weight/weight for length	Normal weight	Under- or overweight
Proteinuria		
Urine protein/creatinine (mg/mg)	<0.6	≥0.6
Urine albumin/creatinine (μg/mg)	< 0	≥30
TKV/BSA	>50th percentile (= 132 mL/m²)	≤10th percentile (=90 mL/m²)
Serum creatinine (mg/dL)	<0.5	≥0.5l
Serum cystatin C (mg/L)	<1.5	≥1.5

BSA, body surface area; *TKV*, total kidney volume.

proteinuria, and hypertension (Fig. 10.3).[80] Hence, excessive weight gain in early childhood and young adulthood in those individuals born preterm is important as outlined previously. This poses a significant challenge in the transition of care to adult nephrology or primary care where the birth history unless clearly stated can be overlooked as a contributing factor to hypertension and early CKD progression. Importantly, this is a modifiable risk factor as studies have shown that weight loss measures such as bariatric surgery have resulted in an improvement in proteinuria and renal function in adult populations.[81] In addition, the use of RAAS blockade for proteinuria and renoprotection as well as newer agents such as the sodium-glucose transporter 2 inhibitors can play a role in slowing the progression of CKD in this unique population.[82]

Follow-up Guidelines After Neonatal Intensive Care Unit Discharge for Prematurity-Related Kidney Disease

The development of standard guidelines for the routine follow-up of preterm or LBW infants at risk for future renal and cardiovascular disease has been limited by a lack of sufficient long-term studies that can clearly outline which subsets of patients should be selectively followed, which biomarkers should be monitored, and at what intervals of frequency biomarker values should these be obtained. There has been a concerted effort in the neonatal and nephrology communities to define reasonable timelines for follow-up after NICU discharge so that these infants can be surveilled for early signs of hypertension, proteinuria, and reduction of kidney function and to allow for closer monitoring and potential intervention such as initiation of RAAS blockade

(>2 years of age after renal maturation is complete) and obesity prevention.[83,84] Table 10.1 is a schematic of considerations for post-NICU discharge follow-up of at-risk infants (i.e., those with AKI, hypertension, those with congenital anomalies of the kidneys and urinary tract, those born very to extremely preterm [28–32 weeks GA and ≤28 weeks, respectively], and/or those with growth restriction). These recommendations are based on current evidence and expert opinion including rough cutoff values for screening within the first year of life into low- and high-risk categories (Fig. 10.6, Table 10.1). These measures are largely noninvasive and low-cost interventions that can help stratify ongoing risk for progressive renal/cardiovascular disease. Age and growth specific calculations and reference ranges should be verified to appropriately assess risk. Feasibility and cost-effectiveness will need to be taken into consideration depending on the center and resources available. The hope is that in the future with more translational studies in preterm and high-risk neonates in the pipeline we can investigate more advanced therapies and interventions to offer for the reprogramming of cardiovascular and kidney disease.

Summary

In conclusion, numerous studies have confirmed that preterm birth as well as LBW infants are at risk of CKD and hypertension in later life. Modifiable risk factors such as nephrotoxic injury and excessive catch-up growth and obesity should be targets for prevention in the NICU and early childhood years. Serial assessment of basic and largely noninvasive measures of renal health such as blood pressure, proteinuria, renal function, and kidney volume is now being considered standard of care for these

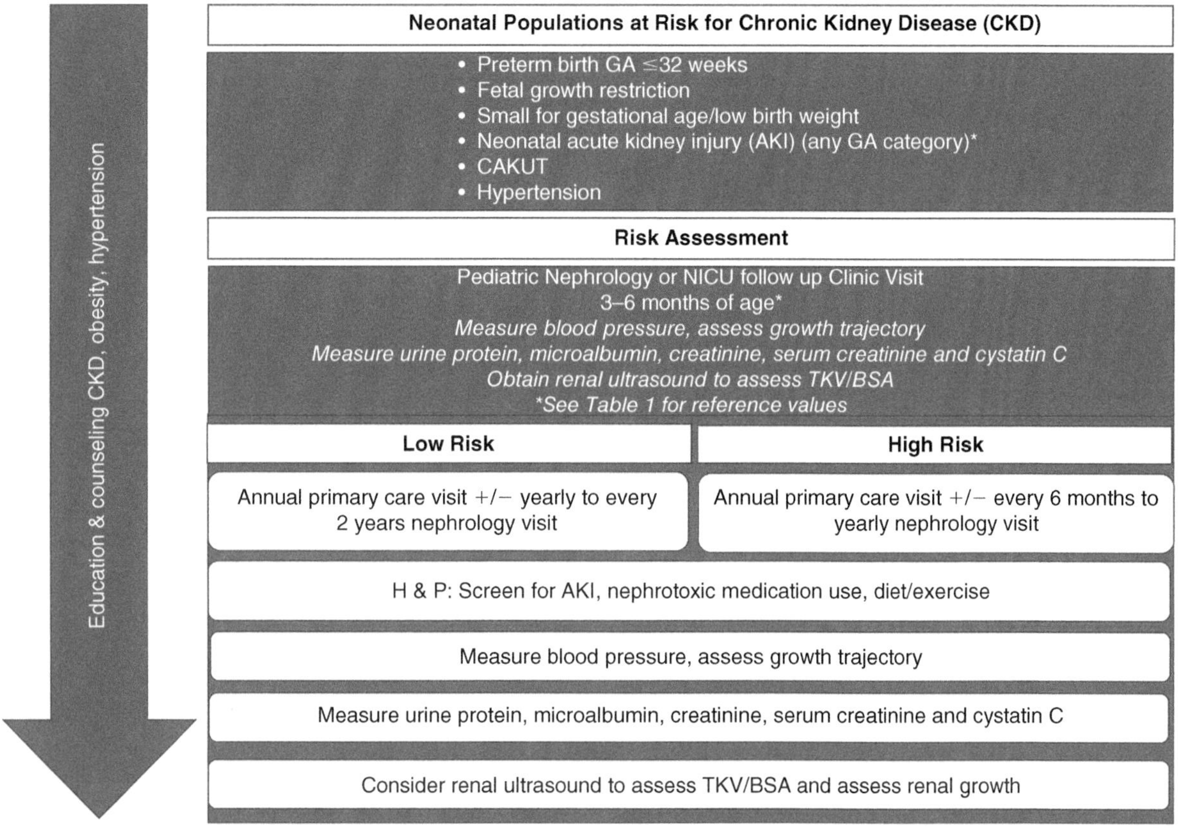

Education & counseling CKD, obesity, hypertension

Neonatal Populations at Risk for Chronic Kidney Disease (CKD)
• Preterm birth GA ≤32 weeks • Fetal growth restriction • Small for gestational age/low birth weight • Neonatal acute kidney injury (AKI) (any GA category)* • CAKUT • Hypertension

Risk Assessment

Pediatric Nephrology or NICU follow up Clinic Visit
3–6 months of age*
Measure blood pressure, assess growth trajectory
Measure urine protein, microalbumin, creatinine, serum creatinine and cystatin C
Obtain renal ultrasound to assess TKV/BSA
*See Table 1 for reference values

Low Risk	High Risk
Annual primary care visit +/− yearly to every 2 years nephrology visit	Annual primary care visit +/− every 6 months to yearly nephrology visit

H & P: Screen for AKI, nephrotoxic medication use, diet/exercise

Measure blood pressure, assess growth trajectory

Measure urine protein, microalbumin, creatinine, serum creatinine and cystatin C

Consider renal ultrasound to assess TKV/BSA and assess renal growth

Fig. 10.6. Follow-up schema for neonatal intensive care unit (*NICU*) graduates at risk of chronic kidney disease (*CKD*). This is derived from current evidence and expert opinion and provides a rough framework to identify infants before NICU discharge who should seek subspecialty care with pediatric nephrology if possible to perform a mostly noninvasive risk assessment within the first 6 months of life and establish primary care and subspecialty follow-up to allow for ongoing assessment of renal health as well as education and anticipatory guidance on avoidance of modifiable risk factors such as obesity and nephrotoxic insults. *AKI*, acute kidney injury; *BMI*, body mass index; *BSA*, body surface area; *CAKUT*, congenital anomalies of the kidney and urinary tract; *GA*, gestational age; *H & P*, history and physical; *TKV*, total kidney volume. *This is a general guide for timing of follow-up and investigations and may need to be modified based on the patient's specific condition at the time of NICU discharge.

vulnerable infants. A concerted effort toward encouraging follow-up of the most at-risk neonates by pediatric nephrologists can facilitate early identification and management of clinically significant CKD and hypertension.

REFERENCES

1. Chawanpaiboon S, Vogel JP, Moller AB, et al. Global, regional, and national estimates of levels of preterm birth in 2014: a systematic review and modelling analysis. *Lancet Glob Health.* 2019;7(1):e37–e46. doi:10.1016/s2214-109x(18)30451-0
2. Crump C. An overview of adult health outcomes after preterm birth. *Early Hum Dev.* 2020;150:105187. doi:10.1016/j.earlhumdev.2020.105187
3. Crump C. Preterm birth and mortality in adulthood: a systematic review. *J Perinatol.* 2020;40(6):833–843. doi:10.1038/s41372-019-0563-y
4. Luyckx VA. Preterm birth and its impact on renal health. *Semin Nephrol.* 2017;37(4):311–319. doi:10.1016/j.semnephrol.2017.05.002
5. Abitbol CL, DeFreitas MJ, Strauss J. Assessment of kidney function in preterm infants: lifelong implications. *Pediatr Nephrol.* 2016;31(12):2213–2222. doi:10.1007/s00467-016-3320-x
6. Crump C, Winkleby MA, Sundquist K, Sundquist J. Risk of hypertension among young adults who were born preterm: a Swedish national study of 636,000 births. *Am J Epidemiol.* 2011;173(7):797–803. doi:10.1093/aje/kwq440
7. Crump C, Sundquist J, Winkleby MA, Sundquist K. Preterm birth and risk of chronic kidney disease from childhood into mid-adulthood: national cohort study. *BMJ.* 2019;365:l1346. doi:10.1136/bmj.l1346

8. Gjerde A, Lillås BS, Marti HP, Reisæter AV, Vikse BE. Intrauterine growth restriction, preterm birth and risk of end-stage renal disease during the first 50 years of life. *Nephrol Dial Transplant.* 2020;35(7):1157–1163. doi:10.1093/ndt/gfaa001

9. Barker DJ, Winter PD, Osmond C, Margetts B, Simmonds SJ. Weight in infancy and death from ischaemic heart disease. *Lancet.* 1989;2(8663):577–580. doi:10.1016/s0140-6736(89)90710-1

10. Hales CN, Barker DJ. Type 2 (non-insulin-dependent) diabetes mellitus: the thrifty phenotype hypothesis. *Diabetologia.* 1992;35(7):595–601. doi:10.1007/bf00400248

11. Faa G, Gerosa C, Fanni D, et al. Morphogenesis and molecular mechanisms involved in human kidney development. *J Cell Physiol.* 2012;227(3):1257–1268. doi:10.1002/jcp.22985

12. Rosenblum S, Pal A, Reidy K. Renal development in the fetus and premature infant. *Semin Fetal Neonatal Med.* 2017;22(2):58–66. doi:10.1016/j.siny.2017.01.001

13. Rodríguez MM, Gómez AH, Abitbol CL, Chandar JJ, Duara S, Zilleruelo GE. Histomorphometric analysis of postnatal glomerulogenesis in extremely preterm infants. *Pediatr Dev Pathol.* 2004;7(1):17–25. doi:10.1007/s10024-003-3029-2

14. Sutherland MR, Gubhaju L, Moore L, et al. Accelerated maturation and abnormal morphology in the preterm neonatal kidney. *J Am Soc Nephrol.* 2011;22(7):1365–1374.

15. Hughson M, Farris AB III, Douglas-Denton R, Hoy WE, Bertram JF. Glomerular number and size in autopsy kidneys: the relationship to birth weight. *Kidney Int.* 2003;63(6):2113–2122. doi:10.1046/j.1523-1755.2003.00018.x

16. Puelles VG, Hoy WE, Hughson MD, Diouf B, Douglas-Denton RN, Bertram JF. Glomerular number and size variability and risk for kidney disease. *Curr Opin Nephrol Hypertens.* 2011;20(1):7–15. doi:10.1097/MNH.0b013e3283410a7d

17. Hinchliffe SA, Sargent PH, Howard CV, Chan YF, van Velzen D. Human intrauterine renal growth expressed in absolute number of glomeruli assessed by the disector method and Cavalieri principle. *Lab Invest.* 1991;64(6):777–784.

18. Luyckx VA, Chevalier RL. Impact of early life development on later onset chronic kidney disease and hypertension and the role of evolutionary trade-offs. *Exp Physiol.* 2022;107(5):410–414. doi:10.1113/ep089918

19. Faa G, Gerosa C, Fanni D, et al. Marked interindividual variability in renal maturation of preterm infants: lessons from autopsy. *J Matern Fetal Neonatal Med.* 2010;23(suppl 3):129–133. doi:10.3109/14767058.2010.510646

20. Abitbol CL, Rodriguez MM. The long-term renal and cardiovascular consequences of prematurity. *Nat Rev Nephrol.* 2012;8(5):265–274. doi:10.1038/nrneph.2012.38

21. Fanos V, Loddo C, Puddu M, et al. From ureteric bud to the first glomeruli: genes, mediators, kidney alterations. *Int Urol Nephrol.* 2015;47(1):109–116. doi:10.1007/s11255-014-0784-0

22. Abitbol CL, DeFreitas MJ, Strauss J. Assessment of kidney function in preterm infants: lifelong implications. *Pediatr Nephrol.* 2016;31(12):2213–2222.

23. Iacobelli S, Guignard JP. Maturation of glomerular filtration rate in neonates and infants: an overview. *Pediatr Nephrol.* 2021;36(6):1439–1446. doi:10.1007/s00467-020-04632-1

24. Tóth-Heyn P, Drukker A, Guignard JP. The stressed neonatal kidney: from pathophysiology to clinical management of neonatal vasomotor nephropathy. *Pediatr Nephrol.* 2000;14(3):227–239. doi:10.1007/s004670050048

25. Drukker A, Guignard JP. Renal aspects of the term and preterm infant: a selective update. *Curr Opin Pediatr.* 2002;14(2):175–182. doi:10.1097/00008480-200204000-00006

26. Askenazi D, Abitbol C, Boohaker L, et al. Optimizing the AKI definition during first postnatal week using Assessment of Worldwide Acute Kidney Injury Epidemiology in Neonates (AWAKEN) cohort. *Pediatr Res.* 2019;85(3):329–338. doi:10.1038/s41390-018-0249-8

27. Abitbol CL, Seeherunvong W, Galarza MG, et al. Neonatal kidney size and function in preterm infants: what is a true estimate of glomerular filtration rate? *J Pediatr.* 2014;164(5):1026–1031.e2. doi:10.1016/j.jpeds.2014.01.044

28. Brenner BM, Chertow GM. Congenital oligonephropathy and the etiology of adult hypertension and progressive renal injury. *Am J Kidney Dis.* 1994;23(2):171–175.

29. Lumbers ER, Kandasamy Y, Delforce SJ, Boyce AC, Gibson KJ, Pringle KG. Programming of renal development and chronic disease in adult life. *Front Physiol.* 2020;11:757. doi:10.3389/fphys.2020.00757

30. Low Birth Weight and Nephron Number Working Group. The impact of kidney development on the life course: a consensus document for action. *Nephron.* 2017;136(1):3–49. doi:10.1159/000457967

31. Luyckx VA, Brenner BM. Clinical consequences of developmental programming of low nephron number. *Anat Rec (Hoboken).* 2020;303(10):2613–2631. doi:10.1002/ar.24270

32. Ruggajo P, Skrunes R, Svarstad E, Skjærven R, Reisæther AV, Vikse BE. Familial factors, low birth weight, and development of ESRD: A Nationwide Registry Study. *Am J Kidney Dis.* 2016;67(4):601–608. doi:10.1053/j.ajkd.2015.11.015

33. Stelloh C, Allen KP, Mattson DL, Lerch-Gaggl A, Reddy S, El-Meanawy A. Prematurity in mice leads to reduction in nephron number, hypertension, and proteinuria. *Transl Res.* 2012;159(2):80–89. doi:10.1016/j.trsl.2011.10.004

34. Cwiek A, Suzuki M, deRonde K, et al. Premature differentiation of nephron progenitor cell and dysregulation of gene pathways critical to kidney development in a model of preterm birth. *Sci Rep.* 2021;11(1):21667. doi:10.1038/s41598-021-00489-y

35. DeFreitas MJ, Katsoufis CP, Infante JC, Granda ML, Abitbol CL, Fornoni A. The old becomes new: advances in imaging techniques to assess nephron mass in children. *Pediatr Nephrol.* 2021;36(3):517–525. doi:10.1007/s00467-020-04477-8

36. Chapman M, Quint LE, Watcharotone K, et al. Pelvic artery aneurysm screening provides value in patients with thoracic aortic aneurysms. *Int J Cardiovasc Imaging.* 2017;33(10):1627–1635. doi:10.1007/s10554-017-1178-z

37. Brennan S, Watson DL, Rudd DM, Kandasamy Y. Kidney growth following preterm birth: evaluation with renal parenchyma ultrasonography. *Pediatr Res.* 2023;93(5):1302–1306. doi:10.1038/s41390-022-01970-8

38. Scholbach T, Weitzel D. Body-surface-area related renal volume: a common normal range from birth to adulthood. *Scientifica (Cairo).* 2012;2012:949164. doi:10.6064/2012/949164

39. Zhang Z, Quinlan J, Hoy W, et al. A common RET variant is associated with reduced newborn kidney size and function. *J Am Soc Nephrol.* 2008;19(10):2027–2034. doi:10.1681/asn.2007101098

40. Abitbol CL, Seeherunvong W, Galarza MG, et al. Neonatal kidney size and function in preterm infants: what is a true estimate of glomerular filtration rate? *J Pediatr.* 2014;164(5):1026–1031.e2.

41. Treiber M, Pečovnik Balon B, Gorenjak M. A new serum cystatin C formula for estimating glomerular filtration rate in newborns. *Pediatr Nephrol.* 2015;30(8):1297–1305. doi:10.1007/s00467-014-3029-7

42. Roseman DA, Hwang SJ, Oyama-Manabe N, et al. Clinical associations of total kidney volume: the Framingham Heart Study. *Nephrol Dial Transplant.* 2017;32(8):1344–1350. doi:10.1093/ndt/gfw237

43. Higashihara E, Nutahara K, Okegawa T, et al. Kidney volume and function in autosomal dominant polycystic kidney disease. *Clin Exp Nephrol.* 2014;18(1):157–165. doi:10.1007/s10157-013-0834-4

44. Kandasamy Y, Smith R, Wright IM, Lumbers ER. Extra-uterine renal growth in preterm infants: oligonephropathy and prematurity. *Pediatr Nephrol.* 2013;28(9):1791–1796. doi:10.1007/s00467-013-2462-3

45. DeFreitas MJ, Mathur D, Seeherunvong W, et al. Umbilical artery histomorphometry: a link between the intrauterine environment and kidney development. *J Dev Orig Health Dis.* 2017;8(3):349–356. doi:10.1017/s2040174417000113

46. Kandasamy Y, Rudd D, Smith R, Lumbers ER, Wright IM. Extra uterine development of preterm kidneys. *Pediatr Nephrol.* 2018;33(6):1007–1012. doi:10.1007/s00467-018-3899-1

47. Iyengar A, Nesargi S, George A, Sinha N, Selvam S, Luyckx VA. Are low birth weight neonates at risk for suboptimal renal growth and function during infancy? *BMC Nephrol.* 2016; 17(1):100. doi:10.1186/s12882-016-0314-7

48. DeFreitas MJ, Abitbol CL. Twin gestation and the burden of adult cardio-renal disease. *Pediatr Nephrol.* 2020;35(12): 2241–2251. doi:10.1007/s00467-019-04418-0

49. Kooijman MN, Bakker H, van der Heijden AJ, et al. Childhood kidney outcomes in relation to fetal blood flow and kidney size. *J Am Soc Nephrol.* 2014;25(11):2616–2624. doi:10.1681/ASN.2013070746

50. Sanderson KR, Chang E, Bjornstad E, et al. Albuminuria, hypertension, and reduced kidney volumes in adolescents born extremely premature. *Front Pediatr.* 2020;8:230. doi:10.3389/fped.2020.00230

51. Rakow A, Johansson S, Legnevall L, et al. Renal volume and function in school-age children born preterm or small for gestational age. *Pediatr Nephrol.* 2008;23(8):1309–1315. doi:10.1007/s00467-008-0824-z

52. Rakow A, Laestadius Å, Liliemark U, et al. Kidney volume, kidney function, and ambulatory blood pressure in children born extremely preterm with and without nephrocalcinosis. *Pediatr Nephrol.* 2019;34(10):1765–1776. doi:10.1007/s00467-019-04293-9

53. Keijzer-Veen MG, Kleinveld HA, Lequin MH, et al. Renal function and size at young adult age after intrauterine growth restriction and very premature birth. *Am J Kidney Dis.* 2007;50(4): 542–551. doi:10.1053/j.ajkd.2007.06.015

54. Kandasamy Y, Rudd D, Lumbers ER, Smith R. An evaluation of preterm kidney size and function over the first two years of life. *Pediatr Nephrol.* 2020;35(8):1477–1482. doi:10.1007/s00467-020-04554-y

55. Starzec K, Klimek M, Grudzień A, Jagła M, Kwinta P. Longitudinal assessment of renal size and function in extremely low birth weight children at 7 and 11 years of age. *Pediatr Nephrol.* 2016;31(11):2119–2126. doi:10.1007/s00467-016-3413-6

56. Charlton JR, Pearl VM, Denotti AR, et al. Biocompatibility of ferritin-based nanoparticles as targeted MRI contrast agents. *Nanomedicine.* 2016;12(6):1735–1745. doi:10.1016/j.nano.2016.03.007

57. Menendez-Castro C, Nitz D, Cordasic N, et al. Neonatal nephron loss during active nephrogenesis - detrimental impact with long-term renal consequences. *Sci Rep.* 2018;8(1):4542. doi:10.1038/s41598-018-22733-8

58. Raming R, Cordasic N, Kirchner P, et al. Neonatal nephron loss during active nephrogenesis results in altered expression of renal developmental genes and markers of kidney injury. *Physiol Genomics.* 2021;53(12):509–517. doi:10.1152/physiolgenomics.00059.2021

59. Parkinson JRC, Emsley R, Adkins JLT, et al. Clinical and molecular evidence of accelerated ageing following very preterm birth. *Pediatr Res.* 2020;87(6):1005–1010. doi:10.1038/s41390-019-0709-9

60. Chevalier RL. Evolution, kidney development, and chronic kidney disease. *Semin Cell Dev Biol.* 2019;91:119–131. doi:10.1016/j.semcdb.2018.05.024

61. Luyckx VA, Compston CA, Simmen T, Mueller TF. Accelerated senescence in kidneys of low-birth-weight rats after catch-up growth. *Am J Physiol Renal Physiol.* 2009;297(6):F1697–F1705. doi:10.1152/ajprenal.00462.2009

62. Hsu CN, Tain YL. Developmental origins of kidney disease: why oxidative stress matters? *Antioxidants (Basel).* 2020;10(1):33. doi:10.3390/antiox10010033

63. Ali MF, Venkatarayappa SKB, Benny M, et al. Effects of Klotho supplementation on hyperoxia-induced renal injury in a rodent model of postnatal nephrogenesis. *Pediatr Res.* 2020;88(4): 565–570. doi:10.1038/s41390-020-0803-z

64. Harer MW, Charlton JR, Tipple TE, Reidy KJ. Preterm birth and neonatal acute kidney injury: implications on adolescent and adult outcomes. *J Perinatol.* 2020;40(9):1286–1295. doi:10.1038/s41372-020-0656-7

65. Starr MC, Charlton JR, Guillet R, et al. Advances in neonatal acute kidney injury. *Pediatrics.* 2021;148(5):e2021051220. doi:10.1542/peds.2021-051220

66. Jetton JG, Boohaker LJ, Sethi SK, et al. Incidence and outcomes of neonatal acute kidney injury (AWAKEN): a multicentre, multinational, observational cohort study. *Lancet Child Adolesc Health.* 2017;1(3):184–194. doi:10.1016/s2352-4642(17)30069-x

67. Charlton JR, Boohaker L, Askenazi D, et al. Incidence and risk factors of early onset neonatal AKI. *Clin J Am Soc Nephrol.* 2019;14(2):184–195. doi:10.2215/cjn.03670318

68. Charlton JR, Boohaker L, Askenazi D, et al. Late onset neonatal acute kidney injury: results from the AWAKEN Study. *Pediatr Res.* 2019;85(3):339–348. doi:10.1038/s41390-018-0255-x

69. Harer MW, Askenazi DJ, Boohaker LJ, et al. Association between early caffeine citrate administration and risk of acute kidney injury in preterm neonates: results from the AWAKEN study. *JAMA Pediatr.* 2018;172(6):e180322. doi:10.1001/jamapediatrics.2018.0322

70. DeFreitas MJ, Griffin R, Sanderson K, et al. Maternal hypertension disorders and neonatal acute kidney injury: results from the AWAKEN study. *American journal of perinatology.* 2022. doi:10.1055/a-1780-2249

71. Stoops C, Stone S, Evans E, et al. Baby NINJA (Nephrotoxic Injury Negated by Just-in-Time Action): reduction of nephrotoxic medication-associated acute kidney injury in the neonatal intensive care unit. *J Pediatr.* 2019;215:223–228.e6. doi:10.1016/j.jpeds.2019.08.046

72. Abitbol CL, Moxey-Mims M. Chronic kidney disease: Low birth weight and the global burden of kidney disease. *Nat Rev Nephrol.* 2016;12(4):199–200. doi:10.1038/nrneph.2016.19

73. Abitbol CL, Chandar J, Rodriguez MM, et al. Obesity and preterm birth: additive risks in the progression of kidney disease in children. *Pediatr Nephrol.* 2009;24(7):1363–1370. doi:10.1007/s00467-009-1120-2

74. Rochow N, Raja P, Liu K, et al. Physiological adjustment to postnatal growth trajectories in healthy preterm infants. *Pediatr Res.* 2016;79(6):870–879. doi:10.1038/pr.2016.15

75. Bartke A. Somatic growth, aging, and longevity. *NPJ Aging Mech Dis.* 2017;3:14. doi:10.1038/s41514-017-0014-y

76. Nüsken E, Voggel J, Fink G, Dötsch J, Nüsken KD. Impact of early-life diet on long-term renal health. *Mol Cell Pediatr.* 2020;7(1):17. doi:10.1186/s40348-020-00109-1

77. Hofman PL, Regan F, Jackson WE, et al. Premature birth and later insulin resistance. *N Engl J Med.* 2004;351(21):2179–2186. doi:10.1056/NEJMoa042275

78. Lurbe E, Ingelfinger J. Developmental and early life origins of cardiometabolic risk factors: novel findings and implications. *Hypertension.* 2021;77(2):308–318. doi:10.1161/hypertensionaha.120.14592

79. Abitbol CL, Bauer CR, Montane B, Chandar J, Duara S, Zilleruelo G. Long-term follow-up of extremely low birth weight infants with neonatal renal failure. *Pediatr Nephrol.* 2003;18(9):887–893.

80. Denic A, Glassock RJ. Obesity-related glomerulopathy and single-nephron GFR. *Kidney Int Rep.* 2020;5(8):1126–1128. doi:10.1016/j.ekir.2020.05.017

81. Docherty NG, le Roux CW. Bariatric surgery for the treatment of chronic kidney disease in obesity and type 2 diabetes mellitus. *Nat Rev Nephrol.* 2020;16(12):709–720. doi:10.1038/s41581-020-0323-4

82. Sarafidis P, Ortiz A, Ferro CJ, et al. Sodium—glucose co-transporter-2 inhibitors for patients with diabetic and nondiabetic chronic kidney disease: a new era has already begun. *J Hypertens.* 2021;39(6):1090–1097. doi:10.1097/hjh.0000000000002776

83. Carmody JB, Charlton JR. Short-term gestation, long-term risk: prematurity and chronic kidney disease. *Pediatrics.* 2013;131(6):1168–1179. doi:10.1542/peds.2013-0009

84. DeFreitas M, Katsoufis, CK, Abitbol CL. Cardio-renal consequences of low birth weight and preterm birth. *Prog Pediatr Cardiol.* 2016;41:83–88.

Chapter 11

Diagnosis and Management of Prenatal Urinary Tract Dilatation

Gina M. Lockwood, MD, MS, FAAP, and C.D. Anthony Herndon, MD, FAAP, FACS

Chapter Outline

Definitions and Scope of Prenatal Urinary Tract Dilation

Abnormal dilation of the fetal urinary tract is a common finding during antenatal screening ultrasound (US) (1%–3% of all pregnancies),[1] second only to cardiac defects. This dilation signifies a spectrum of disease, in some children a transient and physiologic phenomenon and in others an association with significant renal functional impairment. Table 11.1 lists common and impactful causes of prenatal urinary tract dilation (UTD) with their relative incidences. The term "prenatal urinary tract dilation" encompasses a number of commonly used radiographic terms including but not limited to hydronephrosis, pelviectasis, pyelectasis, and pelvicaliectasis, and it does not infer any pathophysiology underlying the imaging finding. Despite being such a common diagnosis, there is significant variability in the evaluation and management of UTD in the fetus and the neonate. With recent creation of a common nomenclature for UTD and increasing prospective research focused on UTD outcomes, UTD management has increasingly been refined.

Both health care providers caring for women with high-risk pregnancies and those caring for the children affected by these abnormalities should be familiar with the effects of UTD on the developing kidney, antenatal management of UTD, its effects on postnatal outcomes, and evidenced-based management strategies.

TABLE 11.1. Important Causes of *Prenatal Urinary Tract Dilation* and Their Incidences

Etiology	Incidence (%)
Transient urinary tract dilation	50–70
Ureteropelvic junction pattern dilation	10–30
Vesicoureteral reflux	10–40
Ureterovesical junction pattern dilation	5–15
Multicystic dysplastic kidney	2–5
Duplex system, ureterocele, ectopic ureter	5–7
Lower urinary tract obstruction (PUV, PBS)	0.1–0.5

PUV, posterior urethral valve; *PBS*, prune belly syndrome.
Modified from Nguyen HT, Herndon CDA, Cooper C, et al. The Society for Fetal Urology Consensus Statement on the evaluation and management of antenatal hydronephrosis. *J Pediatr Urol.* 2010;6(3):217, Table 5.

Antenatal Diagnosis of Urinary Tract Dilation

MATERNAL FETAL ULTRASOUND

The kidneys and bladder can consistently be detected on prenatal US by the end of the first trimester. The most severe urinary tract abnormalities are likely to appear on the first screening US, which in the United States is recommended between 18 and 22 weeks' gestational age.[2] Ultrasonography has a high sensitivity for UTD, with large studies reporting a sensitivity up to 92%.[3] Abnormalities detected on screening US often prompt referral to a specialized high-risk obstetrics practice able to perform a comprehensive US to confirm the abnormality as well as screen other organ systems.

The measurement of anterior-posterior renal pelvis diameter (APD) has traditionally been the most commonly used dimension to communicate severity of UTD on prenatal US (Fig. 11.1). The established normal value for APD prior to 28 weeks' gestation is ≤4 mm and ≤7 mm after 28 weeks' gestation. Notably, this system of classification is highly specific for obstruction in patients with severe dilation, and studies have identified 15 mm of APD detected in the third trimester as a threshold predictive of ureteropelvic junction (UPJ) obstruction.[4,5] The APD system, however, does not address other important elements of UTD including ureteral and bladder abnormalities or the impact of oligohydramnios.

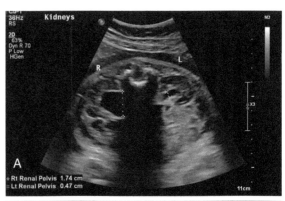

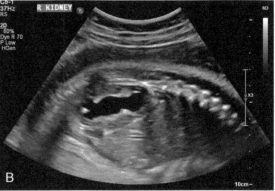

Fig. 11.1 Maternal fetal ultrasound obtained at 32 weeks' gestation. *(A)* Kidneys depicted in the transverse plane. Right renal pelvis diameter 17.4 mm (abnormal) and left renal pelvis diameter 4.7 mm (normal for gestational age). *(B)* Right kidney in sagittal plane showing renal pelvis as well as central and peripheral calyceal dilatation. (Courtesy University of Iowa Hospitals and Clinics.)

In 2014, a multispecialty consensus meeting including representatives from eight professional societies involved in the diagnosis and management of UTD was held to unify grading systems and establish a common language among practitioners.[6] The goals were to develop a standard process for imaging and reporting of US results both antenatally and postnatally. The Urinary Tract Dilation (UTD) Grading System was chosen to describe all degrees of antenatal and postnatal dilation, attempting to limit terms such as hydronephrosis and pelviectasis. This system has both objective and subjective components and measures APD, central calyceal dilation, peripheral calyceal dilation, appearance and thickness of kidney parenchyma, appearance of ureters, appearance of bladder, and unexplained oligohydramnios (Table 11.2).

TABLE 11.2 Prenatal and Postnatal Parameters for Detection of Urinary Tract Dilation for the Urinary Tract Dilation Grading System

Ultrasound Parameter	Measurement/Findings	Notes
Anterior posterior renal pelvis diameter	Millimeters (mm)	Measured on transverse image at maximum diameter of renal pelvis; measured with spine in 6 o'clock or 12 o'clock position Normal ranges by age: • Prenatal <28 weeks: <4 mm • Prenatal ≥28 weeks: <7 mm • Postnatal: <10 mm
Calyceal dilation Central (major calyces) Peripheral (minor calyces) Parenchymal thickness Parenchymal appearance	 Present/absent Present/absent Normal/abnormal Normal/abnormal	 Subjective assessment Subjective assessment Subjective assessment Evaluation of echogenicity and corticomedullary differentiation and for cortical cysts
Ureter	Normal/abnormal	Visualization considered dilated and abnormal, though intermittent visualization of the ureter considered normal postnatally
Bladder	Normal/abnormal	Evaluation of bladder wall thickness, presence of ureterocele, dilated posterior urethra
Unexplained oligohydramnios	Present/absent	

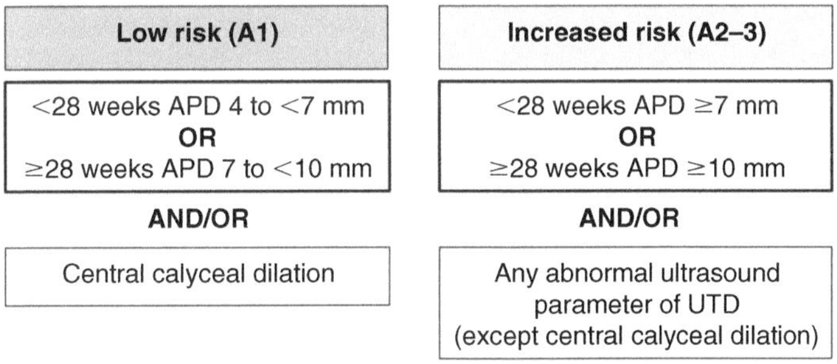

Low risk (A1)	Increased risk (A2–3)
<28 weeks APD 4 to <7 mm **OR** ≥28 weeks APD 7 to <10 mm	<28 weeks APD ≥7 mm **OR** ≥28 weeks APD ≥10 mm
AND/OR	**AND/OR**
Central calyceal dilation	Any abnormal ultrasound parameter of UTD (except central calyceal dilation)

Fig. 11.2 Prenatal urinary tract malformations or dilation UTD Grading System risk stratification. *APD*, anterior posterior renal pelvis diameter; *UTD*, urinary tract dilation.

Using the UTD Grading System, fetuses are classified into a low-risk group (UTD A1, denoted "A" for "antenatal") or an increased risk group (UTD A2–3) (Fig. 11.2). Since its inception, multiple studies have examined the correlation between UTD grade and clinical outcomes.[7–15] These studies have demonstrated a grade-dependent correlation between fetal UTD and postnatal urological abnormalities; higher grades were shown to correlate with lower risk of spontaneous resolution, longer time to resolution, higher risk of urinary tract infections (UTIs), decreased ipsilateral renal function on renal scintigraphy (RS), and higher risk for need for surgical intervention. A caveat to the UTD Grading

System is that it does not specifically refer to those children in whom bladder outlet obstruction is suspected. These children require expedited evaluation and a different management algorithm.

Historically, when a diagnosis of antenatal UTD is made, there has been lack of consensus regarding the frequency and timing of antenatal and postnatal follow-up imaging. A 2006 metaanalysis by Lee et al.[15] found large variability among protocols. Recommendations ranged from vague (e.g., "serially as needed") to specific (e.g., "once at 32–34 weeks") and from infrequent (e.g., "once in the third trimester") to numerous (e.g., "once per month"). Contemporary recommendations for

	Follow-up ultrasound	**Urology/nephrology consultation**
Low risk (A1)	Repeat once prenatally at ≥32 weeks	Not indicated prenatally
Increased risk (A2–3)	Repeat every 4 weeks until delivery	Consider prenatal consult

Fig. 11.3 Suggested prenatal management based on maternal fetal ultrasound < 32 weeks using UTD Grading System risk stratification.

ongoing antenatal management continue to be refined based on prospective research and attempts to minimize unnecessary studies (Fig. 11.3).

FETAL MRI

The use of MRI in diagnosis of fetal UTD is rarely necessary. In situations such as cloacal anomaly, bladder exstrophy, urogenital sinus, and duplication anomalies leading to bladder outlet obstruction in which greater anatomic detail is needed than maternal fetal US can provide, MRI can be useful.

Effects of Urinary Tract Dilation on the Fetal Kidney

The impact of UTD on the fetal kidney ultimately depends on the pathophysiology causing the UTD. It is believed that transient UTD, or UTD that spontaneously resolves prenatally or postnatally with no clinical sequelae, is physiologic and nonpathologic to the developing kidney.

Although the exact pathophysiology of renal maldevelopment associated with vesicoureteral reflux (VUR), or "reflux nephropathy," is not completely understood, it can in part be explained by the theory of Mackie and Stephens that an abnormal origin of the ureteric bud will interact abnormally with the metanephric blastema.[16] Studies have confirmed the association of VUR with a small kidney, reduction in ipsilateral relative renal function, and focal and global areas of poor radiotracer uptake on RS.[17–19]

Obstructive uropathy significantly disrupts normal kidney development, and the effects of obstruction on kidney formation and growth have been well studied. Normal kidney development consists of the acquisition and development of new nephrons (nephrogenesis), the enlargement and growth of existing kidney structures (morphogenesis), and differentiation of the specific functions of the parts of the kidney (segment-specific differentiation). Obstruction is thought to effect all of these processes. Indeed, significant obstructive uropathy results in renal hypodysplasia with a decrease in healthy parenchyma, disrupted architecture often with reduced formation of the medulla, a reduction in the number of glomeruli, cystic transformation of the glomeruli and tubules along the full length of the nephron, remodeling of the developing collecting ducts, and marked expansion and fibrosis of the kidney interstitium.[20–22] Dysplasia is considered irreversible. The small, obstructed kidney is not considered atrophic but hypoplastic, as the obstructed kidney may demonstrate impaired or accelerated growth. The critical factor leading to dysplasia in animal studies has been a complete obstruction early in gestation.[23] Obstructive conditions have been shown to alter expression of growth-regulatory genes and the presence of proteins coded by these genes.[21] Additionally, the role of inappropriate apoptosis in congenital obstruction has become more firmly established in recent years.

The precise effects of obstructive uropathy on fetal kidney function have largely been extrapolated from animal models and from infants born with urinary tract obstruction. There is experimental evidence that obstruction leads to a deficit in nephrons and reduction in fetal glomerular filtration rate (GFR).[24,25] In both human and nonhuman primate fetuses, obstruction causes collecting duct and tubular injury. With obstruction, there is collecting duct epithelial remodeling noted early in fetal development and a reduction in intercalated cells seen by late gestation.[26,27] Proximal tubule epithelial cell injury has been reported in developing rat kidneys. These functional abnormalities are difficult to quantify in the fetus, but in newborns affected by severe posterior urethral valve (PUV), a decrease in GFR, tubular abnormalities leading to a defect in concentrating ability and thus polyuria, urinary salt wasting due to a decrease in tubular sodium reabsorption, and metabolic acidosis due to altered cell expression for collecting duct intercalated cells have all been recognized.[28]

Radiographic findings on prenatal ultrasonography such as hyperechoic renal parenchyma, poor cortico-medullary differentiation, and cystic changes can signify renal dysplasia; however, prenatal radiographic changes are an imperfect measurement of renal function. Amniotic fluid volume can act as a surrogate measure for fetal GFR, as the fetal kidneys become the main source of amniotic fluid production by 20 weeks' gestation. Any impairment of fetal kidney function, including obstructive uropathies, can manifest as oligohydramnios from the second half of pregnancy onward. Fetal blood levels of β_2-microglobulin, the light chain of the class I major histocompatibility complex antigens, have also been used to estimate fetal GFR. Levels are higher in fetuses with urinary tract obstruction, reflecting a decrease in its clearance due to kidney injury.[29] More commonly, fetal urine electrolytes are used to measure fetal kidney function, especially in suspected bladder outlet obstruction. Tubular reabsorption of electrolytes is hypothesized to be impaired, resulting in high fetal urinary sodium and chloride concentrations. Fetal electrolyte levels have been associated with postnatal kidney function[30,31]; however, there is not one clear analyte or threshold level that accurately predicts postnatal kidney function.

Prediction of Postnatal Outcome

Before the advent of antenatal US and diagnosis of UTD, postnatal UTD presentation could range from asymptomatic with diagnosis later in life, symptomatic disease during childhood or adulthood with bladder dysfunction, recurrent UTIs, pyelonephritis or varying degrees of chronic kidney disease (CKD), death in the immediate postnatal period secondary to renal or respiratory insufficiency, or even stillbirth. The value of antenatal diagnosis lies in predicting postnatal outcomes and allowing for consultation of family by subspecialists.

As a general rule, unilateral anomalies, even if there is a high degree of obstruction suspected, are not related to oligohydramnios or fetal or immediate postnatal CKD, as the contralateral kidney compensates. More concerning is the fetus with suspected bilateral kidney obstruction, as is the case in bladder outlet obstruction secondary to PUV, or in a solitary kidney with any degree of abnormality.

In Utero Intervention

Intervention for fetal UTD generally only occurs in the setting of suspected bladder outlet obstruction. Vesicoamniotic shunting and fetal cystoscopy with PUV ablation have been studied, and shunting has been shown to offer a benefit in terms of pulmonary function and fetal survival, but no clear improvement in rate of kidney failure in these patients.[32–34] There is an increased risk with fetal surgery for pregnancy loss and premature rupture of membranes,[32,35] so appropriate counseling is essential in a very select group of patients who may benefit. Reported combined complication rates to both mother and baby are estimated at greater than 40%.[32,36]

The Society of Fetal Urology held a multidisciplinary panel in 2016 to discuss antenatal intervention and to create a discrete classification system to help identify appropriate patients recommended for these interventions.[37] The most favorable outcomes were demonstrated in fetuses with oligohydramnios but not anhydramnios, severe UTD, favorable fetal biochemistry, and absence of renal cortical cysts.[38] Fetal urine testing is considered favorable after 20 weeks' gestation with urinary sodium < 100 mEq/L, chloride < 90 mEq/L, osmolarity < 200 mEq/L, and β_2-microglobulin < 6 mg/L.[39] Serial sampling over 48- to 72-hour intervals was shown in one study to be a more accurate estimator of irreversible renal damage with sequential rises in the urine tests to be more predictive of an unfavorable prognosis.[40] If in utero intervention is considered, prenatal counseling should include a maternal-fetal medicine specialist, pediatric nephrologist, urologist, and neonatologist, and a shared decision-making approach should be taken.

Postnatal Evaluation and Management of Urinary Tract Dilation

PHYSICAL EXAMINATION

If the antenatal diagnosis of UTD has been made, plans for immediate postnatal assessment by neonatology, urology, and nephrology teams should be made, especially if bladder outlet obstruction or UTD in a solitary kidney is suspected. Unexpected physical examination findings or clinical presentation may prompt early imaging or intervention. Severe UTD,

TABLE 11.3 Suggested Postnatal Management Based on Prenatal *Urinary Tract Dilation* Risk Stratification

UTD Classification	Definition	Initial Postnatal US	Urology/Nephrology Consultation
Incomplete or unclear classification Resolved		Follow postnatal evaluation similar to UTD A1 If prior US were all A1 → No postnatal evaluation or surveillance required If any prior US was A2–3 → Manage according to recommendations for "increased risk (A2–3)" below	Follow postnatal evaluation similar to UTD A1
Low risk (A1)	≥28 weeks APD 7 to <10 mm *and/or* central calyceal dilation	≥48 h to 6 weeks of age; need not delay discharge	May consider with outpatient follow-up
Increased risk (A2–3)	≥28 weeks APD ≥ 10 mm *or* any abnormal parameter (except central calyceal dilation)	Prior to discharge, ideally after 48 h of life	Recommended prior to discharge

A1, antenatal low risk; *A2–3,* antenatal increased risk; *APD,* anterior posterior renal pelvis diameter; *US,* ultrasound; *UTD,* urinary tract dilation.

notably UPJ obstruction, can rarely present as a flank mass. Intrinsic compression on surrounding structures can yield feeding intolerance, failure to thrive, and respiratory difficulties in infants, necessitating early surgical intervention.

Infants with bladder outlet obstruction (PUV, urethral atresia, ectopic ureterocele) and oligohydramnios may be affected by pulmonary hypoplasia or have associated stigmata including Potter facies, club feet, deformed hands, and poor visceral muscle tone. They may not urinate within the first 24 hours of life, and if they do urinate, they may have a notably weak or intermittent urinary stream. Bladder distention, urinoma, or forniceal rupture can cause abdominal distention. These findings should prompt immediate bladder decompression with urethral drainage by an experienced practitioner and early kidney and bladder imaging within the first 24 hours of life.

LABORATORY STUDIES

Patients with UTD secondary to bladder outlet obstruction may experience hyponatremia, hyperkalemia, and elevated serum creatinine. Nephrology should be involved early in these patients, as postobstructive diuresis after catheter placement can exacerbate a concentrating defect and lead to fluid underresuscitation.[41] Serum creatinine will be representative of maternal creatinine in the first 48 hours of life and subsequently will reflect the child's kidney function.

Imaging

Renal and Bladder Ultrasound

Renal and bladder ultrasound (RBUS) is the initial imaging study of choice to evaluate children with perinatal UTD. The prenatal degree of UTD dictates the need and timing of postnatal US (Table 11.3). RBUS advantages include that it is noninvasive, widely available, and quickly performed; it lacks ionizing radiation; and it is less costly than other imaging modalities.[42] RBUS can be performed with the infant supine or prone or while being held in the upright position; however, scanning newborns and infants in the prone position may overestimate the degree of dilation in up to 10% of patients.[43] This consideration should be taken into account especially in the first postnatal study, and positioning should be included in the radiology report. For optimal assessment of UTD, RBUS should be performed after 48 hours of life, as studies during the first 48 hours of life might underestimate the degree of dilation.[44–48] RBUS may need to be obtained sooner in some clinical situations, especially with suspicion of bladder outlet obstruction. The postnatal degree of dilation of the pelvicalyceal system and ureters helps guide additional investigations and interventions.[6,49]

The first postnatal US serves as a determinant of risk because, in general, higher levels of dilation correspond with higher need for surgery.[50–52] Under the current postnatal UTD classification (Fig. 11.4),

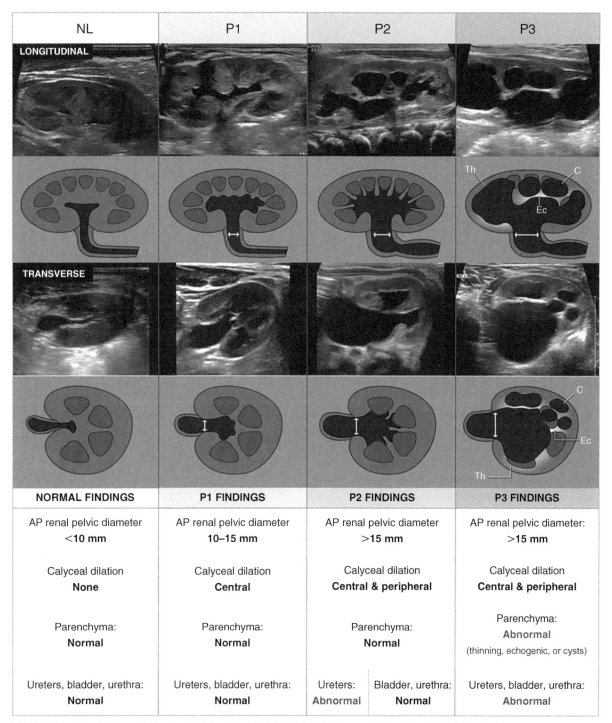

Fig. 11.4 Reproduced with permission from Children's Hospital of Philadelphia. Postnatal Urinary Tract Dilation Grading System. *P1,* postnatal low risk; *P2,* postnatal intermediate risk; *P3,* postnatal high risk; *AP,* anterior posterior; *NL,* normal. (©2021, Children's Hospital of Philadelphia, All Rights Reserved.)

TABLE 11.4   Suggested Postnatal Management Based on Initial Postnatal Ultrasound Using *Urinary Tract Dilation* Postnatal Risk Stratification

UTD Classification	Definition/ Circumstance	Follow-Up (Second) Ultrasound	Antibiotic Prophylaxis	VCUG/CeVUS	MAG3/fMRU	Urology/ Nephrology Consultation
Resolved		3–9 months of age	Not recommended	Not recommended	Not recommended	Not recommended
Low risk (P1)	APD 10 to < 15 mm *and/or* central calyceal dilation	3–6 months of age	Not recommended	Not recommended	Not recommended	Outpatient
Intermediate risk (P2)	APD ≥ 15 mm *and/or* peripheral calyceal dilation	1–3 months of age	Consider upon discharge	May consider	May consider at >6 weeks of age	Inpatient consult or expedited referral
	APD ≥ 15 mm *and/or* ureters abnormal	1–3 months of age	Recommended	Recommended	May consider at >6 weeks of age	Inpatient consult or expedited referral
High risk (P3)	Findings in P2 *and/or* abnormal parenchymal thickness *or* appearance *or* abnormal bladder	1 month of age	Recommended upon discharge	Recommended	Recommended at 6–8 weeks of age	Inpatient consult or expedited referral

APD, anterior posterior renal pelvis diameter; *CeVUS,* contrast-enhanced voiding urosonography; *fMRU,* functional magnetic resonance urography; *MAG3,* mercaptoacetyltriglycine; *UTD,* urinary tract dilation; *VCUG,* voiding cystourethrogram.

patients are stratified into three tiers based on their RBUS: low (UTD P1), intermediate (UTD P2), and high (UTD P3) risk.[6] Recent outcomes research[7–15] has allowed for creation of postnatal recommendations for patients with UTD regarding US surveillance, subspecialist referral, need for additional imaging studies, and need for antibiotic prophylaxis, although there is lack of consensus on some of these topics (Table 11.4).

Voiding Cystourethrogram

Fluoroscopic voiding cystourethrography (VCUG) is the gold standard for diagnosing and grading VUR,[53] which occurs in 15% of children with prenatally diagnosed isolated UTD.[54–56] It can also yield information about bladder or urethral abnormalities contributing to UTD. A VCUG study consists of instilling iodinated contrast material into the bladder via a urinary catheter and imaging with pulsed fluoroscopy (Fig. 11.5). The key images include the bladder at different levels of filling, the urethra during voiding, and the renal fossae immediately after voiding, to document the presence and grade of reflux. Historically, some authors

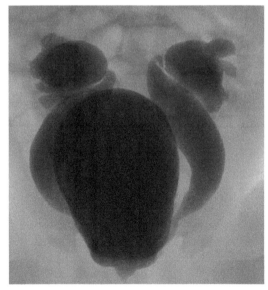

Fig. 11.5 Fluoroscopic voiding cystourethrogram in a child showing a smooth-walled bladder and severe bilateral vesicoureteral reflux with dilated and tortuous ureters and blunting of peripheral renal calyces. The urethra is not adequately visualized in this image. (Courtesy University of Iowa Hospitals and Clinics.)

recommended VCUG in all children with prenatally detected UTD,[57,58] but there is currently great practice variability.[59] Between 26% and 57% of pediatric urologists recommend VCUG and antibiotics for UTD P2 patients, and 85%–88% recommend them for UTD P3 patients.[60] Currently, it is largely accepted that UTD alone should not be considered an indication for VCUG in asymptomatic neonates and infants.[61]

Contrast-Enhanced Voiding Urosonography

Similar information about VUR can be extracted from contrast-enhanced voiding urosonography (CeVUS).[62,63] CeVUS has shown to be more sensitive in detecting VUR than VCUG, with a higher grade of reflux in a majority of patients.[64,65] Instead of iodinated contrast, a US contrast agent is instilled via catheter, and fluoroscopy is avoided. CeVUS is not as sensitive as VCUG for detection of abnormal bladder and urethral morphology. CeVUS is not uniformly available at most institutions, which limits its application.

Functional Renogram—Renal Scintigraphy

Functional nuclear medicine renal scans, also known as renal scintigraphy (RS), follow the uptake of radiotracers by the kidneys and their excretion through the collecting system. The most commonly used radiotracer in the evaluation of UTD is ^{99m}Tc-MAG3 (technetium-99m-labeled-mercaptoacetyltriglycine), which reaches the collecting system via tubular secretion.[66,67] Several other radiotracers can be used to calculate renal function as well, including ^{99m}Tc-DMSA (technetium-99m-labeled-dimercaptosuccinic acid) and ^{99m}Tc-DTPA (technetium-99m-labeled-diethylenetriamine pentaacetic acid). The effective radiation dose of RS is low, and over 95% of the radiotracer is cleared within 3 hours in patients with normal renal function.[68,69]

RS ^{99m}Tc-MAG3 measures two important parameters. First, ^{99m}Tc-MAG3 measures the parenchymal uptake (first pass from the circulation into the kidney), which reflects the split renal function (or differential renal function) and the total renal function. In normal subjects, ^{99m}Tc-MAG3 split renal function values range from 42% to 58%[70]; therefore, a threshold of 40% split function is used to identify those in which renal function is compromised. Second, ^{99m}Tc-MAG3 measures the presence and level of obstruction of the collecting system from the UPJ to the

ureterovesical junction (UVJ) by evaluating clearance over 30 minutes. If there is retained radiotracer in the collecting system after 15 or 20 minutes, a diuretic (furosemide, 1.0 mg/kg; maximum dose of 40 mg) is administered to differentiate dilated systems from those without a critical obstruction.[71] A dilated but unobstructed system will respond to diuretics, and a truly obstructed system will retain radiotracer as it is unable to increase the rate of clearance through the critically narrowed segment.

Accurate RS results in infants with UTD rely on adequate renal blood flow and kidney development, thus tests should ideally be deferred until at least 4–6 weeks of age. During the first months of life, renal immaturity results in low uptake of ^{99m}Tc-MAG3 and slower cortical transit times. Studies performed before 4–6 weeks may over- or underestimate the renal function and are not generally predictive of outcome.[72,73]

Functional Magnetic Resonance Urography

Magnetic resonance urography (MRU) is a reliable and safe diagnostic tool that can substitute RS for the determination of renal function and provide detailed information about the morphology of the kidney with a dilated collecting system.[74] MRU provides excellent morphologic characterization of the renal parenchyma and the entire urinary tract, which can be advantageous in the diagnostic and/or presurgical work up of neonatal UTD.[75,76] Despite advantages related to providing high-quality anatomical and functional data in a single examination that lacks radiation, MRU has ancillary disadvantages including need for sedation or anesthesia for younger children, higher cost, and relatively limited availability.[42]

KEY CONDITIONS

Transient Urinary Tract Dilation

The overall resolution of UTD postnatally ranges in the literature from 41% to 88%; however, the data are fraught because of inconsistent definitions of dilation and lack of universal imaging protocols.[1] A large majority of UTD is thought to be physiologic, spontaneously resolving and of no pathologic significance to the kidneys. Studies have shown a high resolution rate of 90%–98% for "mild dilation" in previous grading systems now accounted for as physiologic in the UTD classification system.[77–79] Most patients with P1 UTD are known to spontaneously resolve within the first 4 years of life.[80,81] The provider must remember that due to the shift to decreased testing postnatally, some of these cases considered to represent transient UTD could actually represent undiagnosed VUR, which is of unclear clinical significance in the absence of other imaging abnormalities and in the absence of urinary tract infection (UTI). Generally, when transient UTD is suspected, it is surveyed with periodic renal US until its resolution.

Ureteropelvic Junction Obstruction Pattern of Dilation

Infantile UPJ obstruction is most commonly caused by an intrinsic narrowing of the UPJ with a segment of abnormally developed circular muscular fibers. This developmental abnormality leads to an insufficient emptying of the renal pelvis, which can, if left untreated, result in renal insufficiency.

Ultrasonography shows significant renal pelvis and often calyceal dilation without hydroureter or bladder anomalies (UTD P2–3). Several studies have reported that the antenatal APD threshold may be predictive of the need for surgery for UPJ obstruction.[5,82] More recently, a review of over 1000 patients identified an APD cutoff of 15 mm to be predictive of the need for intervention and confirmed that postnatal measurements were superior to antenatal measurements.[52] Patients with UTD P2–3 dilation should undergo early US evaluation and lower urinary tract imaging to rule out VUR and visualize urethral abnormalities. In these patients, antibiotic prophylaxis and RS may be considered. Nuclear renogram is recommended especially with renal parenchymal abnormalities.

A few children with prenatal UTD and an ultimate diagnosis of UPJ obstruction will need urgent intervention because of failure to thrive secondary to extrinsic compression of surrounding structures like the diaphragm or stomach. Widely accepted indications for surgical intervention include worsening UTD on US, UTI, decreased differential renal function of <40%, or worsening differential renal function. Only approximately one-third of patients with UPJ obstruction will ultimately be treated with surgery.[4,83] Both open and minimally invasive pyeloplasty for UPJ obstruction demonstrate success in > 90% of cases, even in infants.[84–86]

Vesicoureteral Reflux

VUR is the retrograde flow of urine from the bladder into the ureters and sometimes kidneys. VUR is a risk factor for recurrent pyelonephritis, renal scarring, renal insufficiency, and hypertension and is a cause of end-stage renal disease in children.[87–90] Management of reflux is primarily aimed at reducing the development of these long-term adverse effects through prevention of pyelonephritis, as the presence of persistent reflux alone after birth is not thought to be clinically significant.

In infants, primary VUR is not only attributed to an abnormally short intramural portion of ureter tunnelling through the detrusor muscle at the UVJ but also a delay in maturation of normal voiding. Yeung et al. demonstrated elevated voiding pressures in neonatal VUR patients that decreased to a more normal range over the first year of life.[91] This finding endorses the concept that the natural history of VUR is different in children with prenatal VUR compared with children (predominantly females) that present in early childhood.[92]

In newborns with VUR, scars have been detected in association with high-grade reflux before the occurrence of clinical UTI.[93] These "congenital scars" are thought to be regions of focal dysplasia or hypoplasia resulting from abnormal nephrogenesis as opposed to damaged normal tissue following pyelonephritis. Further acquired scarring can occur with episodes of pyelonephritis as the infant grows. Renal scarring is believed to occur when infected urine comes in contact with renal parenchyma causing an inflammatory reaction; it has been associated with an increased risk of hypertension, proteinuria, and renal insufficiency.[89,94] Screening for VUR has historically been recommended in patients with prenatally diagnosed UTD because VUR has been reported in up to 31% of patients with prenatal UTD; however, prenatal UTD correlates poorly with severity of VUR.[1,95–97] The risk of VUR in patients with a nondilated or a mildly dilated collecting system may be as high as 25%.[96–98] Fortunately, VUR associated with prenatally detected UTD has a high incidence of spontaneous resolution.[99,100] Studies that have assessed whether or not patients with both UTD and VUR are at increased risk for UTI (compared with UTD in the absence of VUR) show conflicting results.[80,101–106]

If VCUG is obtained for patients with prenatal UTD, there is significant practice variability with respect to antibiotic prophylaxis even in the situation of confirmed VUR, as the risk of pyelonephritis and new renal scarring is known to be lower with lower-grade VUR.[107] Antibiotic prophylaxis appears to provide minimal benefit for those with low-grade VUR[108–110] but appears to be beneficial for those with moderate to severe VUR, especially females.[111] If VUR persists and is associated with breakthrough UTI, both open and minimally invasive surgical options are available to correct the reflux and prevent further UTI.

In general, VCUG and antibiotic prophylaxis are best served in patients in whom there is an increased risk of UTI. Until further research can solidify the true value of identifying VUR in patients with prenatal UTD, a shared decision-making approach should be used to counsel families on the risks and benefits of VCUG and antibiotic prophylaxis. Risk factors such as circumcision status, gender, and ureteral dilation on US may increase the risk of UTI in individual patients and make the benefits of antibiotic prophylaxis in reduction of risk of UTI and renal scarring outweigh their risks. It is important for the practitioner to convey that not performing the VCUG does not equate to the absence of VUR. Parents should be made aware that any signs of infection such as fever, lethargy, and foul-smelling urine should be worked up in the context of the history of UTD. Equally, parents should be reassured that in the absence of increased risk factors for infection, patients with VUR can be safely followed off continuous antibiotic prophylaxis (CAP).[112,113]

Megaureter/Ureterovesical Junction Obstruction

Megaureter is a descriptive term to denote dilation of the ureter, regardless of its etiology. This entity has been split into four categories based on etiology: obstructed, refluxing, nonobstructed nonrefluxing, and refluxing with obstruction.[114] Although different thresholds have been used, the term usually refers to a ureter $\geq$ 7 mm in diameter.[115,116] Refluxing megaureter is easily recognized on VCUG, as high-grade VUR by definition is associated with ureteral dilation. Its general evaluation and management are discussed in the previous section. In the absence of VUR, differentiation between megaureter with or without obstruction can be accomplished with RS or MRU.

Megaureter with an orthotopic ureteral insertion should be differentiated from ectopic ureter with insertion into the bladder neck, müllerian or wolffian structures. The primary obstructed megaureter is thought to result from an adynamic segment of ureter at the UVJ. The majority of these cases are asymptomatic but when they do present they can lead to UTI, abdominal pain, hematuria, and decline in ipsilateral kidney function.

As a general rule, VCUG and antibiotic prophylaxis are initiated for megaureter shortly after birth because of increasing risk for UTI with hydroureter. Several studies have confirmed that many patients with megaureter, even if obstructed, can be followed without the need for surgical intervention and that the need for surgery is directly correlated with ureteral diameter.[117–120] Indications for surgery include recurrent UTI, < 40% differential renal function, or worsening differential renal function over time.

Lower Urinary Tract Obstruction/Bladder Outlet Obstruction

These entities encompass abnormalities of the bladder and urethra leading to inadequate bladder emptying and varying degree of ureteral and kidney dilation on prenatal US. They are often associated with oligohydramnios or anhydramnios and bladder distention on prenatal imaging. The most common cause of bladder outlet obstruction in the prenatal period is PUV, affecting between 1.4 and 2.2 per 10,000 births.[121,122] Unfortunately, regardless of prenatal diagnosis, up to 50% of boys with a history of PUV will be diagnosed with end-stage renal disease.[123] Despite this, antenatal consultation with urology and nephrology can be especially helpful for parental counseling, even if in utero intervention is not being considered.

Other causes of bladder outlet obstruction include prune belly syndrome (with megacystis and megalourethra), urethral stenosis or atresia, and congenital megacystis. For all of these diagnoses, early evaluation and management are similar with a primary goal of bladder decompression.

Early urology consultation and bladder decompression is recommended. Catheter placement with a balloon is discouraged because it could obstruct the posterior urethra or ureteral orifices. Catheter placement can sometimes be difficult because of posterior urethral dilation and a high bladder neck, and sometimes upward digital rectal pressure is needed. Catheter placement should be confirmed with abdominal x-ray or pelvic US, as sometimes the catheter tip can be in the posterior urethra and initially drain urine. Alternatively, a suprapubic catheter can be placed with US confirmation by a skilled provider.

Nephrology consultation should also be promptly obtained after bladder decompression for fluid management and monitoring of electrolytes. Many children with bladder outlet obstruction will have kidneys that face a concentrating defect, and intravascular volume depletion can be exacerbated by a postobstructive diuresis after catheter placement.[41] Renal bladder US should be obtained as a baseline after decompression. Once drainage is established, VCUG (Fig. 11.6) can be obtained to make a definitive diagnosis and guide surgical intervention, often with endoscopic valve ablation or cutaneous vesicostomy. Surgical intervention is usually not undertaken until serum creatinine has nadired. Nadir creatinine at 1 year of life appears to be the most accurate predictive tool,

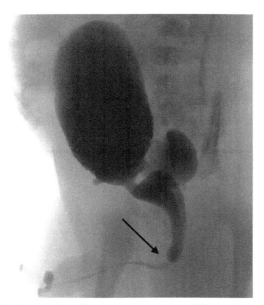

Fig. 11.6. Fluoroscopic voiding cystourethrogram in a child showing a bladder with a few small diverticuli, vesicoureteral reflux, and a dilated posterior urethra. *Arrow* indicates position of posterior urethral valve tissue causing transition point from a dilated posterior urethra to anterior urethra that is decreased in caliber. (Courtesy University of Iowa Hospitals and Clinics.)

with creatinine < 0.8 mg/dL indicating a minimal risk for developing end-stage renal failure and >1.2 mg/dL predicting higher risk.[124–126]

Special Considerations in the Postnatal Management of Urinary Tract Dilation

There is still ambiguity with respect to postnatal management of UTD, especially with regard to use of antibiotic prophylaxis and use of invasive imaging, despite increasing prospective studies. Emerging research has endeavored to determine the frequency of UTI and renal scarring as major preventable outcomes in patients with UTD, to determine which patients are at higher risks, and to determine the patients in whom antibiotics are beneficial.

RISK OF URINARY TRACT INFECTION AND RENAL SCARRING IN CHILDREN WITH URINARY TRACT DILATION: WHICH CHILDREN ARE AT INCREASED RISK?

Rates of UTI in patients with prenatal UTD range from 8% to 22%, with the degree of dilation directly proportional to the risk for UTI.[95] Both recent prospective studies and retrospective studies have shown an increased risk for UTI with high-grade UTD[79,101–104,106,127–129] and/or ureteral dilation,[101,102,128–131] specifically distal ureteral diameter > 7 mm.[132] Other risk factors that have been shown to increase risk of UTI in patients with UTD include female sex,[80,101,103–105,133–135] intact foreskin,[61,80,101–104] and presence of obstructive uropathy.[128] As discussed, risk of UTI with VUR in the setting of UTD is unclear. Of note, most of the mentioned studies excluded patients with known uropathy at birth (e.g., solitary kidney). These frequently excluded patients should also be considered at increased risk. Box 11.1 lists the risk factors that should be taken into consideration when managing children with prenatal UTD.

Timing of UTI will also affect management decisions. The incidence of UTI prior to the first postnatal US is low (1.4%).[136] Zee et al. reported prospective data from the multicenter Society for Fetal Urology registry on 213 patients with antenatal UTD, showing that 89% of UTIs in this cohort occurred before 12 months of age.[79]

The goals of preventing UTIs are to ameliorate symptoms and prevent their short-term sequelae, such

BOX 11.1 RISK FACTORS FOR URINARY TRACT INFECTION IN CHILDREN WITH PRENATALLY DIAGNOSED URINARY TRACT DILATION

Children With UTD and Risk Factors for UTI	Children With Known Uropathy at Birth
Female gender	Ureteropelvic junction obstruction
Intact foreskin	Posterior urethral valves
P3 UTD	Ectopic ureter
Distal ureteral dilation > 1.2 cm	Duplex ureter
Vesicoureteral reflux	Solitary kidney
Obstructive uropathy (suggested by bilateral UTD)	Multicystic dysplastic kidney
	Bladder diverticulum
	Neurogenic bladder
	Bladder exstrophy
	Spina bifida
	Bilateral renal agenesis
	Horseshoe kidney
	Crossed-fused ectopia
	Cloacal exstrophy

P3, high risk; UTD, urinary tract dilation; UTI, urinary tract infection.

as bacteremia, and long-term sequelae, such as renal scarring, hypertension, and end-stage renal disease. The rate of renal scarring is known to increase with increased number of UTIs. Compared with patients with a history of one UTI, having two UTIs increased the odds of renal scarring by a factor of 12, and having three UTIs by a factor of 14.[137] Delaying antibiotic treatment for more than 48–72 hours after onset of fever significantly increases the risk of renal scarring.[138,139]

EFFECTIVENESS OF CONTINUOUS ANTIBIOTIC PROPHYLAXIS IN CHILDREN WITH URINARY TRACT DILATION

Historically, most patients with antenatal UTD were empirically prescribed CAP to prevent UTI and, ultimately, renal damage. To date, no studies have addressed the effect of prophylaxis on renal scarring in patients with UTD. The efficacy of CAP in prevention of UTI in patients with UTD is also unclear. A 2017 metaanalysis found no significant difference in UTI rates between patients that were (9.9%) or were not (7.5%) given CAP.[103] A metaanalysis by Braga et al. found that CAP was associated with decreased UTIs in patients with high-grade UTD (number needed to

treat = 7) but not in patients with low-grade UTD.[127] Notably, neither metaanalysis included any randomized controlled trials. A 2021 study by Holzman et al. also found that CAP prevented UTIs in high-risk patients with UTD with concomitant ureteral dilation > 7 mm regardless of VUR status.[132] However, data from the same year from the SFU Hydronephrosis Registry demonstrated no benefit for CAP for isolated UPJ-like dilation, even adjusted for grade of UTD or other risk factors.[140]

In general, daily antibiotic prophylaxis appears to be safe and well tolerated, but it does incur cost and potential risks. CAP for UTIs has been associated with a 24-fold increased risk of trimethoprim-sulfamethoxazole-resistant *Escherichia coli*.[141] Other studies have demonstrated the emergence of other bacteria with high rates of resistance.[142] In addition to resistance, there are other concerns regarding potential side effects of long-term antibiotics on the gut and urinary microbiome as well as growth.[143–146] Additionally, medication adherence should be considered. A 2010 study suggested that the compliance rate for merely filling the prescription was only 40%, suggesting that many patients placed on CAP never receive the medication.[147]

Some studies have shown circumcision to be an equally preventive alternative to antibiotic prophylaxis for prevention of UTI in boys with UTD.[127,148,149] As mentioned, most UTIs occur within the first year of life, and rates beyond that age are low. Clinicians should therefore consider stopping antibiotic prophylaxis at 12 months of age, unless the child has VUR or ureteral dilation ≥ 7 mm.

Amoxicillin is the primary antibiotic prescribed for UTI prophylaxis in the newborn in the United States. It covers some gram-negative rods and *Enterococcus* species. After 2 months of life, the most commonly prescribed antibiotic for prophylaxis is trimethoprim-sulfamethoxazole, which attains high concentrations in the urine and results in less bacterial resistance. Early in life, trimethoprim-sulfamethoxazole can cause bilirubin displacement, placing the infant at risk for kernicterus. Nitrofurantoin is an equally effective prophylaxis and is excreted primarily in the urine and has poor tissue penetration thus decreasing impact on the gut microbiome. If a cephalosporin is chosen, the clinician should consider using a first-generation cephalosporin as bacterial resistance remains low.[150] Local patterns of resistance should be considered using the hospital antibiogram.

Conclusions

Prenatally diagnosed UTD is a common ultrasonographic finding and can lead to the diagnosis of an array of urologic conditions with varying ultimate outcomes on kidney function. Prenatal diagnosis allows for early counseling of families regarding anticipated postnatal evaluation, management strategies, and outcomes. As ideal treatment continues to be refined, a multidisciplinary and shared decision-making approach should be taken in guiding families with a focus on identifying those children at most risk for UTIs, renal scarring, and renal functional deterioration.

REFERENCES

1. Nguyen HT, Herndon CDA, Cooper C, et al. The Society for Fetal Urology consensus statement on the evaluation and management of antenatal hydronephrosis. *J Pediatr Urol.* 2010; 6(3):212–231. doi:10.1016/J.JPUROL.2010.02.205
2. Practice Bulletin No. 175: Ultrasound in pregnancy. *Obstet Gynecol.* 2016;128(6):e241–e256. doi:10.1097/AOG.0000000000001815
3. Gonçalves LF, Jeanty P, Piper JM. The accuracy of prenatal ultrasonography in detecting congenital anomalies. *Am J Obstet Gynecol.* 1994;171(6):1606–1612. doi:10.1016/0002-9378(94)90411-1
4. Dhillon HK. Prenatally diagnosed hydronephrosis: the Great Ormond Street experience. *Br J Urol.* 1998;81(suppl 2):39–44. doi:10.1046/J.1464-410X.1998.0810S2039.X
5. Coplen DE, Austin PF, Yan Y, Blanco VM, Dicke JM. The magnitude of fetal renal pelvic dilatation can identify obstructive postnatal hydronephrosis, and direct postnatal evaluation and management. *J Urol.* 2006;176(2):724–727. doi:10.1016/J.JURO.2006.03.079
6. Nguyen HT, Benson CB, Bromley B, et al. Multidisciplinary consensus on the classification of prenatal and postnatal urinary tract dilation (UTD classification system). *J Pediatr Urol.* 2014;10(6):982–998. doi:10.1016/j.jpurol.2014.10.002
7. Bratina P, Levart TK. Clinical outcome is associated with the Urinary Tract Dilatation Classification System grade. *Croat Med J.* 2020;61(3):246–251. doi:10.3325/CMJ.2020.61.246
8. Zhang H, Zhang L, Guo N. Validation of "urinary tract dilation" classification system: correlation between fetal hydronephrosis and postnatal urological abnormalities. *Medicine (Baltimore).* 2020;99(2):e18707. doi:10.1097/MD.0000000000018707
9. Kaspar CDW, Lo M, Bunchman TE, Xiao N. The antenatal urinary tract dilation classification system accurately predicts severity of kidney and urinary tract abnormalities. *J Pediatr Urol.* 2017;13(5):485.e1–485.e7. doi:10.1016/J.JPUROL.2017.03.020
10. Nelson CP, Lee RS, Trout AT, et al. The Association of Postnatal Urinary Tract Dilation risk score with clinical outcomes. *J Pediatr Urol.* 2019;15(4):341.e1–341.e6. doi:10.1016/J.JPUROL.2019.05.001
11. Hodhod A, Capolicchio JP, Jednak R, El-Sherif E, El-Doray AEA, El-Sherbiny M. Evaluation of Urinary Tract Dilation Classification System for grading postnatal hydronephrosis. *J Urol.* 2016;195(3):725–730. doi:10.1016/J.JURO.2015.10.089
12. Cakici EK, Aydog O, Eroglu FK, et al. Value of renal pelvic diameter and urinary tract dilation classification in the prediction of urinary tract anomaly. *Pediatr Int.* 2019;61(3):271–277. doi:10.1111/PED.13788
13. Braga LH, McGrath M, Farrokhyar F, Jegatheeswaran K, Lorenzo AJ. Society for Fetal Urology classification vs Urinary Tract Dilation Grading System for prognostication in prenatal hydronephrosis: a time to resolution analysis. *J Urol.* 2018; 199(6):1615–1621. doi:10.1016/J.JURO.2017.11.077
14. Agard H, Massanyi E, Albertson M, et al. The different elements of the Urinary Tract Dilation (UTD) Classification System and their capacity to predict findings on mercaptoacetyltriglycine (MAG3) diuretic renography. *J Pediatr Urol.* 2020;16(5): 686.e1–686.e6. doi:10.1016/J.JPUROL.2020.07.045
15. Lee RS, Cendron M, Kinnamon DD, Nguyen HT. Antenatal hydronephrosis as a predictor of postnatal outcome: a meta-analysis. *Pediatrics.* 2006;118(2):586–593. doi:10.1542/PEDS.2006-0120
16. Mackie GG, Stephens FD. Duplex kidneys: a correlation of renal dysplasia with position of the ureteral orifice. *J Urol.* 1975;114(2):274–280. doi:10.1016/S0022-5347(17)67007-1
17. Najmaldin A, Burge DM, Atwell JD. Reflux nephropathy secondary to intrauterine vesicoureteric reflux. *J Pediatr Surg.* 1990;25(4):387–390. doi:10.1016/0022-3468(90)90376-K
18. Burge DM, Griffiths MD, Malone PS, Atwell JD. Fetal vesicoureteral reflux: outcome following conservative postnatal management. *J Urol.* 1992;148(5 Pt 2):1743–1745. doi:10.1016/S0022-5347(17)37018-0
19. Risdon RA. The small scarred kidney in childhood. *Pediatr Nephrol.* 1993;7(4):361–364. doi:10.1007/BF00857538
20. Peters CA, Carr MC, Lais A, Retik AB, Mandell J. The response of the fetal kidney to obstruction. *J Urol.* 1992;148(2 Pt 2): 503–509. doi:10.1016/S0022-5347(17)36640-5
21. Chevalier RL. Growth factors and apoptosis in neonatal ureteral obstruction. *J Am Soc Nephrol.* 1996;7(8):1098–1105. doi:10.1681/ASN.V781098
22. Tarantal AF, Han VKM, Cochrum KC, Mok A, Dasilva M, Matsell DG. Fetal rhesus monkey model of obstructive renal dysplasia. *Kidney Int.* 2001;59(2):446–456. doi:10.1046/J.1523-1755.2001.059002446.X
23. Beck AD. The effect of intra-uterine urinary obstruction upon the development of the fetal kidney. *J Urol.* 1971;105(6): 784–789. doi:10.1016/S0022-5347(17)61629-X
24. Adzick NS, Harrison MR, Flake AW, Laberge JM. Development of a fetal renal function test using endogenous creatinine clearance. *J Pediatr Surg.* 1985;20(6):602–607. doi:10.1016/S0022-3468(85)80007-5
25. Peters CA, Carr MC, Lais A, Retik AB, Mandell J. The response of the fetal kidney to obstruction. *J Urol.* 1992;148(2 Pt 2): 503–509. doi:10.1016/S0022-5347(17)36640-5
26. Butt MJ, Tarantal AF, Jimenez DF, Matsell DG. Collecting duct epithelial–mesenchymal transition in fetal urinary tract obstruction. *Kidney Int.* 2007;72(8):936–944. doi:10.1038/SJ.KI.5002457

27. Hiatt MJ, Ivanova L, Toran N, Tarantal AF, Matsell DG. Remodeling of the fetal collecting duct epithelium. *Am J Pathol.* 2010;176(2):630–637. doi:10.2353/AJPATH.2010.090389

28. Matsell DG. Congenital urinary tract obstruction—diagnosis and management in the fetus. In: Oh W, Baum M, Polin R, eds. *Nephrology and Fluid/Electrolyte Physiology: Neonatology Questions and Controversies.* 3rd ed. Elsevier; 2019:391–409.

29. Dommergues M, Muller F, Ngo S, et al. Fetal serum β2-microglobulin predicts postnatal renal function in bilateral uropathies. *Kidney Int.* 2000;58(1):312–316. doi:10.1046/J.1523-1755.2000.00167.X

30. Miguelez J, Bunduki V, Yoshizaki CT, et al. Fetal obstructive uropathy: is urine sampling useful for prenatal counselling? *Prenat Diagn.* 2006;26(1):81–84. doi:10.1002/PD.1360

31. Guez S, Assael BM, Melzi ML, Tassis B, Nicolini U. Shortcomings in predicting postnatal renal function using prenatal urine biochemistry in fetuses with congenital hydronephrosis. *J Pediatr Surg.* 1996;31(10):1401–1404. doi:10.1016/S0022-3468(96)90838-6

32. Morris RK, Malin GL, Quinlan-Jones E, et al. Percutaneous vesicoamniotic shunting versus conservative management for fetal lower urinary tract obstruction (PLUTO): a randomised trial. *Lancet.* 2013;382(9903):1496–1506. doi:10.1016/S0140-6736(13)60992-7

33. Clark TJ, Martin WL, Divakaran TG, Whittle MJ, Kilby MD, Khan KS. Prenatal bladder drainage in the management of fetal lower urinary tract obstruction: a systematic review and meta-analysis. *Obstet Gynecol.* 2003;102(2):367–382. doi:10.1016/S0029-7844(03)00577-5

34. Ruano R. Fetal surgery for severe lower urinary tract obstruction. *Prenat Diagn.* 2011;31(7):667–674. doi:10.1002/PD.2736

35. Holmes N, Harrison MR, Baskin LS. Fetal surgery for posterior urethral valves: long-term postnatal outcomes. *Pediatrics.* 2001;108(1):E7. doi:10.1542/PEDS.108.1.E7

36. Elder JS, Duckett JW, Snyder HM. Intervention for fetal obstructive uropathy: has it been effective? *Lancet.* 1987;2(8566):1007–1010. doi:10.1016/S0140-6736(87)92567-0

37. Farrugia MK, Braun MC, Peters CA, Ruano R, Herndon CD. Report on The Society for Fetal Urology panel discussion on the selection criteria and intervention for fetal bladder outlet obstruction. *J Pediatr Urol.* 2017;13(4):345–351. doi:10.1016/J.JPUROL.2017.02.021

38. Ruano R, Sananes N, Wilson C, et al. Fetal lower urinary tract obstruction: proposal for standardized multidisciplinary prenatal management based on disease severity. *Ultrasound Obstet Gynecol.* 2016;48(4):476–482. doi:10.1002/UOG.15844

39. Nicolini U, Spelzini F. Invasive assessment of fetal renal abnormalities: urinalysis, fetal blood sampling and biopsy. *Prenat Diagn.* 2001;21(11):964–969. doi:10.1002/pd.212

40. Johnson MP, Bukowski TP, Reitleman C, Isada NB, Pryde PG, Evans MI. In utero surgical treatment of fetal obstructive uropathy: a new comprehensive approach to identify appropriate candidates for vesicoamniotic shunt therapy. *Am J Obstet Gynecol.* 1994;170(6):1770–1779. doi:10.1016/S0002-9378(94)70353-1

41. Dinneen MD, Duffy PG, Barratt TM, Ransley PG. Persistent polyuria after posterior urethral valves. *Br J Urol.* 1995;75(2):236–240. doi:10.1111/J.1464-410X.1995.TB07318.X

42. Viteri B, Calle-Toro JS, Furth S, Darge K, Hartung EA, Otero H. State-of-the-art renal imaging in children. *Pediatrics.* 2020;145(2):e20190829. doi:10.1542/PEDS.2019-0829

43. Calle-Toro JS, Maya CL, Gorfu Y, Dunn E, Darge K, Back SJ. Supine versus prone positioning for ultrasound evaluation of postnatal urinary tract dilation in children. *Pediatr Radiol.* 2020;50(3):357–362. doi:10.1007/S00247-019-04546-7

44. Zhang L, Liu C, Li Y, Sun C, Li X. Determination of the need for surgical intervention in infants diagnosed with fetal hydronephrosis in China. *Med Sci Monit.* 2016;22:4210–4217. doi:10.12659/MSM.897665

45. Djahangirian O, Young I, Dorgalli C, et al. Safe discharge parameters for patients with isolated antenatal hydronephrosis. *J Pediatr Urol.* 2018;14(4):321.e1–321.e5. doi:10.1016/J.JPUROL.2018.04.016

46. Wiener JS, O'Hara SM, Voigt R, Brock J. Optimal timing of initial postnatal ultrasonography in newborns with prenatal hydronephrosis. *J Urol.* 2002;168(4 Pt 2):1826–1829. doi:10.1097/01.JU.0000030859.88692.DD

47. Laing FC, Burke VD, Wing VW, Jeffrey RB, Hashimoto B. Postpartum evaluation of fetal hydronephrosis: optimal timing for follow-up sonography. *Radiology.* 1984;152(2):423–424. doi:10.1148/RADIOLOGY.152.2.6539930

48. Dejter SW, Gibbons MD. The fate of infant kidneys with fetal hydronephrosis but initially normal postnatal sonography. *J Urol.* 1989;142(2 Pt 2):661–662. doi:10.1016/S0022-5347(17)38846-8

49. Ismail A, Elkholy A, Zaghmout O, et al. Postnatal management of antenatally diagnosed ureteropelvic junction obstruction. *J Pediatr Urol.* 2006;2(3):163–168. doi:10.1016/J.JPUROL.2005.07.005

50. Passerotti CC, Kalish LA, Chow J, et al. The predictive value of the first postnatal ultrasound in children with antenatal hydronephrosis. *J Pediatr Urol.* 2011;7(2):128–136. doi:10.1016/J.JPUROL.2010.09.007

51. Dias CS, Silva JMP, Pereira AK, et al. Diagnostic accuracy of renal pelvic dilatation for detecting surgically managed ureteropelvic junction obstruction. *J Urol.* 2013;190(2):661–666. doi:10.1016/J.JURO.2013.02.014

52. Arora S, Yadav P, Kumar M, et al. Predictors for the need of surgery in antenatally detected hydronephrosis due to UPJ obstruction—a prospective multivariate analysis. *J Pediatr Urol.* 2015;11(5):248.e1–248.e5. doi:10.1016/J.JPUROL.2015.02.008

53. Frimberger D, Mercado-Deane MG, McKenna PH, et al. Establishing a standard protocol for the voiding cystourethrography. *Pediatrics.* 2016;138(5)e20162590. doi:10.1542/PEDS.2016-2590

54. Phan V, Traubici J, Hershenfield B, Stephens D, Rosenblum ND, Geary DF. Vesicoureteral reflux in infants with isolated antenatal hydronephrosis. *Pediatr Nephrol.* 2003;18(12):1224–1228. doi:10.1007/S00467-003-1287-X

55. Gloor JM, Ramsey PS, Ogburn PL, Danilenko-Dixon DR, DiMarco CS, Ramin KD. The association of isolated mild fetal hydronephrosis with postnatal vesicoureteral reflux. *J Matern Fetal Neonatal Med.* 2002;12(3):196–200. doi:10.1080/JMF.12.3.196.200

56. Van Eerde AM, Meutgeert MH, De Jong TPVM, Giltay JC. Vesico-ureteral reflux in children with prenatally detected hydronephrosis: a systematic review. *Ultrasound Obstet Gynecol.* 2007;29(4):463–469. doi:10.1002/UOG.3975

57. Brophy MM, Austin PF, Yan Y, Coplen DE, Herndon A, Rushton HG. Vesicoureteral reflux and clinical outcomes in infants with prenatally detected hydronephrosis. *J Urol.* 2002;168(4 Pt 2):1716–1719. doi:10.1097/01.JU.0000026907.65728.6E

58. Estrada CR, Peters CA, Retik AB, Nguyen HT. Vesicoureteral reflux and urinary tract infection in children with a history of prenatal hydronephrosis—should voiding cystourethrography be performed in cases of postnatally persistent grade II hydronephrosis? *J Urol.* 2009;181(2):801–807. doi:10.1016/J.JURO.2008.10.057

59. Vemulakonda VM, Chiang G, Corbett ST. Variability in use of voiding cystourethrogram during initial evaluation of infants with congenital hydronephrosis. *Urology.* 2014;83(5):1135–1138. doi:10.1016/J.UROLOGY.2013.11.011

60. Jackson JN, Zee RS, Martin AN, Corbett ST, Herndon CDA. A practice pattern assessment of members of the Society of Pediatric Urology for evaluation and treatment of urinary tract dilation. *J Pediatr Urol.* 2017;13(6):602–607. doi:10.1016/J.JPUROL.2017.03.032

61. Sencan A, Carvas F, Hekimoglu IC, et al. Urinary tract infection and vesicoureteral reflux in children with mild antenatal hydronephrosis. *J Pediatr Urol.* 2014;10(6):1008–1013. doi:10.1016/J.JPUROL.2014.04.001

62. Papadopoulou F, Ntoulia A, Siomou E, Darge K. Contrast-enhanced voiding urosonography with intravesical administration of a second-generation ultrasound contrast agent for diagnosis of vesicoureteral reflux: prospective evaluation of contrast safety in 1,010 children. *Pediatr Radiol.* 2014;44(6):719–728. doi:10.1007/S00247-013-2832-9

63. Riccabona M, Vivier PH, Ntoulia A, et al. ESPR uroradiology task force imaging recommendations in paediatric uroradiology, part VII: standardised terminology, impact of existing recommendations, and update on contrast-enhanced ultrasound of the paediatric urogenital tract. *Pediatr Radiol.* 2014;44(11):1478–1484. doi:10.1007/S00247-014-3135-5

64. Papadopoulou F, Anthopoulou A, Siomou E, Efremidis S, Tsamboulas C, Darge K. Harmonic voiding urosonography with a second-generation contrast agent for the diagnosis of vesicoureteral reflux. *Pediatr Radiol.* 2009;39(3):239–244. doi:10.1007/S00247-008-1080-X

65. Darge K. Voiding urosonography with US contrast agents for the diagnosis of vesicoureteric reflux in children. II. Comparison with radiological examinations. *Pediatr Radiol.* 2008;38(1):54–63. doi:10.1007/S00247-007-0528-8

66. Taylor A, Nally JV. Clinical applications of renal scintigraphy. *AJR Am J Roentgenol.* 1995;164(1):31–41. doi:10.2214/AJR.164.1.7998566

67. Taylor AT. Radionuclides in nephrourology, part 1: radiopharmaceuticals, quality control, and quantitative indices. *J Nucl Med.* 2014;55(4):608–615. doi:10.2967/JNUMED.113.133447

68. Stabin M, Taylor A, Eshima D, Wooter W. Radiation dosimetry for technetium-99m-MAG3, technetium-99m-DTPA, and iodine-131-OIH based on human biodistribution studies. *J Nucl Med.* 1992;33(1):33–40.

69. Durand E, Chaumet-Riffaud P, Grenier N. Functional renal imaging: new trends in radiology and nuclear medicine. *Semin Nucl Med.* 2011;41(1):61–72. doi:10.1053/J.SEMNUCLMED.2010.08.003

70. Esteves FP, Taylor A, Manatunga A, Folks RD, Krishnan M, Garcia EV. 99mTc-MAG3 renography: normal values for MAG3 clearance and curve parameters, excretory parameters, and residual urine volume. *AJR Am J Roentgenol.* 2006;187(6):W610–W617. doi:10.2214/AJR.05.1550

71. Shulkin BL, Mandell GA, Cooper JA, et al. Procedure guideline for diuretic renography in children 3.0. *J Nucl Med Technol.* 2008;36(3):162–168. doi:10.2967/JNMT.108.056622

72. Treves ST, Baker A, Fahey FH, et al. Nuclear medicine in the first year of life. *J Nucl Med.* 2011;52(6):905–925. doi:10.2967/JNUMED.110.084202

73. Gordon I, Piepsz A, Sixt R. Guidelines for standard and diuretic renogram in children. *Eur J Nucl Med Mol Imaging.* 2011;38(6):1175–1188. doi:10.1007/S00259-011-1811-3

74. Pavicevic PK, Saranovic DZ, Mandic MJ, et al. Efficacy of magnetic resonance urography in detecting crossing renal vessels in children with ureteropelvic junction obstruction. *Ann Ital Chir.* 2015;86(5):443–449.

75. McMann LP, Kirsch AJ, Scherz HC, et al. Magnetic resonance urography in the evaluation of prenatally diagnosed hydronephrosis and renal dysgenesis. *J Urol.* 2006;176(4 Pt 2):1786–1792. doi:10.1016/J.JURO.2006.05.025

76. Leppert A, Nadalin S, Schirg E, et al. Impact of magnetic resonance urography on preoperative diagnostic workup in children affected by hydronephrosis: should IVU be replaced? *J Pediatr Surg.* 2002;37(10):1441–1445. doi:10.1053/JPSU.2002.35408

77. Barbosa JABA, Chow JS, Benson CB, et al. Postnatal longitudinal evaluation of children diagnosed with prenatal hydronephrosis: insights in natural history and referral pattern. *Prenat Diagn.* 2012;32(13):1242–1249. doi:10.1002/PD.3989

78. Maayan-Metzger A, Lotan D, Jacobson JM, et al. The yield of early postnatal ultrasound scan in neonates with documented antenatal hydronephrosis. *Am J Perinatol.* 2011;28(8):613–617. doi:10.1055/S-0031-1276735/ID/19

79. Zee RS, Herbst KW, Kim C, et al. Urinary tract infections in children with prenatal hydronephrosis: a risk assessment from the Society for Fetal Urology Hydronephrosis Registry. *J Pediatr Urol.* 2016;12(4):261.e1–261.e7. doi:10.1016/J.JPUROL.2016.04.024

80. Zee RS, Herndon CDA, Cooper CS, et al. Time to resolution: a prospective evaluation from the Society for Fetal Urology hydronephrosis registry. *J Pediatr Urol.* 2017;13(3):316.e1–316.e5. doi:10.1016/J.JPUROL.2016.12.012

81. Braga LH, McGrath M, Farrokhyar F, Jegatheeswaran K, Lorenzo AJ. Society for Fetal Urology classification vs Urinary Tract Dilation grading system for prognostication in prenatal hydronephrosis: a time to resolution analysis. *J Urol.* 2018;199(6):1615–1621. doi:10.1016/J.JURO.2017.11.077

82. Dhillon HK. Prenatally diagnosed hydronephrosis: the Great Ormond Street experience. *Br J Urol.* 1998;81(suppl 2):39–44. doi:10.1046/J.1464-410X.1998.0810S2039.X

83. Koff SA. Neonatal management of unilateral hydronephrosis. Role for delayed intervention. *Urol Clin North Am.* 1998;25(2):181–186. doi:10.1016/S0094-0143(05)70006-9

84. Avery DI, Herbst KW, Lendvay TS, et al. Robot-assisted laparoscopic pyeloplasty: multi-institutional experience in infants. *J Pediatr Urol.* 2015;11(3):139.e1–139.e5. doi:10.1016/J.JPUROL.2014.11.025

85. Song SH, Lee C, Jung J, et al. A comparative study of pediatric open pyeloplasty, laparoscopy-assisted extracorporeal pyeloplasty, and robot-assisted laparoscopic pyeloplasty. *PLoS One.* 2017;12(4):e0175026. doi:10.1371/JOURNAL.PONE.0175026

86. Murthy P, Cohn JA, Gundeti MS. Evaluation of robotic-assisted laparoscopic and open pyeloplasty in children: single-surgeon experience. *Ann R Coll Surg Engl.* 2015;97(2):109–114. doi:10.1308/003588414X14055925058797

87. Mathews R, Carpenter M, Chesney R, et al. Controversies in the management of vesicoureteral reflux: the rationale for the

RIVUR study. *J Pediatr Urol.* 2009;5(5):336–341. doi:10.1016/J.JPUROL.2009.05.010

88. Kaefer M, Curran M, Treves ST, et al. Sibling vesicoureteral reflux in multiple gestation births. *Pediatrics.* 2000;105(4 Pt 1):800–804. doi:10.1542/PEDS.105.4.800

89. Smellie JM, Poulton A, Prescod NP. Retrospective study of children with renal scarring associated with reflux and urinary infection. *BMJ.* 1994;308(6938):1193–1196.

90. Garin EH, Olavarria F, Nieto VG, Valenciano B, Campos A, Young L. Clinical significance of primary vesicoureteral reflux and urinary antibiotic prophylaxis after acute pyelonephritis: a multicenter, randomized, controlled study. *Pediatrics.* 2006;117(3):626–632. doi:10.1542/PEDS.2005-1362

91. Yeung CK, Godley ML, Dhillon HK, Duffy PG, Ransley PG. Urodynamic patterns in infants with normal lower urinary tracts or primary vesico-ureteric reflux. *Br J Urol.* 1998;81(3):461–467. doi:10.1046/J.1464-410X.1998.00567.X

92. Herndon CDA, DeCambre M, McKenna PH. Changing concepts concerning the management of vesicoureteral reflux. *J Urol.* 2001;166(4):1439–1443. doi:10.1016/S0022-5347(05)65804-1

93. Nguyen HT, Bauer SB, Peters CA, et al. 99m Technetium dimercapto-succinic acid renal scintigraphy abnormalities in infants with sterile high grade vesicoureteral reflux. *J Urol.* 2000;164(5):1674–1679. doi:10.1016/S0022-5347(05)67081-4

94. Ransley PG, Risdon RA. Reflux nephropathy: effects of antimicrobial therapy on the evolution of the early pyelonephritic scar. *Kidney Int.* 1981;20(6):733–742. doi:10.1038/KI.1981.204

95. Lee RS, Cendron M, Kinnamon DD, Nguyen HT. Antenatal hydronephrosis as a predictor of postnatal outcome: a meta-analysis. *Pediatrics.* 2006;118(2):586–593. doi:10.1542/PEDS.2006-0120

96. Herndon CDA, McKenna PH, Kolon TF, Gonzales ET, Barker LA, Docimo SG. A multicenter outcomes analysis of patients with neonatal reflux presenting with prenatal hydronephrosis. *J Urol.* 1999;162(3 Pt 2):1203–1208. doi:10.1097/00005392-199909000-00096

97. Upadhyay J, McLorie GA, Bolduc S, Bägli DJ, Khoury AE, Farhat W. Natural history of neonatal reflux associated with prenatal hydronephrosis: long-term results of a prospective study. *J Urol.* 2003;169(5):1837–1841. doi:10.1097/01.JU.0000062440.92454.CF

98. Berrocal T, Pinilla I, Gutiérrez J, Prieto C, Pablo L, Hoyo ML. Mild hydronephrosis in newborns and infants: can ultrasound predict the presence of vesicoureteral reflux. *Pediatr Nephrol.* 2007;22(1):91–96. doi:10.1007/S00467-006-0285-1

99. Farhat W, Mclorie G, Geary D, et al. The natural history of neonatal vesicoureteral reflux associated with antenatal hydronephrosis. *J Urol.* 2000;164(3 Pt 2):1057–1060. doi:10.1097/00005392-200009020-00033

100. St. Aubin M, Willihnganz-Lawson K, Varda BK, et al. Society for Fetal Urology recommendations for postnatal evaluation of prenatal hydronephrosis—will fewer voiding cystourethrograms lead to more urinary tract infections? *J Urol.* 2013;190(suppl 4):1456–1461. doi:10.1016/J.JURO.2013.03.038

101. Braga LH, Farrokhyar F, D'Cruz J, Pemberton J, Lorenzo AJ. Risk factors for febrile urinary tract infection in children with prenatal hydronephrosis: a prospective study. *J Urol.* 2015;193(suppl 5):1766–1771. doi:10.1016/J.JURO.2014.10.091

102. Silay MS, Undre S, Nambiar AK, et al. Role of antibiotic prophylaxis in antenatal hydronephrosis: a systematic review

from the European Association of Urology/European Society for Paediatric Urology Guidelines Panel. *J Pediatr Urol.* 2017;13(3):306–315. doi:10.1016/J.JPUROL.2017.02.023

103. Easterbrook B, Capolicchio JP, Braga LH. Antibiotic prophylaxis for prevention of urinary tract infections in prenatal hydronephrosis: an updated systematic review. *Can Urol Assoc J.* 2017;11(1-2 suppl 1):S3–S11. doi:10.5489/CUAJ.4384

104. Zareba P, Lorenzo AJ, Braga LH. Risk factors for febrile urinary tract infection in infants with prenatal hydronephrosis: comprehensive single center analysis. *J Urol.* 2014;191(suppl 5):1614–1619. doi:10.1016/J.JURO.2013.10.035

105. Coelho GM, Bouzada MCF, Pereira AK, et al. Outcome of isolated antenatal hydronephrosis: a prospective cohort study. *Pediatr Nephrol.* 2007;22(10):1727–1734. doi:10.1007/S00467-007-0539-6

106. Szymanski KM, Al-Said AN, Pippi Salle JL, Capolicchio JP. Do infants with mild prenatal hydronephrosis benefit from screening for vesicoureteral reflux? *J Urol.* 2012;188(2):576–581. doi:10.1016/J.JURO.2012.04.017

107. Alsaywid BS, Saleh H, Deshpande A, Howman-Giles R, Smith GHH. High grade primary vesicoureteral reflux in boys: long-term results of a prospective cohort study. *J Urol.* 2010;184(suppl 4):1598–1603. doi:10.1016/J.JURO.2010.04.021

108. Wang ZT, Wehbi E, Alam Y, Khoury A. A reanalysis of the RIVUR trial using a risk classification system. *J Urol.* 2018;199(6):1608–1614. doi:10.1016/J.JURO.2017.11.080

109. Garcia-Roig M, Travers C, McCracken CE, Kirsch AJ. National trends in the management of primary vesicoureteral reflux in children. *J Urol.* 2018;199(1):287–293. doi:10.1016/J.JURO.2017.09.073

110. Roussey-Kesler G, Gadjos V, Idres N, et al. Antibiotic prophylaxis for the prevention of recurrent urinary tract infection in children with low grade vesicoureteral reflux: results from a prospective randomized study. *J Urol.* 2008;179(2):674–679. doi:10.1016/J.JURO.2007.09.090

111. Holmdahl G, Brandström P, Läckgren G, et al. The Swedish Reflux Trial in children: II. vesicoureteral reflux outcome. *J Urol.* 2010;184(1):280–285. doi:10.1016/J.JURO.2010.01.059

112. Cooper CS, Chung BI, Kirsch AJ, Canning DA, Snyder HM. The outcome of stopping prophylactic antibiotics in older children with vesicoureteral reflux. *J Urol.* 2000;163(1):269–273. doi:10.1016/S0022-5347(05)68034-2

113. Kitchens DM, Herndon A, Joseph DB. Outcome after discontinuing prophylactic antibiotics in children with persistent vesicoureteral reflux. *J Urol.* 2010;184(suppl 4):1594–1597. doi:10.1016/J.JURO.2010.04.020

114. King LR. Megaloureter: definition, diagnosis and management. *J Urol.* 1980;123(2):222–223. doi:10.1016/S0022-5347(17)55867-X

115. Cussen LJ. Dimensions of the normal ureter in infancy and childhood. *Invest Urol.* 1967;5(2):164–178.

116. Hellstrom M, Hjalmas K, Jacobsson B, Jodal U, Odén A. Normal ureteral diameter in infancy and childhood. *Acta Radiol Diagn (Stockh).* 1985;26(4):433–439. doi:10.1177/028418510502600412

117. Shukla AR, Cooper J, Patel RP, et al. Prenatally detected primary megaureter: a role for extended followup. *J Urol.* 2005;173(4):1353–1356. doi:10.1097/01.JU.0000152319.72909.52

118. McLellan DL, Retik AB, Bauer SB, et al. Rate and predictors of spontaneous resolution of prenatally diagnosed primary

nonrefluxing megaureter. *J Urol.* 2002;168(5):2177–2180. doi:10.1097/01.JU.0000034943.31317.2F

119. Chertin B, Pollack A, Koulikov D, et al. Long-term follow up of antenatally diagnosed megaureters. *J Pediatr Urol.* 2008;4(3):188–191. doi:10.1016/J.JPUROL.2007.11.013

120. Braga LH, D'Cruz J, Rickard M, Jegatheeswaran K, Lorenzo AJ. The fate of primary nonrefluxing megaureter: a prospective outcome analysis of the rate of urinary tract infections, surgical indications and time to resolution. *J Urol.* 2016;195(4):1300–1305. doi:10.1016/J.JURO.2015.11.049

121. Anumba DO, Scott JE, Plant ND, Robson SC. Diagnosis and outcome of fetal lower urinary tract obstruction in the northern region of England. *Prenat Diagn.* 2005;25(1):7–13. doi:10.1002/PD.1074

122. Malin G, Tonks AM, Morris RK, Gardosi J, Kilby MD. Congenital lower urinary tract obstruction: a population-based epidemiological study. *BJOG.* 2012;119(12):1455–1464. doi:10.1111/J.1471-0528.2012.03476.X

123. Smith JM, Stablein DM, Munoz R, Hebert D, McDonald RA. Contributions of the Transplant Registry: The 2006 Annual Report of the North American Pediatric Renal Trials and Collaborative Studies (NAPRTCS). *Pediatr Transplant.* 2007; 11(4):366–373. doi:10.1111/J.1399-3046.2007.00704.X

124. Drozdz D, Drozdz M, Gretz N, Möhring K, Mehls O, Schärer K. Progression to end-stage renal disease in children with posterior urethral valves. *Pediatr Nephrol.* 1998;12(8): 630–636. doi:10.1007/S004670050517

125. Heikkilä J, Holmberg C, Kyllönen L, Rintala R, Taskinen S. Long-term risk of end stage renal disease in patients with posterior urethral valves. *J Urol.* 2011;186(6):2392–2396. doi:10.1016/j.juro.2011.07.109

126. DeFoor W, Clark C, Jackson E, Reddy P, Minevich E, Sheldon C. Risk factors for end stage renal disease in children with posterior urethral valves. *J Urol.* 2008;180(suppl 4):1705–1708. doi:10.1016/J.JURO.2008.03.090

127. Braga LH, Mijovic H, Farrokhyar F, Pemberton J, DeMaria J, Lorenzo AJ. Antibiotic prophylaxis for urinary tract infections in antenatal hydronephrosis. *Pediatrics.* 2013;131(1):e251–e261. doi:10.1542/PEDS.2012-1870

128. Lee JH, Choi HS, Kim JK, et al. Nonrefluxing neonatal hydronephrosis and the risk of urinary tract infection. *J Urol.* 2008;179(4):1524–1528. doi:10.1016/J.JURO.2007.11.090

129. Herz D, Merguerian P, McQuiston L. Continuous antibiotic prophylaxis reduces the risk of febrile UTI in children with asymptomatic antenatal hydronephrosis with either ureteral dilation, high-grade vesicoureteral reflux, or ureterovesical junction obstruction. *J Pediatr Urol.* 2014;10(4):650–654. doi:10.1016/J.JPUROL.2014.06.009

130. Chandran L, Latorre P. Neonatal circumcisions performed by pediatric residents: implementation of a training program. *Ambul Pediatr.* 2002;2(6):470–474.

131. Braga LH, Pemberton J, Heaman J, Demaria J, Lorenzo AJ. Pilot randomized, placebo controlled trial to investigate the effect of antibiotic prophylaxis on the rate of urinary tract infection in infants with prenatal hydronephrosis. *J Urol.* 2014;191(suppl 5):1501–1507. doi:10.1016/J.JURO.2013.10.033

132. Holzman SA, Braga LH, Zee RS, et al. Risk of urinary tract infection in patients with hydroureter: an analysis from the Society of Fetal Urology Prenatal Hydronephrosis Registry. *J Pediatr Urol.* 2021;17(6):775–781. doi:10.1016/J.JPUROL.2021.09.001

133. Braga LH, McGrath M, Farrokhyar F, Jegatheeswaran K, Lorenzo AJ. Associations of initial Society for Fetal Urology grades and urinary tract dilatation risk groups with clinical outcomes in patients with isolated prenatal hydronephrosis. *J Urol.* 2017;197(3 Pt 2):831–837. doi:10.1016/J.JURO.2016.08.099

134. Leigh J, Rickard M, Sanger S, Petropoulos J, Braga LH, Chanchlani R. Antibiotic prophylaxis for prevention of urinary tract infections in the first year of life in children with vesicoureteral reflux diagnosed in the workup of antenatal hydronephrosis: a systematic review. *Pediatr Nephrol.* 2020;35(9):1639–1646. doi:10.1007/S00467-020-04568-6

135. Walsh TJ, Hsieh S, Grady R, Mueller BA. Antenatal hydronephrosis and the risk of pyelonephritis hospitalization during the first year of life. *Urology.* 2007;69(5):970–974. doi:10.1016/J.UROLOGY.2007.01.062

136. Varda BK, Finkelstein JB, Wang HH, Logvinenko T, Nelson CP. The association between continuous antibiotic prophylaxis and UTI from birth until initial postnatal imaging evaluation among newborns with antenatal hydronephrosis. *J Pediatr Urol.* 2018; 14(6):539.e1–539.e6. doi:10.1016/J.JPUROL.2018.04.022

137. Shaikh N, Haralam MA, Kurs-Lasky M, Hoberman A. Association of renal scarring with number of febrile urinary tract infections in children. *JAMA Pediatr.* 2019;173(10):949–952. doi:10.1001/JAMAPEDIATRICS.2019.2504

138. Finnell SME, Carroll AE, Roberts KB, et al. Technical report—diagnosis and management of an initial UTI in febrile infants and young children. *Pediatrics.* 2011;128(3):e749–e770. doi:10.1542/PEDS.2011-1332

139. Shaikh N, Mattoo TK, Keren R, et al. Early antibiotic treatment for pediatric febrile urinary tract infection and renal scarring. *JAMA Pediatr.* 2016;170(9):848–854. doi:10.1001/JAMAPEDIATRICS.2016.1181

140. Chamberlin JD, Braga LH, Davis-Dao CA. Continuous antibiotic prophylaxis in isolated prenatal hydronephrosis. *J Pediatr Urol.* 2022; 18(3):363. doi: 10.1016/j.jpurol.2022.03.027

141. Allen UD, MacDonald N, Fuite L, Chan F, Stephens D. Risk factors for resistance to "first-line" antimicrobials among urinary tract isolates of *Escherichia coli* in children. *CMAJ.* 1999;160(10):1436–1440.

142. Cheng C-H, Tsai M-H, Huang Y-C, et al. Antibiotic resistance patterns of community-acquired urinary tract infections in children with vesicoureteral reflux receiving prophylactic antibiotic therapy. *Pediatrics.* 2008;122(6):1212–1217. doi:10.1542/peds.2007-2926

143. Cooper CS. Fat, demented and stupid: an unrecognized legacy of pediatric urology? *J Pediatr Urol.* 2017;13(4):341–344. doi:10.1016/J.JPUROL.2017.04.027

144. Guidos PJ, Arlen AM, Leong T, Bonnett MA, Cooper CS. Impact of continuous low-dose antibiotic prophylaxis on growth in children with vesicoureteral reflux. *J Pediatr Urol.* 2018;14(4): 325.e1–325.e7. doi:10.1016/J.JPUROL.2018.07.007

145. Gaither TW, Cooper CS, Kornberg Z, Baskin LS, Copp HL. Predictors of becoming overweight among pediatric patients at risk for urinary tract infections. *J Pediatr Urol.* 2019;15(1): 61.e1–61.e6. doi:10.1016/J.JPUROL.2018.09.002

146. Akagawa Y, Kimata T, Akagawa S, et al. Impact of long-term low dose antibiotic prophylaxis on gut microbiota in children. *J Urol.* 2020;204(6):1320–1325. doi:10.1097/JU.0000000000001227

147. Copp HL, Nelson CP, Shortliffe LD, Lai J, Saigal CS, Kennedy WA. Compliance with antibiotic prophylaxis in children with

vesicoureteral reflux: results from a national pharmacy claims database. *J Urol.* 2010;183(5):1994–2000. doi:10.1016/J.JURO.2010.01.036

148. Davenport MT, Merguerian PA, Koyle M. Antenatally diagnosed hydronephrosis: current postnatal management. *Pediatr Surg Int.* 2013;29(3):207–214. doi:10.1007/S00383-012-3258-4

149. Kose E, Yavascan O, Turan O, et al. The effect of circumcision on the frequency of urinary tract infection, growth and nutrition status in infants with antenatal hydronephrosis. *Ren Fail.* 2013;35(10):1365–1369. doi:10.3109/0886022X.2013.828263

150. Fusco NM, Islam S, Polischuk E. Optimal antibiotics at hospital discharge for children with urinary tract infection. *Hosp Pediatr.* 2020;10(5):438–442. doi:10.1542/HPEDS.2019-0301

Chapter 12

Dialysis and Kidney Transplantation in Infancy

Heather A. Morgans, DO, MS, and Bradley A. Warady, MD

Chapter Outline

Introduction

Although the provision of dialysis and the need for a kidney transplant during infancy is rare, medical advancements have led to increased availability and efficacy of these treatments when needed worldwide. Data from the US Renal Data System (USRDS) show that the overall incidence of pediatric end-stage kidney disease (ESKD) requiring dialysis or transplantation has decreased slightly from 12 cases per million people in 2009 to 11 cases per million people in 2019. Despite this decrease, the <1-year-old age group remains the highest pediatric incidence group with an adjusted ESKD incidence rate of 27 cases per million people in 2019.[1] As more medically complex infants with severe kidney disorders are surviving with the help of prenatal diagnoses, in utero interventions, and multidisciplinary maternal fetal medicine teams with detailed postnatal plans for treatment, it is not surprising that a growing number of these infants will require dialysis and kidney transplantation in the future. With the need for optimal management strategies for these infants, novel treatment regimens and the introduction of new technology have been incorporated as part of complex patient care with a goal of reducing overall morbidity and mortality. Despite these improvements, there continues to be a higher morbidity and mortality rate in infants compared to older children with ESKD, reinforcing the need for continued improvement in therapies associated with the care of infants with acute and chronic kidney disease (CKD).

Indications for Kidney Replacement Therapy

Kidney replacement therapy (KRT) encompasses treatment with any dialysis modality including peritoneal dialysis (PD), hemodialysis (HD), or continuous kidney replacement therapy (CKRT). Both PD and HD can be used for the management of either acute kidney injury (AKI) or ESKD, whereas CKRT is reserved for intensive care unit (ICU) care. The specific dialysis modality chosen for treatment is typically based on the underlying condition and characteristics of the patient such as size, comorbidities, and overall hemodynamic stability, in addition to the resources and expertise available at the treating institution.

KIDNEY REPLACEMENT THERAPY FOR THE MANAGEMENT OF ACUTE KIDNEY INJURY

AKI occurs in up to 25% of all neonatal and pediatric ICU admissions and is associated with elevated rates of morbidity and mortality. Risk factors for the development of AKI in neonates and infants include immature development of the kidneys combined with exposure to nephrotoxic medications, renal hypoperfusion related to sepsis or hypovolemia, or direct injury to the kidneys from infection, a hypoxic event, or thrombosis.[2-4] Special populations including very low birth weight infants and those requiring cardiopulmonary bypass or extracorporeal membrane oxygenation have also been shown to be at higher risk for the development of AKI.[5]

The initial treatment of AKI consists of medical management with a focus on supportive therapy and resolution of the inciting event. For sequela of AKI unresponsive to medical management, such as electrolyte disturbances (hyperkalemia, acidosis), fluid overload and the associated cardiovascular manifestations, or an inability to provide full nutrition, KRT is indicated.[2,4] Another indication for KRT is an infant born with an inborn error of metabolism leading to hyperammonemia. Elevated ammonia levels (>200 μmol/L) are neurotoxic and associated with poor neurocognitive outcomes, whereas rising levels (>800 μmol/L) can lead to cerebral edema and death. Acute management of hyperammonemia, for which consensus guidelines have been published, includes cessation of protein intake and introduction of intravenous glucose and lipids for neonates with ammonia levels that are elevated for age.[5] Initiation of a nitrogen

scavenger medication is indicated for ammonia levels > 150 μmol/L or rapidly rising levels or for neonates with neurologic sequela. For neonates with ammonia levels > 400 μmol/L, levels < 400 μmol/L but not responding to medical therapies, or with clinical concern for the development of neurologic involvement, rapid reduction with the use of KRT is necessary to prevent neurologic damage. Ammonia levels should be reduced to <200 μmol/L with the use of KRT prior to discontinuation of the treatment. Close monitoring for rebound hyperammonemia is essential, especially when using HD. Ammonia is a small, non-protein-bound molecule (17 Da) that is readily removed with KRT. Depending on the patient characteristics and the resources available at the treating facility, treatment may be initiated with HD followed by continuous clearance with CKRT if needed, or CKRT can be used preferentially to effectively decrease ammonia levels. In centers where extracorporeal KRT is not available, PD should be used initially to decrease ammonia levels, with consideration for transfer to a center with HD or CKRT if levels are not decreasing rapidly.[5,6]

KIDNEY REPLACEMENT THERAPY FOR THE MANAGEMENT OF CHRONIC KIDNEY DISEASE

The main etiology resulting in ESKD in children < 1 year of age is congenital anomalies of the kidneys and urinary tract (CAKUT), which makes up approximately 55% of all infantile ESKD diagnoses.[1] This includes infants with obstructive uropathy (e.g., posterior urethral valves), renal dysplasia or hypoplasia, and reflux nephropathy. The second most common etiology consists of cystic or genetic diseases such as congenital nephrotic syndrome and autosomal dominant or recessive polycystic kidney disease.[1] Indications for the provision of KRT for management of CKD/ESKD are similar to those for AKI and include the inability to medically manage fluid balance and nutritional status, as well as treatment resistant electrolyte and acid-base abnormalities.

Ethical Considerations for Kidney Replacement Therapy in Infants With Chronic Kidney Disease

Despite continued improvements in dialysis equipment and overall morbidity and mortality in infants with ESKD, there are several ethical dilemmas to consider in this population. Chronic dialysis during infancy, regardless of the modality, is associated with a significant burden on the family (e.g., parents) related to increased mental stress, financial needs, and time requirements. Parents are expected to give multiple medications several times per day, keep track of vital signs such as weight and blood pressure, and either conduct nightly PD at home or travel to the dialysis unit 3–6 times per week for their child to receive a 3- to 4-hour HD session. Not only are the patient and parents affected by the burdens of dialysis, but siblings are also often impacted by the necessity for so much parental attention being directed to the ill child.[7]

For infants with multiple comorbidities, especially severe neurologic disorders, it is important to discuss the parents' wishes for overall quality of life for their child. Establishing goals for quality of life can help guide treatment options, such as chronic dialysis, and determine if and when these treatments become futile.[8–11] Honest conversations regarding daily life with chronic dialysis and transplant, along with potential complications, is also imperative. For infants on chronic dialysis, life is often complicated by frequent hospital visits, repeated blood draws, dialysis complications and infections, and frequent nutrition assessments with formula modifications. Developmental delay is common for infants on chronic dialysis due to many factors including long hospitalizations, suboptimal nutrition, and the uremic milieu, which generally requires the support of physical, occupational, and speech therapy. Even after kidney transplantation, children require frequent clinic visits, blood draws, a variety of daily medications, multiple kidney transplants and/or additional courses of dialysis in the future.

Due to the complexities that often exist, not only is making decisions regarding initiation of chronic dialysis in infants difficult for the family, but it can also be challenging for the medical team. A survey completed in 2011 found that only 30% of nephrologists would always offer KRT to neonates < 1 month of age and that the majority of medical providers would consider parental refusal of dialysis as an acceptable alternative during the neonatal period. This is especially true in the setting of significant comorbidities and emphasizes the need for detailed discussions between the health-care providers and family members regarding the benefits and risks of long-term KRT.[12]

In many cases, the prenatal diagnosis of congenital kidney anomalies such as CAKUT or other significant genetic or cystic renal disorders is made following a prenatal ultrasound. Although the findings are most often distressing to the family, early detection allows for an in-depth discussion of the possible clinical course, treatment plans, and likely outcomes between the family and a multidisciplinary medical team (e.g., neonatologist, nephrologist, social worker, ethicist) before the baby is born. Despite differing ethical opinions that may arise pertaining to the provision of chronic dialysis to neonates and young infants with ESKD, the necessity for these initial and reoccurring multidisciplinary meetings with families is undisputed by pediatric kidney groups worldwide. Through the use of frequent communication and full discussion of current clinical status, prognosis, and treatment options, families can feel supported and informed as they are called upon to make lifelong decisions on behalf of their child.[13]

Dialysis Modalities

CONTINUOUS KIDNEY REPLACEMENT THERAPY

CKRT is a 24-hour continuous extracorporeal form of dialysis utilized in ICUs for infants and children who may be hemodynamically unstable or who may require an extracorporeal dialysis therapy for other reasons (e.g., recent abdominal surgery, omphalocele). With this modality, a CKRT machine is set up at the patient's bedside and can be connected to an extracorporeal membrane oxygenation circuit or directly to the patient through a double-lumen HD catheter. The CKRT machine pulls blood from the patient at a slow, constant rate, which decreases the risk of hypotension that can occur secondary to abrupt or large fluid shifts with HD. The blood is then run through a filter for removal of fluid and solute (e.g., potassium, urea, phosphorus) via diffusion and/or convection, based on one of three types of CKRT prescriptions, and returned back to the patient. Continuous venovenous hemofiltration utilizes convection to clear solute without the use of dialysis fluid. Continuous venovenous hemodialysis incorporates the use of dialysis fluid to clear solute via diffusion, whereas continuous venovenous hemodiafiltration combines the two methods to use both diffusion and convection (Fig. 12.1).

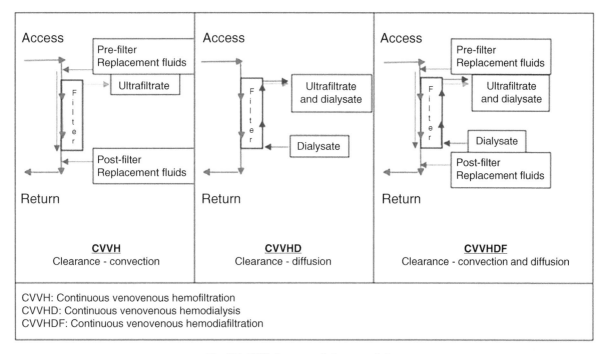

Fig. 12.1 CKRT diagram and clearance choices.

Diffusion is the movement of small to intermediate molecular weight molecules across a semipermeable membrane from an area of higher concentration to lower concentration. Convection is the mass movement of solute that accompanies fluid across a semipermeable membrane (termed solvent drag) from an area of high pressure to low pressure. More intermediate and large molecular weight molecules can be cleared with convection compared with diffusion (Fig. 12.2). In all types of CKRT, fluid removal (termed ultrafiltration) can be managed precisely by the medical team for gradual alterations in fluid balance to maintain cardiovascular stability and adequacy of nutritional support. CKRT is utilized for management of AKI until signs of kidney recovery are present or in patients with ESKD as a bridge to long-term dialysis with either HD or PD.[2,4]

Despite the benefits, there are several disadvantages of CKRT. Clearance is nonselective; therefore, beneficial electrolytes and nutrients accompany the waste products that are removed throughout the treatment. Although this is the case for all dialysis modalities, the impact is more significant with CKRT as a result of the continuous nature of the therapy, leading to potential difficulties with nutrition and bone and mineral management. Typically, protein, electrolyte, and vitamin (B_1, B_6, B_9, C) supplementation is required along with close monitoring of trace elements.[14] When not optimally managed, the protein-energy wasting related to CKRT can lead to poor weight gain and ultimately malnutrition, which in turn has been associated with higher mortality rates than what is experienced by those with an ideal body weight.[15,16] Ideally, CKRT should be used for a short duration to prevent excessive removal of these products, with special care taken in the design of the nutrition plan for each patient to ensure that the appropriate replacement nutrients are provided.

Other disadvantages of CKRT include the need for central venous access and anticoagulation. An effective central venous access that facilitates the performance of dialysis can be difficult to obtain and maintain in infants due to their small vessel size. It may result in long-term vascular injury and requires close

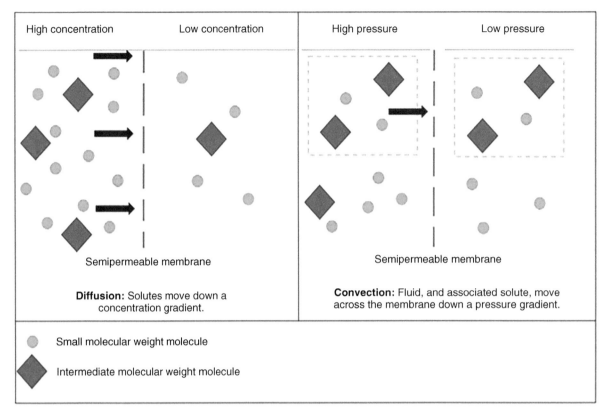

High concentration   Low concentration   High pressure   Low pressure

Semipermeable membrane   Semipermeable membrane

Diffusion: Solutes move down a
concentration gradient.

Convection: Fluid, and associated solute, move
across the membrane down a pressure gradient.

Small molecular weight molecule

Intermediate molecular weight molecule

Fig. 12.2 Diffusive and convective clearance.

monitoring for signs of infection or thrombosis. The therapy is time intensive and requires specially trained nurses, generally in a one-to-one patient-to-nurse ratio. To prevent blood clotting in the CKRT circuit during treatment, anticoagulation is generally required (except in the case of infants with substantial alterations of their coagulation status) and can lead to hematologic complications. A commonly used anticoagulation regimen consists of regional citrate and calcium, which has the advantage of acting locally only in the CKRT circuit but cannot be used in certain circumstances (e.g., infants with liver failure). Alternatives include systemic anticoagulation with continuous heparin or bivalirudin, therapies that may be associated with an increased risk for bleeding in critically ill infants. Initiation of CKRT can also precipitate hypotension or a bradykinin release syndrome, which is associated with certain filter membranes and can

lead to tachycardia, hypotension, anaphylaxis, and possible death. Strategies to decrease the risk for these potential complications have been published.[17]

Lastly, despite the frequent off-label use of CKRT in infants and young children, the current CKRT machines in the United States are only approved by the Food and Drug Administration for pediatric patients ≥ 20 kg. The majority of the CKRT circuit volumes far exceed 10% of the total blood volume for infants and require a blood prime to be used during the initiation of each CKRT circuit to prevent hemodynamic instability. Smaller filters are now available for children 8–20 kg in weight (HF20 filter), which decreases the need for a blood prime in some, but not all, infants. Newer technology has, thankfully, resulted in the development of three small but highly effective extracorporeal volume CKRT machines made specifically for neonates and infants. The Cardiac and Renal Pediatric

Dialysis Emergency Circuit (CARPEDIEM), Newcastle Infant Dialysis Ultrafiltration System (NIDUS), and the Aquadex dialysis machine all significantly decrease the need for blood product exposure in small infants.[2,4,18-20]

HEMODIALYSIS

HD is an efficient form of dialysis that is able to clear solute and remove fluid in short treatment sessions. Treatments are generally 3–4 hours in duration and are typically performed three times per week or more, depending on the individualized needs of the patient. The performance of HD in an infant requires central venous access with a double-lumen HD catheter. Similar to CKRT, blood flows from the patient through the catheter, passes through an HD filter against a countercurrent flow of dialysis fluid, and is returned back to the patient. Fluid removal, titrated by the medical team, occurs through the application of hydrostatic pressure. Since the treatment durations are short and are associated with a limited time for fluid removal, fluid shifts are larger with HD compared with CKRT and therefore are associated with a greater risk for hemodynamic instability in infants. Solute clearance, which occurs by diffusion and convection, is primarily controlled by the blood flow, with higher blood flow rates leading to higher clearance. HD can be utilized in hemodynamically stable infants with AKI or as part of long-term management in infants with ESKD (Fig. 12.3).[2,4]

The efficient solute clearance and fluid removal characteristic of HD alleviates fluid restrictions for nutrition and helps control uremia, electrolytes, and acid-base status. In addition, HD provides a means of chronic dialysis for those infants who do not have a functional peritoneal cavity (e.g., recent abdominal surgery or a history of severe peritonitis), which precludes the performance of PD (see later discussion). With treatments being completed in a dialysis unit, there is also less burden on the family with respect to completing dialysis tasks at home, although there continues to be a significant time- and stress-related burden on the family.

Challenges associated with HD during infancy are mainly associated with small patient size. Infants need to be large enough to tolerate placement of a double-lumen central venous catheter for vascular access.

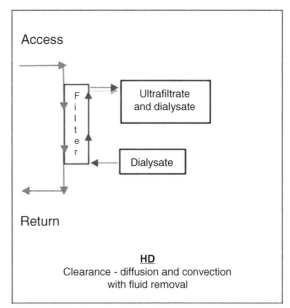

HD
Clearance - diffusion and convection
with fluid removal

Fig. 12.3 **HD diagram and clearance.** *HD*, hemodialysis.

These catheters are typically inserted into the right internal jugular vein to ensure a large enough vessel size to permit the required blood flow during HD treatments. Catheter malfunction from thrombosis or displacement and the development of bacteremia are common complications of HD catheters and mandate effective monitoring and the institution of evidence-based infection prevention strategies to mitigate these risks.[21,22] On average, HD catheter survival in patients < 2 years of age was approximately 3 months in one pediatric dialysis center, emphasizing the frequent need for catheter interventions and replacement in this age group.[23]

HD treatments require monitoring by a trained HD nurse, generally with a one-to-one patient-to-nurse ratio for infants, especially to ensure that intradialytic hemodynamic stability is maintained. As an extracorporeal therapy, HD requires anticoagulation to prevent blood clotting in the circuit. Generally, a bolus of heparin followed by a continuous heparin infusion is utilized throughout the HD treatment. General bleeding risks associated with anticoagulation use and patient-specific risk factors need to be monitored with each treatment.

It is also important to recognize the need to limit blood exposure in all infants with ESKD, so as to avoid developing antibodies, which makes finding an acceptable kidney donor for transplantation in the future more difficult. HD circuits have varying filter and tubing sizes designed to meet the needs of the patient, although the majority of neonates and small infants will still require a blood prime with each treatment if the circuit volume is >10% of their total blood volume. This requirement limits the use of HD as a preferred long-term dialytic option for ESKD management in a large proportion of neonates and infants.

Lastly, HD has been shown to cause myocardial stunning, defined as decreased myocardial blood flow with a reversible decrease in myocardial contractility during HD treatments. This is thought to be caused by intradialytic changes in blood pressure and is worsened by removing large amounts of fluid during HD treatments. Myocardial stunning during HD was first documented in pediatric patients in 2009 and because cardiovascular disease is the most common cause of death in people with ESKD, a great deal of attention has been directed to the prevention of this complication. Currently, control of intradialytic blood pressure along with closely monitoring and limiting fluid removal during any single dialysis session has been recommended to prevent excessive myocardial stunning with a goal of decreasing cardiovascular morbidity and mortality.[24,25]

PERITONEAL DIALYSIS

PD is the dialysis modality of choice for the majority (>90%) of neonates and infants requiring KRT for management of AKI or ESKD.[1] PD utilizes the peritoneal membrane as a dialyzing membrane across which fluid and solute are removed via convection and diffusion. The PD access consists of a catheter inserted through the abdominal wall, generally on the right side away from the diaper area and any stomas. A chronic catheter should ideally be placed by a surgeon experienced in the operation, as failure of catheter function and the need for revision is very common in the young infant.[26] Typically, the catheter will have two Dacron cuffs and a downward or lateral facing exit site to optimize healing and decrease infection risk; an upgoing exit site is a significant risk factor for infection.[27] In small infants or neonates where there is minimal subcutaneous tissue, single-cuff catheters with the cuff situated adjacent to the peritoneum are sometimes required. In preterm neonates who are too small for a single-cuff PD catheter, an abdominal drain can be used for temporary access, although it requires replacement as soon as the baby is big enough for a cuffed catheter to decrease the risk of infection.[28]

During PD, dextrose-containing dialysis fluid is instilled through the PD catheter into the peritoneal cavity. A variety of dextrose concentrations are available, all creating an osmotic gradient to facilitate fluid removal (ultrafiltration). As fluid is removed, solute also moves across the peritoneal membrane down a concentration gradient allowing for diffusion of electrolytes and solute. The dialysis fluid dwells in the peritoneal cavity for a prescribed amount of time allowing for solute clearance and fluid removal to occur and is then drained from the abdomen via the PD catheter, completing a single dialysis exchange or cycle. This is repeated a prescribed number of times over 24 hours with each exchange conducted either manually or by an automated cycling machine (Fig. 12.4). Clearance is nonselective, therefore beneficial electrolytes and nutrients are also removed during treatment and may mandate replacement. The weight-related loss of protein with PD is the greatest during infancy and requires specific attention when developing and assessing nutrition regimens.

A PD catheter should ideally be allowed to heal for 2 weeks following placement prior to initiating

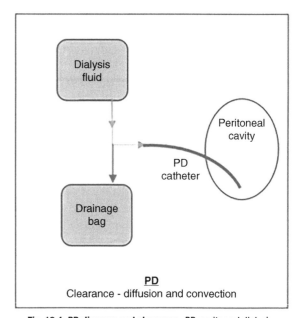

Fig. 12.4 PD diagram and clearance. *PD*, peritoneal dialysis.

dialysis to help optimize healing and prevent leakage of dialysis fluid through the PD catheter exit site. However, the delay in usage is often not possible, especially in the neonate or infant for whom an extracorporeal therapy may not be available, because of the need to institute dialysis promptly for AKI or ESKD management. In turn, a low fill volume of dialysis fluid, usually 10 mL/kg per exchange, is used at PD initiation and is gradually increased to a goal volume of around 35–40 mL/kg or 600 mL/m^2, as tolerated by the patient. Infants with small initial fill volumes require a one-to-one patient-to-nursing ratio with a nurse trained to conduct manual PD as the treatments are time intensive and require close monitoring for complications. Depending on the tolerance of the individual patient, fill volumes are advanced every few days by the managing team. Patients typically require manual PD until fill volumes reach 120–150 mL per cycle, at which time an automated PD cycler can be used to conduct the dialysis exchanges. The final PD prescription for young infants with ESKD generally consists of 6–10 cycles each night and a fill volume of 600–800 mL/m^2 per exchange delivered by an automated cycling device. PD treatments are generally completed by caregivers at home over 10 hours nightly, while the patient is sleeping.[29] Parents undergo rigorous training on how to initiate, manage, and discontinue PD treatments at home, with a focus on infection prevention, identification of potential complications, and emergency protocols.

Benefits of PD for the neonate and infant with kidney failure include the ability to utilize this modality for hospital management of AKI as well as for the long-term management of ESKD at home. It is conducted without the need for central venous access, repeated blood transfusions, or anticoagulation. The fact that it can be conducted at home also reduces the time the patient and parents need to spend at a medical facility, which may decrease the overall burden of care on the family. Since PD treatments are completed nightly with fluid and solute removal, nutrition restrictions can frequently be liberalized to allow more fluid and electrolytes (e.g., special infant formula) to be provided. PD is also the most cost-efficient dialysis modality. Patients requiring dialysis in resource limited areas are more likely to utilize PD than either CKRT or HD for management of AKI and ESKD.

Although PD is generally the preferred method of dialysis during infancy, there are several challenges

associated with the therapy. Infection, most commonly peritonitis, is the most serious complication and is the primary factor resulting in patient morbidity and mortality in infants. The frequency of peritonitis is greatest in the younger age groups, and it is one of the most common reasons for hospitalization of infants on PD.[30,31] Infants also have a higher risk compared with older children of developing an early PD catheter leak, which further increases the risk for infection.[32] In a study of children < 2 years of age and receiving PD, PD catheter survival was approximately 9.1 months prior to needing some type of intervention or replacement for either infection-related complications or catheter dysfunction.[23] In addition, the need for catheter revision within the initial 3 months of dialysis has been associated with an increased risk for PD technique failure.[26]

Peritonitis can lead to peritoneal membrane scarring and less effective or ineffective PD. Likewise, the development of peritonitis during the neonate's initial hospitalization when PD is initiated has been associated with an increased mortality risk.[33] This has led to several initiatives focused on decreasing peritonitis rates in this population such as the multicenter Standardizing Care to Improve Outcomes in Pediatric ESKD (SCOPE) quality improvement collaborative. SCOPE has developed several catheter care bundles aimed to decrease infection rates and has documented significant success with a decrease in peritonitis rates in children on PD from 0.53 infections per patient-year to 0.30 infections per patient-year at 84 months after initiation of the collaborative.[34]

Additional complications of PD include PD catheter malfunction, the development of umbilical or inguinal hernias due to increased intraperitoneal pressure resulting from the presence of dialysis fluid, or hyperglycemia related to the dextrose concentration of the dialysate. Higher dextrose concentrations in the dialysis fluid leads to a higher osmotic gradient, which can produce more fluid removal than may be necessary in some infants. Ideally, use of the lowest dextrose concentration possible that results in adequate ultrafiltration is preferred to prevent hyperglycemia and to decrease the risk of peritoneal membrane injury, which can ultimately lead to PD failure.

Finally, for safe and reliable home-based PD treatments to occur, most dialysis centers require two trained caregivers in an attempt to avoid burnout of the primary caregiver. Nevertheless, there is a significant burden of care experienced by the family as the caregivers must learn how to manage PD at home, regularly monitor vital signs, administer medications, and frequently oversee enteral tube feeding, all of which is very time intensive. For single-parent households without significant external support, PD may not be the best modality choice for the patient because of these requirements for the parent. Accordingly, discussions between the medical team, dietitian, social worker, and family prior to the initiation of this long-term dialysis modality is imperative so as to educate family members on the treatment expectations, the usual course of treatment, and potential complications, so that following a philosophy of shared decision-making, the best treatment option for the patient and family is selected (Table 12.1).

Due to the complexity of dialysis in children, several international collaborations have written guidelines for the optimal management of both acute and chronic PD. Some of these collaborations include the Kidney Disease Outcomes Quality Initiative (KDOQI), the International Society for Peritoneal Dialysis, the Canadian Association of Pediatric Nephrologists, and the European Pediatric Dialysis Working Group.[35–39] These guidelines include evidenced and expert opinion-based recommendations for optimal pediatric PD prescription management, evaluation of dialysis adequacy, monitoring for comorbidities, and treatment recommendations for common complications.

Comorbidities Associated With End-Stage Kidney Disease

NUTRITION

Nutrition and growth are two factors that are negatively affected in infants with ESKD requiring KRT. Since adequate nutrition has the greatest influence on achieved growth velocity in infants with ESKD, it is a significant area of focus in the management of these

TABLE 12.1   Comparison of Kidney Replacement Therapy Modalities

Dialysis Modality	CKRT	HD	PD
Benefits	• Can be used in hemodynamically unstable infants o Gradual fluid removal and continuous clearance • Newer options with small extracorporeal circuit volumes may decrease blood prime needs • Used in AKI or as a bridge to long-term dialysis management	• Shorter treatment duration • Performed at pediatric dialysis centers, which can decrease burden on families • Used in AKI or CKD	• Can be used in hemodynamically unstable infants • No need for central venous access • Treatments can be completed at home by caregivers • No blood prime exposures • Used in AKI or CKD
Potential complications in infants	• Blood exposure if circuit volume is > 10% of patient blood volume • Requires anticoagulation • Need for central venous access • Vascular access complications: thrombosis, infection, displacement	• May require up to daily treatments to control fluid balance and electrolytes • Requires anticoagulation • Blood exposure if circuit volume is >10% of patient blood volume • Need for central venous access • Vascular access complications: thrombosis, infection, displacement • Myocardial stunning	• Requires training and adequate support at home to complete treatment daily • Risk of peritonitis • PD catheter complications, migration, infection, malfunction

AKI, acute kidney injury; *CKD*, chronic kidney disease; *CKRT*, continuous kidney replacement therapy; *HD*, hemodialysis; *PD*, peritoneal dialysis.

patients.[40] Factors that may predispose to poor nutrition and growth include decreased appetite and recurrent emesis, renal salt wasting in polyuric kidney disease, renal osteodystrophy related to secondary hyperparathyroidism, chronic metabolic acidosis, and growth hormone resistance. Due to these factors and because infancy is typically a period of rapid growth, the growth and nutritional status of infants with ESKD should be monitored at least monthly, as recently recommended by the Pediatric Renal Nutrition Taskforce.[41] Many infants require assistance to reliably receive the necessary formula intake, generally in the form of gastrostomy tube feedings. It is imperative to note that gastrostomy tubes should be placed before or at the time of PD catheter placement for infants receiving PD to decrease the risk of developing peritonitis subsequent to the procedure.[37,42]

Both KDOQI and the Pediatric Renal Nutrition Taskforce have developed nutrition guidelines for children with CKD/ESKD, which summarize important requirements and modifications needed based on CKD stage and dialysis modality.[43–46] Infants with CKD/ESKD should receive 100% of daily estimated energy requirements for age, 100% of daily required intake (DRI) of protein (plus a supplement to account for protein and amino acid losses through dialysis), 100%–200% of DRI of calcium for age, and a daily water-soluble renal multivitamin. Sodium supplementation due to sodium wasting is also frequently required to promote growth, especially for infants with polyuria. Infants receiving PD require sodium supplementation as well due to sodium losses in the drained dialysate. Appropriate supplementation is also imperative as sodium depletion caused by dialysis can result in hypotension and acute onset of blindness secondary to anterior ischemic optic neuropathy.[47,48] Potassium, phosphorus, and vitamin A are frequently restricted in patients with ESKD to avoid hyperkalemia, hyperphosphatemia, and vitamin A toxicity, respectively. It is also recommended to monitor and supplement as needed several micronutrients including the B vitamins, vitamin C, vitamin E, vitamin K, folic acid, cooper, and zinc. Whereas the most recent KDOQI nutrition guidelines do not recommend routine supplementation of carnitine in patients with ESKD for lack of evidence, several studies have suggested that carnitine deficiency can lead to erythropoietin-resistant anemia, muscle weakness, and cardiomyopathy.[43,49] With recognition of the complexity of nutritional requirements in infants with ESKD, it is necessary to collaborate with a pediatric renal dietician to ensure that optimal nutritional requirements are being met on a regular basis.[50]

In 2018, the USRDS reported that approximately 55% of infants met the criteria for short stature at ESKD diagnosis.[51] For infants with continued poor growth despite optimal management of nutrition, chronic kidney disease-mineral bone disorder (CKD-MBD), and correction of acidosis, initiation of recombinant growth hormone (rhGH) supplementation is warranted. In most cases during infancy, rhGH is prescribed starting at >1 year of age. The need for rhGH in the setting of ESKD is a result of decreased clearance of insulin growth factor-1 (IGF-1) binding protein, which leads to an increased percentage of IGF-1 being bound to protein and therefore inactive. The decrease in free IGF-1 in the body mimics growth hormone resistance leading to poor linear growth. Supplementation with exogenous growth hormone leads to increased levels of free IGF-1 and improved growth velocity. Short stature related to ESKD has been shown to decrease quality of life in adults with childhood-onset ESKD, which emphasizes the need to be vigilant and treat short stature early in life to improve long-term outcomes.[28,52,53]

CHRONIC KIDNEY DISEASE-MINERAL BONE DISORDER

Patients with ESKD develop CKD-MBD related to imbalances in the calcium, phosphorus, parathyroid hormone (PTH), and fibroblast growth factor-23 axis, which can result in bone and cardiovascular disease. As previously discussed, infants with CKD/ESKD require 100%–200% DRI of total calcium for age. The higher calcium requirements are due to the rapid growth and bone turnover characteristics of the infant age group, along with poor enteral calcium absorption. CKD-MBD can manifest with inadequate bone turnover as adynamic bone disease if calcium levels are elevated and PTH is suppressed. Conversely, it can be characterized by excessive bone turnover via secondary hyperparathyroidism, with elevated PTH and generally normal calcium and phosphorus levels. With CKD/ESKD, there is inadequate activation of vitamin D in the kidneys by α-1-hydroxylase. Therefore, supplementation with

25-OH vitamin D and 1-25 OH vitamin D are often needed to maintain bone health. Uncontrolled CKD-MBD increases the risk for poor growth, fractures, and bony malformations. Treatment goals include maintaining normal calcium and phosphorus levels for age and titrating medications to maintain PTH levels less than twice the upper limit of normal for age for infants with ESKD.[28]

CARDIOVASCULAR

The leading cause of death in all pediatric ESKD patients, including infants, is cardiovascular disease.[1] Therefore, significant attention is placed on monitoring blood pressure both during dialysis and between treatments. Infants can develop either hypotension or hypertension leading to arrhythmias or long-term cardiac damage. Hypotension can result from inadequate sodium supplementation or decreased intravascular volume related either to dehydration or overaggressive ultrafiltration or it may be secondary to prescribed medications such as antihypertensive agents. Hypertension is generally seen in infants with excess sodium supplementation or intravascular fluid overload. Treatment goals include maintaining normotension and monitoring cardiac function with routine echocardiograms.[28]

HEMATOLOGIC

Anemia is a frequent comorbidity of ESKD, largely due to iron deficiency and decreased native erythropoietin production from the kidneys. Maintenance iron supplementation along with the use of erythropoiesis-stimulating agents (ESAs) should be prescribed to help maintain hemoglobin in the ideal range of 11–12 gm/dL based on the Kidney Disease: Improving Global Outcomes guidelines.[54] Concerns with persistent anemia in infants with ESKD include potential detrimental effects on neurodevelopmental outcomes, although evidence supporting this relationship is limited. Most importantly, it should be recognized that infants require higher doses of ESAs than older children to achieve target hemoglobin levels. At the same time, excessive dosing of ESAs and hemoglobin < 11 g/dL have both been associated with an increased mortality risk for patients on PD and therefore need to be monitored closely with treatment modifications instituted as deemed necessary.[28,55]

Outcomes Associated With Infant Dialysis

Despite improvements in the prevention and treatment of comorbidities, infants with ESKD continue to have higher hospitalization, morbidity, and mortality rates compared with children > 1 year of age with ESKD. The majority of hospitalizations in the youngest infants with ESKD are related to infection during the first year of ESKD diagnosis; 1.06 hospitalizations per person-year equating to approximately 10.9 hospitalization days per person-year.[1] Although first-year mortality rates in infants with ESKD (dialysis and transplant) continue to improve, they continue to be the highest based on age group; 68.1 per 1000 person-years with an 80% 5-year survival probability in infants < 1 year of age at ESKD diagnosis, with the highest survival probability in the transplant group.[1] Specific to PD, survival rates for infants < 1 year at ESKD diagnosis are significantly improved when comparing outcomes from the USRDS database from 1990–1999 and 2000–2014 with 1- and 5-year survival rates in the latter era of 86.8% and 74.6% in infants who started PD at <1 month of age and 89.6% and 79.3% in older infants (PD initiation at 1–12 months), respectively. Risk for mortality in this cohort was greatest in the first 2 years after dialysis initiation (Fig. 12.5).[56] Similarly, a recent study evaluating mortality risk factors in infants who received dialysis during their neonatal ICU hospitalization found that 74% of the 273 patients across 415 neonatal ICUs in North America survived to discharge. Factors associated with increased mortality included patients without congenital kidney anomalies, those of Black race, and those with characteristics consistent with severe illness including necrotizing enterocolitis, gestational age < 32 weeks, the need for dialysis within 7 days of life, and the use of paralytics or vasopressors.[57] Thankfully, other long-term outcome parameters such as developmental status have shown improvements with the majority of infants who require dialysis at an early age meeting criteria for normal development later on in life and as candidates for kidney transplantation.[29,58]

Kidney Transplantation in Infancy
RECIPIENT CHARACTERISTICS

The goal for virtually all patients who receive KRT in infancy is to receive a kidney transplant early in life.

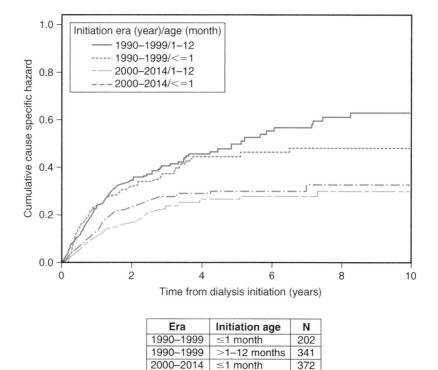

Era	Initiation age	N
1990–1999	≤1 month	202
1990–1999	>1–12 months	341
2000–2014	≤1 month	372
2000–2014	>1–12 months	808

Fig. 12.5 The cumulative cause-specific hazard plot of death on dialysis for infants initiated on chronic peritoneal dialysis (CPD) at age ≤ 12 months, stratified by age at CPD initiation and era of initiation. (Reprinted with permission from Sanderson KR, Yu Y, Dai H, Willig LK, Warady BA. Outcomes of infants receiving chronic peritoneal dialysis: an analysis of the USRDS registry. *Pediatr Nephrol.* 2018;34(1):155–162.)

Although not a cure, patient outcomes including growth, neurocognitive development, and quality of life are greatly improved after kidney transplantation compared with outcomes with chronic dialysis.[59] A limiting factor for receiving a kidney transplant during infancy is small patient size. Patients with ESKD generally need to be approximately 10–12 kg in weight and close to 2 years of age to have sufficient abdominal space to accept a transplanted kidney. Exact specifications and requirements vary between centers based on transplant surgeon experience and potentially the size of the donor kidney. Although kidney transplants have been performed in infants < 10 kg, the risk of complications such as thrombosis of the transplanted kidney's vessels due to their small size is increased.[59–61]

DONOR CHARACTERISTICS

The North American Pediatric Renal Trials and Collaborative Studies (NAPRTCS) previously found that deceased donors of both young and old age increased the risk of graft loss and that the ideal donor age is 20–25 years.[62] This has led to the majority of pediatric patients receiving adult kidneys for their kidney transplant. Two options are available for pediatric patients in need of a kidney transplant. A living donor kidney, either related or unrelated, is generally preferred over a deceased donor kidney for optimal matching and the shortest cold ischemia time, both of which are associated with improved long-term outcomes. Of the approximately 12,000 pediatric patients in the NAPRTCS database, 5.5% of transplanted patients were <1 year of age at transplantation and the majority received a living donor kidney transplant.[63] Infants frequently receive kidney donations from their parents, although nonrelated living kidney donations are increasing in frequency as well. Since pediatric kidney transplant recipients are likely going to require multiple kidney transplants in their lifetime as the average transplant half-life ranges between

12.5 and 15.3 years, finding the best match to allow the longest graft survival is imperative.[64] Both human leukocyte antigen and epitope matching between donors and recipients are evaluated prior to transplant to ensure the lowest risk of the patient developing significant antibodies against the transplanted kidney leading to acute or chronic kidney rejection.[59–61,65]

PRESURGICAL EVALUATION

There are several pediatric-specific considerations when evaluating a young patient for kidney transplant. Since CAKUT is the main etiology for kidney failure in infants and young children, pretransplant urologic evaluation is essential to ensure appropriate drainage and function of the urinary tract and bladder after kidney transplant. The presence of a low-pressure system is necessary for optimal function of the newly transplanted kidney. Subspecialty evaluation should also be completed based on comorbid conditions. This includes developmental and behavioral screening to assess baseline achievements and to establish a long-term relationship for ongoing care. Finally, children should receive all scheduled vaccines prior to transplantation to optimize antibody response and protection prior to the initiation of immunosuppressive medications.

INTRAOPERATIVE CONSIDERATIONS

In children < 2 years of age, time to transplant is similar for those receiving HD or PD, with the majority of procedures taking place approximately 20 months after dialysis initiation (Fig. 12.6).[66] To accommodate the large size of an adult kidney in small infants and children, the transplanted kidney is most often placed in the abdominal cavity in contrast to older children in whom it is placed retroperitoneally in the right or left pelvic region. Fluid management is a key aspect of intraoperative care with a goal to provide the patient with the volume required to ensure that the transplanted kidney is appropriately perfused, especially when the infant receives

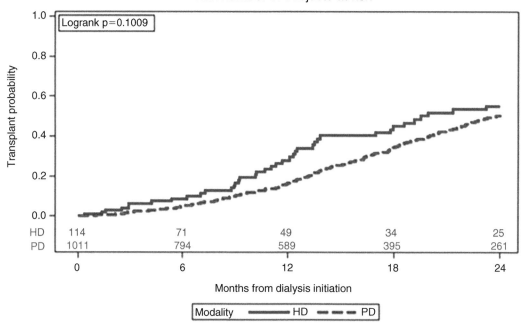

Fig. 12.6 Kaplan-Meier curves showing probability of transplantation postinitiation of dialysis, $P = .100$. *HD*, hemodialysis; *PD*, peritoneal dialysis. (Reprinted with permission from Yu ED, Galbiati S, Munshi R, Smith JM, Menon S. Practice patterns and outcomes of maintenance dialysis in children < 2 years of age: a report of the North American Pediatric Renal Trials and Collaborative Studies (NAPRTCS). *Pediatr Nephrol.* 2022;37(5):1117–1124.)

an adult kidney, while also aiming to avoid fluid over-load and a subsequent compromised cardiopulmonary status. There are several guidelines for immunosuppression regimens following kidney transplantation, which should be tailored to each individual patient with close monitoring for efficacy and toxicity.[59–61]

GRAFT AND PATIENT OUTCOME

Overall, the USRDS reports excellent kidney transplant graft outcomes in children with a 1-year adjusted incidence of graft failure of only 4.5% and 2.7% for deceased and living donors, respectively, in 2018.[1] Likewise, NAPRTCS reports significant improvement in kidney transplant survival in children < 2 years of age with a 1-year graft survival of approximately 98% and 5-year graft survival above 90% for both living and deceased donor recipients.[63] A recent report using the Organ Procurement and Transplantation Network Database evaluated kidney transplant in infants compared with older children. Fewer than 1% of transplants (27 total) were performed in infants, and although the graft failure rate in the first year posttransplant was higher in infants compared with older children (10.4% and 3.8%, respectively), 5-year outcomes (16.4%) were comparable to the older age groups (Fig. 12.7).[67] Excellent results have also been shown in the Scientific Registry of Transplant Recipients database with a 100% 5-year graft and overall patient survival in infants < 1 year at ESKD diagnosis from 2012 to 2014.[68] Posttransplant multidisciplinary visits, which include providers from nephrology, urology, social work, nutrition, pharmacy, and others as required by the individual patient, continue to be important to help ensure that appropriate care is being provided to these patients and families so that they experience the best possible outcome.[59–61]

Conclusion

Significant improvements have been made in the management of infants with AKI and ESKD who require dialysis and kidney transplantation. Attention to a variety of clinical issues that impact patient outcome by a multidisciplinary team of health-care providers is essential. The associated burden of care

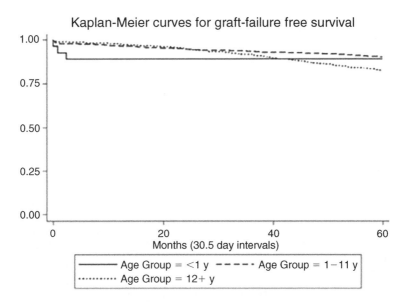

Kaplan-Meier curves for graft-free survival in various age groupings.

Fig. 12.7 Kaplan-Meier curves for graft-failure free survival in various age groupings. (Reprinted with permission from Tancredi D, Butani L. Uncovering a long-term graft survival advantage afforded by infant renal transplants—an organ procurement and Transplantation Network Database Analysis. *Transplant Direct.* 2021;8(1):e1267.)

on the family must also be appreciated and revisited on a regular basis with the required support provided. This is most evident in the infant with CKD who, along with the patient's family, must navigate a course of chronic dialysis therapy while working toward the ultimate goal of a successful kidney transplant.

REFERENCES

1. United States Renal Data System. *USRDS Annual Data Report: Epidemiology of Kidney Disease in the United States.* National Institutes of Health, National Institute of Diabetes and Digestive and Kidney Diseases; 2021.
2. Sanderson KR, Harshman LA. Renal replacement therapies for infants and children in the ICU. *Curr Opin Pediatr.* 2020;32(3):360–366. Available at: https://doi.org/10.1097/mop.0000000000000894
3. Noh J, Kim CY, Jung E, et al. Challenges of acute peritoneal dialysis in extremely-low-birth-weight infants: a retrospective cohort study. *BMC Nephrol* 21, 437 (2020). https://doi.org/10.1186/s12882-020-02092-1
4. Spector BL, Misurac JM. Renal replacement therapy in neonates. *Neoreviews.* 2019;20(12):e697–e710. Available at: https://doi.org/10.1542/neo.20-12-e697
5. Raina R, Bedoyan JK, Lichter-Konecki U, et al. Consensus guidelines for management of hyperammonaemia in paediatric patients receiving continuous kidney replacement therapy. *Nat Rev Nephrol.* 2020;16(8):471–482. Available at: https://doi.org/10.1038/s41581-020-0267-8
6. Kaddourah A, Goldstein SL. Renal replacement therapy in neonates. *Clin Perinatol.* 2014;41(3):517–527. doi:10.1016/j.clp.2014.05.003
7. Agerskov H, Thiesson HC, Pedersen BD. Siblings of children with chronic kidney disease: a qualitative study of everyday life experiences. *J Ren Care.* 2021;47(4):242–249. doi:10.1111/jorc.12389
8. Lantos JD, Warady BA. The evolving ethics of infant dialysis. *Pediatr Nephrol.* 2012;28(10):1943–1947. Available at: https://doi.org/10.1007/s00467-012-2351-1
9. Ranchin B, Plaisant F, Demède D, Guillebon JM, Javouhey E, Bacchetta J. Review: neonatal dialysis is technically feasible but ethical and global issues need to be addressed. *Acta Paediatr.* 2020;110(3):781–788. Available at: https://doi.org/10.1111/apa.15539
10. Wightman A. Caregiver burden in pediatric dialysis. *Pediatr Nephrol.* 2019;35(9):1575–1583. Available at: https://doi.org/10.1007/s00467-019-04332-5
11. Van Stralen KJ, Borzych-Duzałka D, Hataya H, et al. Survival and clinical outcomes of children starting renal replacement therapy in the neonatal period. *Kidney Int.* 2014;86(1):168–174. doi:10.1038/ki.2013.561
12. Teh JC, Frieling ML, Sienna JL, Geary DF. Attitudes of caregivers to management of end-stage renal disease in infants. *Perit Dial Int.* 2011;31(4):459–465. doi:10.3747/pdi.2009.00265
13. Rees L. Infant dialysis—what makes it special? *Nat Rev Nephrol.* 2012;9(1):15–17. Available at: https://doi.org/10.1038/nrneph.2012.263
14. Jonckheer J, Vergaelen K, Spapen H, Malbrain MLNG, De Waele E. Modification of nutrition therapy during continuous renal replacement therapy in critically ill pediatric patients: a narrative review and recommendations. *Nutr Clin Pract.* 2019;34(1):37–47. doi:10.1002/ncp.10231
15. Castillo A, Santiago MJ, López-Herce J, et al. Nutritional status and clinical outcome of children on continuous renal replacement therapy: a prospective observational study. *BMC Nephrol.* 2012;13:125. Published 2012 Sep 27. doi:10.1186/1471-2369-13-125
16. Lozano MJS, Álvarez CA, Heidbüchel CA, Lafever SF, García MJS, Cid JL-H. Nutrición en niños tratados con técnicas de depuración extrarrenal continua. *An Pediatr (Barc).* 2020;92:208–214.
17. Brophy PD, Mottes TA, Kudelka TL, et al. AN-69 membrane reactions are pH-dependent and preventable. *Am J Kidney Dis.* 2001;38(1):173–178. doi:10.1053/ajkd.2001.25212
18. Ronco C, Garzotto F, Brendolan A, et al. Continuous renal replacement therapy in neonates and small infants: development and first-in-human use of a miniaturised machine (CARPEDIEM). *Lancet.* 2014;383(9931):1807–1813.
19. Coulthard MG, Crosier J, Griffiths C, et al. Haemodialysing babies weighing <8 kg with the Newcastle infant dialysis and ultrafiltration system (Nidus): comparison with peritoneal and conventional haemodialysis. *Pediatr Nephrol.* 2014;29(10):1873–1881.
20. Askenazi D, Ingram D, White S, et al. Smaller circuits for smaller patients: improving renal support therapy with Aquadex™. *Pediatr Nephrol.* 2015;31(5):853–860. Available at: https://doi.org/10.1007/s00467-015-3259-3.
21. Das CJ, Razik A, Sharma S. Hemodialysis in infants: challenges and new paradigms. *J Vasc Interv Radiol.* 2020;31(5):787. Available at: https://doi.org/10.1016/j.jvir.2020.02.011
22. Marsenic O, Rodean J, Richardson T, et al. Tunneled hemodialysis catheter care practices and blood stream infection rate in children: results from the Scope Collaborative. *Pediatr Nephrol.* 2019;35(1):135–143. Available at: https://doi.org/10.1007/s00467-019-04384-7
23. Paul A, Fraser N, Manoharan S, Williams AR, Shenoy MU. The challenge of maintaining dialysis lines in the under twos. *J Pediatr Urol.* 2011;7(1):48–51. Available at: https://doi.org/10.1016/j.jpurol.2010.01.018
24. Hothi DK, Rees L, Marek J, Burton J, McIntyre CW. Pediatric myocardial stunning underscores the cardiac toxicity of conventional hemodialysis treatments. *Clin J Am Soc Nephrol.* 2009;4(4):790–797. Available at: https://doi.org/10.2215/cjn.05921108
25. Geer JJ, Shah S, Williams E, Arikan AA, Srivaths P. Faster rate of blood volume change in pediatric hemodialysis patients impairs cardiac index. *Pediatr Nephrol.* 2017;32(2):341–345. doi:10.1007/s00467-016-3486-2
26. Borzych-Duzalka D, Aki TF, Azocar M, et al. Peritoneal dialysis access revision in children: causes, interventions, and outcomes. *Clin J Am Soc Nephrol.* 2016;12(1):105–112. Available at: https://doi.org/10.2215/cjn.05270516
27. Sethna CB, Bryant K, Munshi R, et al. Risk factors for and outcomes of catheter-associated peritonitis in children: the SCOPE Collaborative. *Clin J Am Soc Nephrol.* 2016;11(9):1590–1596. doi:10.2215/CJN.02540316
28. Sanderson KR, Warady BA. End-stage kidney disease in infancy: an educational review. *Pediatr Nephrol.* 2018;35(2):229–240. Available at: https://doi.org/10.1007/s00467-018-4151-8
29. Zaritsky J, Warady BA. Peritoneal dialysis in infants and young children. *Semin Nephrol.* 2011;31(2):213–224. Available at: https://doi.org/10.1016/j.semnephrol.2011.01.009

30. Vidal E. Peritoneal dialysis and infants: further insights into a complicated relationship. *Pediatr Nephrol.* 2017;33(4):547–551. Available at: https://doi.org/10.1007/s00467-017-3857-3

31. Ploos van Amstel S, Noordzij M, Borzych-Duzalka D, et al. Mortality in children treated with maintenance peritoneal dialysis: findings from the International Pediatric Peritoneal Dialysis Network Registry. *Am J Kidney Dis.* 2021;78(3): 380–390. doi:10.1053/j.ajkd.2020.11.031

32. Stewart CL, Acker SN, Pyle LL, et al. Factors associated with peritoneal dialysis catheter complications in children. *J Pediatr Surg.* 2016;51(1):159–162. Available at: https://doi.org/10.1016/j.jpedsurg.2015.10.035

33. Zaritsky JJ, Hanevold C, Quigley R, et al. Epidemiology of peritonitis following maintenance peritoneal dialysis catheter placement during infancy: a report of the SCOPE collaborative. *Pediatr Nephrol.* 2018;33(4):713–722. doi:10.1007/s00467-017-3839-5

34. Neu AM, Richardson T, De Souza HG, et al. Continued reduction in peritonitis rates in pediatric dialysis centers: results of the Standardizing Care to Improve Outcomes in Pediatric End Stage Renal Disease (SCOPE) Collaborative. *Pediatr Nephrol.* 2021;36(8):2383–2391. doi:10.1007/s00467-021-04924-0

35. KDOQI Pediatric Peritoneal Dialysis guideline and CPRS. *Am J Kidney Dis.* 2006;48(1):165–166. Available at: https://doi.org/10.1053/j.ajkd.2006.05.017

36. Nourse P, Cullis B, Finkelstein F, et al. ISPD guidelines for peritoneal dialysis in acute kidney injury: 2020 Update (paediatrics). *Perit Dial Int.* 2021;41(2):139–157. doi:10.1177/0896860820982120

37. Warady BA, Bakkaloglu S, Newland J, et al. Consensus guidelines for the prevention and treatment of catheter-related infections and peritonitis in pediatric patients receiving peritoneal dialysis: 2012 update. *Perit Dial Int.* 2012;32(suppl 2):32–86. Available at: https://doi.org/10.3747/pdi.2011.00091

38. White CT, Gowrishankar M, Feber J, Yiu V. Clinical practice guidelines for pediatric peritoneal dialysis. *Pediatr Nephrol.* 2006;21(8):1059–1066. Available at: https://doi.org/10.1007/s00467-006-0099-1

39. Schmitt CP, Bakkaloglu SA, Klaus G, Schröder C, Fischbach M. Solutions for peritoneal dialysis in children: recommendations by the European Pediatric Dialysis Working Group. *Pediatr Nephrol.* 2011;26(7):1137–1147. Available at: https://doi.org/10.1007/s00467-011-1863-4

40. Betts PR, Magrath G. Growth pattern and dietary intake of children with chronic renal insufficiency. *Br Med J.* 1974; 2(5912):189–193. doi:10.1136/bmj.2.5912.189

41. Nelms CL, Shaw V, Greenbaum LA, et al. Assessment of nutritional status in children with kidney diseases—clinical practice recommendations from the Pediatric Renal Nutrition Taskforce. *Pediatr Nephrol.* 2020;36(4):995–1010. Available at: https://doi.org/10.1007/s00467-020-04852-5

42. Rees L. Long-term peritoneal dialysis in infants. *Perit Dial Int.* 2007;27(suppl 2):180–184. Available at: https://doi.org/10.1177/089686080702702s31

43. National Kidney Foundation. KDOQI Clinical Practice guideline for nutrition in children with CKD: 2008 update. *Am J Kidney Dis.* 2009;53(3):11–104. Available at: https://doi.org/10.1053/j.ajkd.2008.11.017

44. Rees L, Shaw V, Qizalbash L, et al. Delivery of a nutritional prescription by enteral tube feeding in children with chronic kidney disease stages 2–5 and on dialysis—clinical practice recommendations from the Pediatric Renal Nutrition Taskforce.

Pediatr Nephrol. 2020;36(1):187–204. Available at: https://doi.org/10.1007/s00467-020-04623-2

45. Shaw V, Polderman N, Renken-Terhaerdt J, et al. Energy and protein requirements for children with CKD stages 2-5 and on dialysis—clinical practice recommendations from the Pediatric Renal Nutrition Taskforce. *Pediatr Nephrol.* 2019;35(3):519–531. Available at: https://doi.org/10.1007/s00467-019-04426-0

46. McAlister L, Pugh P, Greenbaum L, et al. The dietary management of calcium and phosphate in children with CKD stages 2-5 and on dialysis—clinical practice recommendation from the Pediatric Renal Nutrition Taskforce. *Pediatr Nephrol.* 2019;35(3):501–518. Available at: https://doi.org/10.1007/s00467-019-04370-z

47. Bunchman TE. Chronic dialysis in the infant less than 1 year of age. *Pediatr Nephrol.* 1995;9(suppl 1):S18–S22. Available at: https://doi.org/10.1007/bf00867678

48. Donaldson L, Freund P, Aslahi R, Margolin E. Dialysis-associated nonarteritic anterior ischemic optic neuropathy. A case series and review. *J Neuroophthalmol.* 2022;42(1):e116–e123. doi:10.1097/WNO.0000000000001493

49. Morgans HA, Chadha V, Warady BA. The role of carnitine in maintenance dialysis therapy. *Pediatr Nephrol.* 2021;36(8): 2545–2551. doi:10.1007/s00467-021-05101-z

50. Rönnholm K, Holmberg C. Peritoneal dialysis in infants. *Pediatr Nephrol.* 2006;21:751–756.

51. United States Renal Data System. *USRDS Annual Data Report: Epidemiology of Kidney Disease in the United States.* National Institutes of Health, National Institute of Diabetes and Digestive and Kidney Diseases; 2020.

52. Flynn JT, Warady BA. Peritoneal dialysis in children: challenges for the new millennium. *Adv Ren Replace Ther.* 2000;7(4):347–354. Available at: https://doi.org/10.1053/jarr.2000.16271

53. Al-Uzri A, Matheson M, Gipson DS, et al. The impact of short stature on health-related quality of life in children with chronic kidney disease. *J Pediatr.* 2013;163(3):736–741.e1. doi:10.1016/j.jpeds.2013.03.016

54. Chapter 3: Use of ESAs and other agents to TREAT anemia in CKD. *Kidney Int Suppl.* 2012;2(4):299–310. doi:10.1038/kisup.2012.35

55. Borzych-Duzalka D, Bilginer Y, Ha IS, et al. Management of anemia in children receiving chronic peritoneal dialysis. *J Am Soc Nephrol.* 2013;24(4):665–676. doi:10.1681/ASN.2012050433

56. Sanderson KR, Yu Y, Dai H, Willig LK, Warady BA. Outcomes of infants receiving chronic peritoneal dialysis: an analysis of the USRDS registry. *Pediatr Nephrol.* 2018;34(1):155–162. Available at: https://doi.org/10.1007/s00467-018-4056-6

57. Sanderson KR, Warady B, Carey W, et al. Mortality risk factors among infants receiving dialysis in the neonatal intensive care unit. *J Pediatr.* 2022;242:159–165. doi:10.1016/j.jpeds.2021.11.025

58. Madden SJ, Ledermann SE, Guerrero-Blanco M, Bruce M, Trompeter RS. Cognitive and psychosocial outcome of infants dialysed in infancy. *Child Care Health Dev.* 2003;29(1):55–61. doi:10.1046/j.1365-2214.2003.00311.x

59. Fernandez HE, Foster BJ. Long-term care of the pediatric kidney transplant recipient. *Clin J Am Soc Nephrol.* 2022;17(2):296–304. doi:10.2215/CJN.16891020

60. Cho MH. Pediatric kidney transplantation is different from adult kidney transplantation. *Korean J Pediatr.* 2018;61(7):205–209. Available at: https://doi.org/10.3345/kjp.2018.61.7.205

61. Hebert SA, Swinford RD, Hall DR, Au JK, Bynon JS. Special considerations in pediatric kidney transplantation. *Adv Chronic Kidney Dis.* 2017;24(6):398–404. Available at: https://doi.org/10.1053/j.ackd.2017.09.009

62. Harmon WE, Alexander SR, Tejani A, Stablein D. The effect of donor age on graft survival in pediatric cadaver renal transplant recipients—a report of the North American Pediatric Renal Transplant Cooperative Study. *Transplantation*. 1992;54(2):232–237. doi:10.1097/00007890-199208000-00008

63. Chua A, Cramer C, Moudgil A, et al. Kidney transplant practice patterns and outcome benchmarks over 30 years: the 2018 report of the NAPRTCS. *Pediatr Transplant*. 2019;23(8):e13597. Available at: https://doi.org/10.1111/petr.13597

64. Matas AJ, Smith JM, Skeans MA, et al. OPTN/SRTR 2012 annual data report: kidney. *Am J Transplant*. 2014;14(suppl 1):11–44. Available at: https://doi.org/10.1111/ajt.12579

65. Bryan CF, Chadha V, Warady BA. Donor selection in pediatric kidney transplantation using DR and DQ eplet mismatching: a new histocompatibility paradigm. *Pediatr Transplant*. 2016;20(7):926–930. doi:10.1111/petr.12762

66. Yu ED, Galbiati S, Munshi R, Smith JM, Menon S. NAPRTCS Investigators. Practice patterns and outcomes of maintenance dialysis in children <2 years of age: a report of the North American Pediatric Renal Trials and Collaborative Studies (NAPRTCS). *Pediatr Nephrol*. 2022;37(5):1117–1124. doi:10.1007/s00467-021-05287-2

67. Tancredi D, Butani L. Uncovering a long-term graft survival advantage afforded by infant renal transplants—an organ procurement and Transplantation Network Database Analysis. *Transplant Direct*. 2021;8(1):e1267. Available at: https://doi.org/10.1097/txd.0000000000001267

68. Hart A, Lentine KL, Smith JM, et al. OPTN/SRTR 2019 annual data report: kidney. *Am J Transplant*. 2021;21(suppl 2):21–137. doi:10.1111/ajt.16502

Chapter 13

Renal Tubular Acidosis

Silvia Iacobelli, MD, PhD and Jean-Pierre Guignard MD, PhD (Deceased)

Renal Acid-Base Regulation

Since birth, the kidney represents the crucial ultimate line of defense against disturbances of acid-base balance, which is performed by the tubular reabsorption of bicarbonate and the excretion of fixed hydrogen ions.[1] The glomerulus contributes to renal acid-base homeostasis by the filtration of urea (the major end-product of protein catabolism) and by providing the filtered load of bicarbonates to the proximal tubule. Up to 85% of the filtered load of bicarbonates is then reabsorbed by the proximal tubule, with the remainder reabsorbed by the thick ascending limb of Henle, and a small portion reabsorbed by distal nephron segments. The distal tubule and the collecting duct contribute to acid-base homeostasis through the excretion of fixed hydrogen ions and ammonia, which yields for terminal urinary acidification.

The key sites of the acidification process in the nephron are shown in Fig. 13.1.

HCO_3^- reabsorption mostly occurs via transcellular ion transport in the S1 and S2 convoluted segments of the proximal tubule. Protons are secreted into luminal fluid by the apical membrane antiporter Na^+/H^+ (NHE3, ① in Fig. 13.1) and the H^+-ATPase pump (② in Fig. 13.1). The driving force of proton secretion is the low intracellular sodium generated by the basolateral membrane Na^+/K^+-ATPase pump and the twin-pore domain acid-sensing TASK2 K^+ channels.[2] Secreted protons add hydrogen ion to intraluminal HCO_3^- and H_2CO_3 is formed. This is rapidly dehydrated to form H_2O and CO_2, freely diffusible and reabsorbed, with the contribution of aquaporin-1, along proximal tubule cells. Inside the proximal tubule cell, H_2CO_3 is formed from CO_2 and H_2O and rapidly dissociated to H^+ and HCO_3. Apical and intracellular carbonic anhydrases catalyze the interconversion of CO_2 and HCO_3^-. Intracellular HCO_3^- exits the cell via the basolateral membrane Na^+/HCO_3^- cotransporter (NBC1, ③ in Figs. 13.1).

Fixed hydrogen ions and ammonia are excreted in the distal tubule and in the collecting duct (Figs. 13.1 and 13.2). In the collecting duct active proton secretion is carried by the apical H^+-ATPase pump (⑤ in Fig. 13.1 and Fig. 13.2) of α-intercalated cells. The H^+/K^+-ATPase

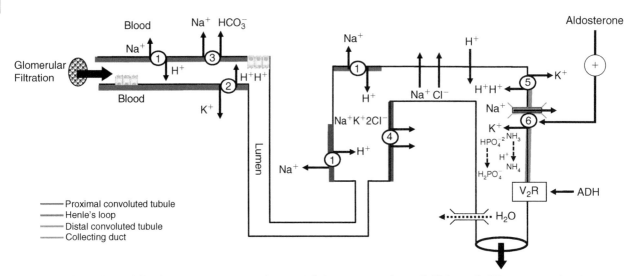

Fig. 13.1 Sites of the acidification process along the nephron. ①, Apical membrane antiporter Na$^+$/H$^+$; ②, H$^+$-ATPase pump; ③, basolateral membrane Na$^+$/HCO$_3^-$ cotransporter; ④, sodium potassium chloride cotransporter (furosemide receptor); ⑤, H$^+$-ATPase pump (α-intercalated cells); ⑥, amiloride-sensitive epithelial Na$^+$ channels (principal cells). *ADH*, antidiuretic hormone; *V$_2$R*, arginine vasopressin receptor.

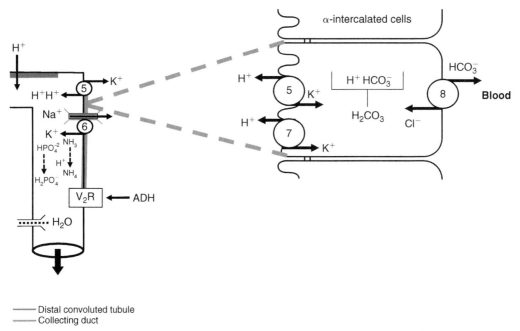

Fig. 13.2. Proton and ammonia excretion in the distal tubule and in the collecting duct. ⑤, H$^+$-ATPase pump (α-intercalated cells); ⑥, amiloride-sensitive epithelial Na$^+$ channels (principal cells); ⑦, H$^+$/K$^+$-ATPase pump (α-intercalated cells); ⑧, basolateral membrane Cl$^-$/HCO$_3^-$ exchanger. *ADH*, antidiuretic hormone, *V$_2$R*, arginine vasopressin receptor.

pump (⑦ in Fig. 13.2) contributes to proton secretion at the apical membrane level. The intracellular bicarbonate generated with proton excretion exits the α-intercalated cell via the basolateral membrane Cl^-/HCO_3^- exchanger (AE1, ⑧ in Fig. 13.2). This band-3 protein is also critically important for continued acid excretion via the apical H^+-ATPase and H^+/K^+-ATPase pumps.[3]

Proton excretion by α-intercalated cells is enhanced by Na^+ reabsorption and electronegative intraluminal gradient effected by amiloride-sensitive epithelial Na^+ channels (ENaC, ⑥ in Fig. 13.1 and Fig. 13.2) of the principal cells, under the control of aldosterone (Figs. 13.1 and 13.2). The integrity of the mineralocorticoid receptor and of all subunits of ENaC is necessary for the aldosterone action. Aldosterone has other effects on renal acidification, which have been extensively studied.[4] These include (1) direct stimulatory action on α-intercalated cells, causing them to increase H^+ secretion; (2) ammonia excretion (direct or secondary to the aldosterone effects on serum potassium levels).

Proton excretion into the lumen titrates luminal NH_3, forming NH_4^+. This allows maintaining a low luminal NH_3 concentration, necessary for ammonia excretion.

Several conditions affect the production of NH_3 by the kidney: chronic metabolic acidosis increases NH_3 production and potassium homeostasis (such that hyperkalemia suppresses and hypokalemia increases NH_3 formation). The decrease in NH_4^+ excretion that accompanies hyperkalemia is a major mechanism through which chronic hyperkalemia is associated with chronic metabolic acidosis (see later discussion of type 4 renal tubular acidosis [RTA]).

RENAL ACID-BASE REGULATION IN THE DEVELOPING KIDNEY

A tight control of pH is relatively efficient since birth. However, it is well established that the renal bicarbonate threshold is lower in neonates compared with older infants and children. The plasma concentration of bicarbonate is within the range of 20–22 mmol/L in term healthy infants and in the range of 18–20 mmol/L in preterm infants. Bicarbonate concentrations as low as 14 mmol/L can be observed in extremely preterm infants.[5] Adult values are achieved during the first year of life. This "physiological acidosis" observed in neonates can be explained by the immaturity of glomerular filtration rate (GFR)[6] and tubular function[7] during the transition from a fetal to an extrauterine environment.

Retracing the steps of the acidification process at different nephron levels, several mechanisms that reduce the kidneys' ability to maintain acid-base homeostasis can be identified in neonates (Table 13.1).[7–9]

The postnatal maturation of tubular transporters is under hormonal control. Experimental studies show that prenatal glucocorticoids stimulate neonatal juxtamedullary proximal convoluted tubule acidification.[10] The postnatal rise of thyroid hormones and glucocorticoids increases messenger RNA expression and the activity of NHE3 and Na^+/K^+-ATPase pumps.[7]

In very preterm infants, the state of relative expansion of the extracellular fluid volume, the disparate

TABLE 13.1 Factors and Mechanisms That Limit the Kidney Acidification Capacity in Neonates at Different Nephron Levels	
Proximal Nephron	**Determinant Mechanisms**
Low glomerular filtration rate Extracellular volume expansion Proximal tubule immaturity	Reduced filtered load of $HCO3^-$ Low renal $HCO3^-$ threshold Apical Na^+/H^+ exchanger immaturity Lack of H^+-ATPase activity Low rate of Na^+/K^+-ATPase activity
Distal Nephron	
Distal tubule and collecting duct immaturity	Reduced number of α-intercalated cells (cortical collecting duct) Low excretion of titratable acids and ammonium salts Aldosterone resistance

maturity of nephrons, as well as some glomerulotubular imbalance during postnatal development are responsible for a greater difficulty to maintain high levels of plasma bicarbonate. The urinary excretion of titratable acids (mostly in the form of phosphates) and ammonia is lower in preterm infants compared with infants born at term and increases as a function of gestational age. This maturation process is quite abrupt and occurs by the age of 1 month, regardless of the gestational age at birth.[11] Human studies showed that the renal mechanisms for preserving bicarbonate to compensate for the acid load delivered by milk intake are normally effective enough in preterm infants.[12] However, considering the age-specific low capacity for renal acidification, attention has been given traditionally to reducing acid load of preterm formula, as this prevents the development of "incipient late metabolic acidosis" in formula-fed preterm babies. This entity, which is rare nowadays, was characterized by persistent maximum renal acid excretion (urinary pH < 5.4), with normal or almost normal systemic acid–base status, in premature infants receiving alimentation with cow milk–based formulas. As the development of late metabolic acidosis lasted several days, exposed infants exhibited compensating mechanisms (volume contraction, hyperventilation, increased renal bicarbonate threshold), ensuring that their acid-base status in the blood remained within the normal values. "Incipient late metabolic acidosis" was accompanied by increased phosphaturia, decreased nitrogen assimilation, and impaired weight gain.[13] More recently, a randomized controlled trial[14] in breast milk–fed preterm infants showed that the addition of a milk fortifier with an acidic composition created a high renal acid load and induced the occurrence of metabolic acidosis, with consequent effects on growth and bone mineralization.

Finally, several drugs administered in neonatal intensive care units may be responsible for RTA, as they can increase base loss or decrease renal acid excretion: (1) both dopamine[15] and carbonic-anhydrase inhibitors (acetazolamide)[16] lower the renal bicarbonate threshold by decreasing the apical sodium ion (Na^+/H^+) exchanger activity; (2) K^+-sparing diuretics reduce the excretion of H^+ into distal tubular fluid[16]; (3) gentamicin interferes with the conversion of ADP to ATP, thus inhibiting the Na^+/K^+-ATPase pump, and also inhibits NHE3 pump activity[17]; and (4) amphotericin B might lead to pores in collecting duct cell membranes. This results in K^+ waste and a back-flux of H^+ into the cells, which inhibits collecting duct urinary H^+ excretion.[17]

Renal Tubular Acidosis

The term "renal tubular acidosis" is applied to a group of tubule defects in the reabsorption of bicarbonate, excretion of hydrogen ions, or both.[18] These defects occur with a normal or only slightly decreased GFR.

In metabolic acidosis of renal tubular origin, hyperchloremia compensates for the loss of bicarbonate or the deficient urinary acidification. So RTA is characterized by a normal anion gap hyperchloremic metabolic acidosis. Metabolic acidosis is defined by a pH less than 7.35, a PCO_2 in the normal range of 35–45 mmHg, and a base excess less than or equal to 5 mmol/L. The serum anion gap ($Na^+ - [Cl^- + HCO_3^-]$) remains within the normal value of 10–12 mEq/L.

RTA can be categorized into four types (numbered in the order of discovery): proximal (RTA type 2); distal (RTA type 1); combined proximal and distal RTA (type 3); type 4 RTA (also called hyperkalemic RTA). Each type can be inherited or acquired. Children with inherited RTA can present with early onset of the disease during the first month of life or somewhat later.

PROXIMAL RENAL TUBULAR ACIDOSIS (TYPE 2 AND FANCONI SYNDROME)

Proximal renal tubular acidosis (pRTA) (RTA type 2) is caused by a defect in tubular transport of bicarbonate and characterized by a low renal threshold of bicarbonate. The defect may present as a single dysfunction of the proximal tubule, which relates exclusively to the reabsorption of bicarbonate and occurs without alterations in the transport of other solutes. This form, called isolated pRTA, can be inherited or acquired. The acquired form is essentially due to the administration of carbonic-anhydrase inhibitors (acetazolamide). These diuretics are occasionally used in the treatment of posthemorrhagic hydrocephalus in newborn infants, but more often as a treatment of congenital glaucoma until surgery can be performed. Inherited, isolated pRTA is a very rare

TABLE 13.2 Inherited Renal Tubular Acidosis: Defective Genes, Mode of Inheritance, Involved Cotransporters and Exchangers, Cell Type Involvement and Localization

Disorder	Mode of inheritance and frequent extra-renal features	Gene	Defective Protein	Cell Type Involvement, Localization	Outset of Clinical Symptoms
pRTA (type 2)	AR (with ocular abnormalities)	SLC4A4	Na$^+$-HCO3$^-$ cotransporter (NBC1)	Proximal, Basolateral	Infancy
dRTA (type 1)	AD	SLC4A1	AE1	α-intercalated, Basolateral	Childhood Adolescence Adulthood
	AR	SLC4A1	AE1	α-intercalated, Basolateral	Infancy, childhood
	AR (with deafness)	ATP6V0A4	A^4 subunit of H$^+$-ATPase	α-intercalated, Luminal	Infancy
	AR (with deafness)	ATP6V1B1	B$_1$ subunit of H$^+$-ATPase	α-intercalated, Luminal	Infancy
	AR (with deafness)	FOXI1	AE1 B$_1$ subunit of H$^+$-ATPase	α-intercalated, Basolateral and luminal	Childhood
	AR (with dental abnormalities)	WDR72	H$^+$-ATPase trafficking	α-intercalated, cytoplasm	Childhood
	AR	ATP6V1C2	C subunit of H$^+$-ATPase	α-intercalated, luminal	Childhood
Type 4 RTA	AD pseudohypoaldosteronism type 1A	MLR	Mineralocorticoid receptor	Principal, cytoplasm	Infancy
	AR pseudohypoaldosteronism type 1B	SCNN1A SCNN1B SCNN1C	Na$^+$ channel ENaC subunit α Na$^+$ channel ENaC subunit β Na$^+$ channel ENaC subunit γ	Principal, luminal	Infancy
Combined p/dRTA (type 3)	AR	CA2	CAII	PT and α-intercalated, Cytoplasm	Infancy

AD, autosomal dominant; AE1, anion exchanger 1; AR, autosomal recessive; CAII, carbonic-anhydrase II: dRTA, distal renal tubular acidosis; ENaC, Epithelial Na$^+$ channel; p/dRTA, combined proximal and distal RTA; pRTA, proximal renal tubular acidosis; PT, proximal tubule.

disease that can present at birth. The implicated gene is the *SLC4A4*, encoding the membrane Na$^+$/HCO$_3^-$ cotransporter (NBC1) (Table 13.2).[19,20] The mutation can be autosomal recessive, autosomal dominant, or sporadic. The autosomal recessive trait should be suspected in the presence of severe failure to thrive and with ocular abnormalities such as band keratopathy, glaucoma, or cataracts, and it is associated with intellectual developmental disability.[2,21] The autosomal dominant form has been reported in two distinct families showing similar clinical features, but the involved gene has not yet been identified.[22] The sporadic isolated pRTA has been reported as a transient

disease in infants, affecting renal and intestinal bicarbonate reabsorption.[23]

In pRTA there is a low renal threshold for bicarbonate, and bicarbonate begins to appear in the urine at serum concentration of 15 mEq/L. At the outset of the disease, when the serum HCO$_3^-$ concentration is within the normal range, the filtered load of bicarbonates escaping proximal reabsorption will reach the distal tubule and will be excreted into the urine, thus producing an alkaline urine. Once the serum bicarbonate level has lowered below the renal threshold, HCO$_3^-$ lost by the defective proximal tubule can be reabsorbed by the intact distal tubule, thus the urinary pH decreases to less than 6.2 and urinary pH can be as low as <5.5. In addition, the delivery of the bicarbonate to the collecting duct occurs in the form of sodium bicarbonate, where some of the sodium is exchanged for potassium. This leads to increase in serum aldosterone concentration, mild volume depletion, and enhanced potassium excretion, which is responsible for significant hypokalemia. Newborn and young infants with isolated pRTA can present with mild or severe disease. The clinical manifestations of mild disease are usually limited to growth failure and lethargy. Severe symptoms are often related to untreated hypokalemia and patients present with dehydration, vomiting, polyuria, and feeding difficulties.

pRTA can be part of a generalized proximal tubule dysfunction (Fanconi syndrome), which includes pRTA, phosphaturia, glycosuria, and aminoaciduria. Fanconi syndrome is usually due to hereditary disorders, such as cystinosis (the most common cause of congenital Fanconi), galactosemia, tyrosinemia, hereditary fructose intolerance, and mitochondrial cytopathies. A discussion of inherited causes of Fanconi syndrome is beyond the scope of this review. The reader is referred to Quigley and Wolf[4] for a more detailed description. Drug-induced Fanconi syndrome is exceptionally rare in neonates.[24]

The treatment of pRTA consists of the administration of large amounts of oral alkali in the form of sodium salts (bicarbonate, citrate, or lactate), correction of water depletion, and potassium supplementation. As above previously, when serum bicarbonate levels are normalized, bicarbonaturia occurs, and supplements of HCO_3^- as high as 15 mEq/kg per day can be required. Thiazides can be used to create mild hypovolemia, which encourages salt and bicarbonate uptake by the proximal tubule and in the loop of Henle. This may allow for a reduction of daily intakes of bicarbonate. Hypokalemia can be aggravated by the combination of sodium bicarbonate and thiazides, as their administration increases the K^+ secretion in the collecting duct. Therefore, potassium supplementation should be given together with these treatments, and careful monitoring of K serum concentration is needed. With proper treatment the prognosis of pRTA is good, but associated extrarenal features impact on patient outcomes. The correction of chronic acidosis is critical to avoid failure to thrive, and this can be

avoided with proper treatment. In Fanconi syndrome, the long-term outcome is affected by associated extrarenal manifestations and underlying disease.

DISTAL RENAL TUBULAR ACIDOSIS (TYPE 1)

Distal renal tubular acidosis (dRTA) (RTA type 1) is the most common form of RTA. The hallmark of dRTA is failure of proton (H^+) secretion by the α-intercalated cells of the cortical collecting duct, in the presence of moderate to severe metabolic acidosis. The primary, or inherited dRTA, may present in infancy, childhood, or young adulthood and is transmitted as a dominant or recessive trait. Progress in genetics has allowed identification of six pathogenic variants in genes encoding the basolateral membrane Cl^-/HCO_3^- exchanger (AE1) or proteins/subunits of the apical H^+-ATPase pump of α-intercalated cells (see Table 13.2).[25,26] The clinical manifestations of dRTA are growth retardation, anorexia, vomiting, polyuria, polydipsia, dehydration, constipation, and other symptoms of hypokalemia. Different underlying genetic mutations causing dRTA are associated with nephrocalcinosis and extrarenal symptoms, such as early or late deafness (see Table 13.2).[25,26] The biochemical characteristic of dRTA is a metabolic hyperchloremic acidosis, with a urinary pH remaining always higher than 6.2. Hypokalemia (from mild to severe) is present, due to urinary potassium loss, as potassium is the only proton exchanged with sodium, when distal secretion of H^+ is diminished. Hypercalciuria and hypocitraturia are seen in the forms with nephrocalcinosis.

Acquired forms of dRTA are rare in pediatric patients but can occur secondary to obstructive uropathies, drugs or toxin exposures, and autoimmune diseases.

The goal of the treatment in dRTA is the early correction of metabolic acidosis, which should start from the first months of life to ensure normal growth, and the prevention of complications, such as nephrocalcinosis and chronic kidney disease (CKD). Treatment by alkali is advised, and the amount of bases is modulated according to patient's weight and needs. In general, forms with defective H^+-ATPase protein require more oral alkalizers than those with defective AE1.[25] The control of hypercalciuria is strongly facilitated by the correction of metabolic acidosis, as this raises urinary citrate. Bases are given in the form of sodium and potassium salts. In case of hypercalciuria, potassium citrate is the preferred treatment, as it reduces calcium excretion. The described treatments may not be well tolerated, because they cause gastrointestinal discomfort. A recent multicenter, open-label trial in adult patients and infants with dRTA showed the noninferiority, better palatability, and gastrointestinal safety of a new prolonged-release formulation, called ADV7103, compared with standard-of-care oral alkalizers.[27]

COMBINED PROXIMAL AND DISTAL RENAL TUBULAR ACIDOSIS (TYPE 3)

This pattern has been described in very rare cases of congenital carbonic anhydrase deficiency. It associates impaired renal bicarbonate reabsorption with the inability to acidify the urine (decreased NH_4^+ excretion). Urinary pH remains always higher than 6.2 and serum potassium is low, as in RTA type 1.

This variant of RTA has an autosomal recessive transmission due to a mutation in the gene for carbonic anhydrase II (CAII)[28] (see Table 13.2) and is associated with additional clinical signs: osteopetrosis, cerebral calcifications, and mental retardation. Other clinical features include bone fractures (due to increased bone fragility) and growth failure. Excessive facial bone growth leads to facial dysmorphism, conductive hearing loss, and blindness due to nerve compression.[29]

TYPE 4 RENAL TUBULAR ACIDOSIS

Aldosterone stimulates sodium reabsorption through the ENaC in principal cells, thus creating the electronegative gradient, which facilitates proton secretion by neighboring intercalated cells. As noted previously, this mineralocorticoid has other effects on renal acidification. In type 4 RTA (also called hyperkalemic RTA), aldosterone deficiency (hypoaldosteronism) or resistance (pseudohypoaldosteronism [PHA]) results in impaired distal H^+ and K^+ secretion.

Due to hypoaldosteronism, Na^+ reabsorption by the principal cells is reduced in the cortical collecting duct, leading to diminished transepithelial voltage and reduced proton excretion. In the proximal tubule, hyperkalemia inhibits ammoniagenesis, and this further reduces distal net acid excretion.

In type 4 RTA, metabolic hyperchloremic acidosis is associated with severe hyperkalemia, hyponatremia, salt wasting, and hypotension.

Aldosterone deficiency may occur in the context of congenital adrenal hyperplasia or as an isolated defect of aldosterone synthesis. Both these diseases may present in neonatal life as inherited forms of mineralocorticoid deficiency.

PHA can be congenital or acquired

Congenital Pseudohypoaldosteronism Type 1

In congenital PHA type 1 symptoms and biological disturbances may appear early in postnatal life. They are associated with elevated plasma renin activity and aldosterone excretion. The mutation can be autosomal dominant, recessive, or spontaneous (see Table 13.2).[4,30] In the autosomal dominant form—as in spontaneous mutation—the lack of response to mineralocorticoid affects only the kidneys, and the recessive form leads to severe symptoms in other organs (kidneys, lungs, colon, and salivary and sweat glands) in which aldosterone and ENaC play a crucial role in controlling Na^+ and fluid reabsorption.

Congenital Pseudohypoaldosteronism Type 2

A clinical form of congenital PHA, also called PHA type 2 or Gordon syndrome,[31] has been described in familial cases with hyperchloremic acidosis, hyperkalemia, normal or low aldosterone levels, and suppressed renin activity. Clinical and biological manifestations of PHA can again appear early in postnatal life,[32] with inconstant features such as arterial hypertension, short stature, abnormal dentition, and neurodevelopment impairment. The underlying mechanism is chloride-dependent Na^+ retention caused by mutations in genes encoding the with-no-lysine family of kinases.[33] Other genetic mutations have been further identified, some of those presenting early in infancy with hyperkalemia, hypertension, and metabolic acidosis.[4]

Acquired Pseudohypoaldosteronism

Acquired, transient PHA may occur due to urinary tract infection in infants with or without urinary tract malformations or after renal vein thrombosis, and it may be drug induced. Renal ultrasonography and urinary culture are useful for exclusion of acquired PHA. PHA usually resolves after recovery from the underlying disease or drug discontinuation.[34]

Management of Type 4 RTA

Initial management of type 4 RTA involves prompt correction of electrolyte imbalances and restoration of intravascular fluid volume. A blood sample for the essential hormonal investigations should be collected before any steroid treatment is given in cases of suspected aldosterone insufficiency.[35] In general, the treatment of congenital form of type 4 RTA requires alkali supplementation and compensation for electrolyte abnormalities in case of salt loss. The correction of metabolic acidosis is aided by the treatment of hyperkalemia.

Laboratory Testing in Suspected Renal Tubular Acidosis

As noted previously, RTA is suspected in patients with a normal anion gap hyperchloremic metabolic acidosis. Thus the first step is to determine that a normal anion gap metabolic acidosis exists and to rule out other causes of normal anion gap metabolic acidosis, especially bicarbonate gastrointestinal loss. Multiple etiologies of metabolic acidosis can sometimes occur in combination. Patients who are septic or in shock, for instance, are often dehydrated or volume depleted. These clinical changes can make the blood draws difficult and may impact the results of serum chemistries, thus the complete evaluation of an infant with suspected RTA should be performed after stabilization of the critical illness.

Once a nonanion gap metabolic acidosis without extra renal cause is established, workup of these patients begins with evaluation of the renal acid secreting capacity and to differentiate proximal and distal RTA.[36]

URINARY pH

Urinary pH measurement is useful in the assessment of normal serum anion gap metabolic acidosis. Urinary pH measurement can be inappropriately high in diluted urine. For the best precision, urinary pH should be measured in a sample of urine collected by bladder puncture or catheterization. If bladder puncture or catheterization are not possible, a bagged urinary sample can be used provided that urinary pH is measured immediately after collection.

In patients with a normal GFR and without urinary tract infection, a urinary pH higher than 6.2, in the presence of moderate to severe metabolic acidosis (serum bicarbonate <17 mEq/L), is suggestive of a defective distal renal acidification. If there is no systemic acidosis and plasma bicarbonate concentration is within the normal range, a test of urinary acidification (see following details) is required to evaluate the renal acidification capacity.

THE URINARY ANION GAP

In normal serum anion gap metabolic acidosis, the assessment of the urinary excretion of ammonium can be used as an index of the distal acidification and thus points to the renal origin of the acidosis. The normal value of urinary ammonium is 57.0 ± 4.3 mEq/min per 1.73 m^2 (age 1–16 month).[37] The measurement of ammonium in the urine is not easily available in all medical centers. Information on urinary ammonium excretion can be obtained by measuring the urinary anion gap: urinary anion gap = $(Na^+ + K^+ - Cl^-)$. This concept assumes that during metabolic acidosis the major cations in the urine are Na^+, K^+, and NH_4^+ and the major anion is Cl^-. Consequently, a negative urinary anion gap indicates that adequate amounts of NH_4^+ are being excreted. The presence of a positive value of urinary anion gap indicates a defect in the production and urinary excretion of NH_4^+ by the kidney. Such is for instance the case in dRTA (type 1) and in type 4 RTA. Unfortunately, the correlation between urinary NH_4^+ and urinary anion gap during the first weeks of life is absent or very weak, thus urinary anion gap is not reliable in neonates.

TRADITIONAL TESTS FOR THE DIAGNOSIS OF RENAL TUBULAR ACIDOSIS

Traditionally, several tests have been used to diagnose RTA, such as bicarbonate load, ammonium chloride load, and the combination of a mineralocorticoid with furosemide.[38] The bicarbonate load test consists of the administration of an oral sodium bicarbonate load to achieve a normal serum bicarbonate concentration and an alkaline urine, followed by the assessment of urine to blood CO_2 difference. This test is based on the assumption that urinary CO_2 excretion is an indicator of H^+ secretion. Thus in the presence of normal blood bicarbonate, a low urine to blood CO_2 difference (<10 mm Hg) suggests distal defect of renal acidification. The main limitation of this test is the technical difficulty of measuring urinary pCO_2. The oral ingestion of a load of ammonium chloride followed by serial measurements of urinary pH is not currently performed, because it is not well tolerated. At this time, a useful alternative to ammonium chloride is the assessment of urinary acidification after administration of furosemide and fludrocortisone.

In infants with a suspected inherited RTA, most of these laboratory approaches and traditional tests have been replaced by molecular genetic tests using next-generation sequencing techniques. The reader is referred to Giglio et al.[26] for a more detailed description of these genetic evaluations in RTA and to Chapter 8 of this textbook for a more detailed description of these genetic evaluations in renal anomalies in general.

Long-Term Consequences of Metabolic Acidosis in Infants With Renal Tubular Acidosis

Chronic acidosis due to RTA can have substantial adverse effects. These longer-term adverse effects include altered protein synthesis, increased muscle wasting, development or exacerbation of bone disease, and chronic hypokalemia. The associated clinical complications (anorexia, vomiting, growth retardation) may be absent during neonatal life and during early stages of the disease, but they should be anticipated as soon as the diagnosis is made. In particular failure to thrive and nutritional deficits are a major challenge in newborn and young infants suffering from chronic metabolic acidosis. Current nutritional guidelines in children with CKD, including pRTA or dRTA, recommend measurement and monitoring of the serum bicarbonate level and advocate measures to keep the bicarbonate level above 22 mmol/L for the neonate and young infant below 2 years of age to improve bone histology and linear growth.[39]

In addition to nutritional concerns, overall decreased renal function and CKD are regular long-term consequences of RTAs. Recently, the long-term follow-up of a large European cohort of pediatric and adult patients with primary dRTA was published.[40] The authors reported a prevalence rate of CKD stage $\geq$ 2 of 35% and 88%, respectively, in children and adult patients. The rate of nephrocalcinosis was 88%. In this cohort, more than 30 different alkali formulations were used and median prescribed doses of alkali equivalent were significantly higher in younger patients compared with older ones. At follow-up, patients with plasma or serum bicarbonate $\geq$ 22.0 mmol/L and without hypercalciuria had significantly better growth (higher height) and renal function (estimated GFR). These results highlight the importance of adequate treatment to maintain metabolic control to improve the long-term outcome of patients with RTA. Further investigations are clearly warranted with regard to the long-term effects of alkali therapy, the optimal type of alkali supplement, the influence of dietary habits, and the factors explaining the variability in the treatment dose needed in each disease.

REFERENCES

1. Hamm LL, Nakhoul N, Hering-Smith KS. Acid-base homeostasis. *Clin J Am Soc Nephrol.* 2015;10(12):2232–2242.
2. Kurtz I, Zhu Q. Proximal renal tubular acidosis mediated by mutations in NBCe1-A: unraveling the transporter's structure-functional properties. *Front Physiol.* 2013;4:350. doi:10.3389/fphys.2013.00350
3. Alper SL, Darman RB, Chernova MN, Dahl NK. The AE gene family of Cl/HCO3- exchangers. *J Nephrol.* 2002;15(suppl 5):S41–S53.
4. Quigley R, Wolf TFM. Renal tubular acidosis in children. In: *Pediatric Nephrology.* Springer-Verlag; 2014:1-40. doi:10.1007/978-3-642-27843-3_35-1
5. Guignard JP, John EG. Renal function in the tiny, premature infant. *Clin Perinatol.* 1986;13:377–401.
6. Iacobelli S, Guignard JP. Maturation of glomerular filtration rate in neonates and infants: an overview. *Pediatr Nephrol.* 2021;36(6):1439-1446. doi:10.1007/s00467-020-04632-1
7. Gattineni J, Baum M. Developmental changes in renal tubular transport-an overview. *Pediatr Nephrol.* 2015;30(12):2085–2098. doi:10.1007/s00467-013-2666-6
8. Iacobelli S, Guignard JP. Renal aspects of metabolic acid-base disorders in neonates. *Pediatr Nephrol.* 2020;35(2):221–228. doi:10.1007/s00467-018-4142-9
9. Bourchier D, Weston PJ. Metabolic acidosis in the first 14 days of life in infants of gestation less than 26 weeks. *Eur J Pediatr.* 2015;174:49–54. doi:10.1007/s00431-014-2364-9
10. Baum M. Developmental changes in rabbit juxtamedullar proximal convoluted tubule acidification. *Pediatr Res.* 1992;31(4):411–414. doi:10.1203/00006450-199204000-00021
11. Sulyok E, Guignard JP. Relationship of urinary anion gap to urinary ammonium excretion in the neonate. *Biol Neonate.* 1990;57:98–106. doi:10.1159/000243169
12. Kalhoff H, Manz F, Kiwull P, Kiwull-Schöne H. Food mineral composition and acid-base balance in preterm infants. *Eur J Nutr.* 2007;46:188–195. doi:10.1093/jn/138.2.431S
13. Kalhoff H, Diekmann L, Hettrich B, et al. Modified cow's milk formula with reduced renal acid load preventing incipient late metabolic acidosis in premature infants. *J Pediatr Gastroenterol Nutr.* 1997;25(1):46–50. doi:10.1097/00005176-199707000-00007

14. Rochow N, Jochum F, Redlich A, et al. Fortification of breast milk in VLBW infants: metabolic acidosis is linked to the composition of fortifiers and alters weight gain and bone mineralization. *Clin Nutr.* 2011;30(1):99–105. doi:10.1016/j.clnu.2010.07.016

15. Seri I. Cardiovascular, renal, and endocrine actions of dopamine in neonates and children. *J Pediatr.* 1995;126(3):333–344.

16. Guignard JP, Iacobelli S. Use of diuretics in the neonatal period. *Pediatr Nephrol.* 2021;36(9):2687–2695. doi:10.1007/s00467-021-04921-3

17. Kitterer D, Schwab M, Alscher MD, Braun N, Latus J. Drug-induced acid-base disorders. *Pediatr Nephrol.* 2015;30(9):1407–1423. doi:10.1007/s00467-014-2958-5

18. Rodríguez-Soriano J. Renal tubular acidosis: the clinical entity. *J Am Soc Nephrol.* 2002;13:2160–2170.

19. Enerbäck S, Nilsson D, Edwards N, et al. Acidosis and deafness in patients with recessive mutations in FOXI1. *J Am Soc Nephrol.* 2018;29(3):1041–1048. doi:10.1681/ASN.2017080840

20. Igarashi T, Sekine T, Inatomi J, Seki G. Unraveling the molecular pathogenesis of isolated proximal renal tubular acidosis. *J Am Soc Nephrol.* 2002;13(8):2171–2177. doi:10.1097/01.asn.0000025281.70901.30

21. Demirci FY, Chang MH, Mah TS, Romero MF, Gorin MB. Proximal renal tubular acidosis and ocular pathology: a novel missense mutation in the gene (SLC4A4) for sodium bicarbonate cotransporter protein (NBCe1). *Mol Vis.* 2006;10;12:324–330.

22. Haque SK, Ariceta G, Batlle D. Proximal renal tubular acidosis: a not so rare disorder of multiple etiologies. *Nephrol Dial Transplant.* 2012;27(12):4273–4287. doi:10.1093/ndt/gfs493

23. Kashoor I, Batlle D. Proximal renal tubular acidosis with and without Fanconi syndrome. *Kidney Res Clin Pract.* 2019;38(3):267–281. doi:10.23876/j.krcp.19.056

24. Hall AM, Bass P, Unwin RJ. Drug-induced renal Fanconi syndrome. *QJM.* 2014;107(4):261–269. doi:10.1093/qjmed/hct258

25. Besouw MTP, Bienias M, Walsh P, et al. Clinical and molecular aspects of distal renal tubular acidosis in children. *Pediatr Nephrol.* 2017;32(6):987–996. Available at: https://doi.org/10.1007/s00467-016-3573-4

26. Giglio S, Montini G, Trepiccione F, Gambaro G, Emma F. Distal renal tubular acidosis: a systematic approach from diagnosis to treatment. *J Nephrol.* 2021;34(6):2073–2083. doi:10.1007/s40620-021-01032-y

27. Bertholet-Thomas A, Guittet C, Manso-Silván MA, et al. Safety, efficacy, and acceptability of ADV7103 during 24 months of treatment: an open-label study in pediatric and adult patients with distal renal tubular acidosis. *Pediatr Nephrol.* 2021;36(7):1765–1774. doi:10.1007/s00467-020-04873-0

28. Sly WS, Hewett-Emmett D, Whyte MP, Yu YS, Tashian RE. Carbonic anhydrase II deficiency identified as the primary defect in the autosomal recessive syndrome of osteopetrosis with renal tubular acidosis and cerebral calcification. *Proc Natl Acad Sci U S A.* 1983;80(9):2752–2756.

29. Mustaqeem R, Aggarwal S. Renal tubular acidosis. In: *StatPearls.* StatPearls Publishing; 2018. Available at: https://pubmed.ncbi.nlm.nih.gov/30085586/. Accessed August 11, 2022.

30. Batlle D, Arruda J. Hyperkalemic forms of renal tubular acidosis: clinical and pathophysiological aspects. *Adv Chronic Kidney Dis.* 2018;25(4):321–333. doi:10.1053/j.ackd.2018.05.004

31. Gordon RD. Syndrome of hypertension and hyperkalemia with normal glomerular filtration rate. *Hypertension.* 1986;8:93–102.

32. Gereda JE, Bonilla-Felix M, Kalil B, Dewitt SJ. Neonatal presentation of Gordon syndrome. *J Pediatr.* 1996;129(4):615–617. doi:10.1016/s0022-3476(96)70131-2

33. Proctor G, Linas S. Type 2 pseudohypoaldosteronism: new insights into renal potassium, sodium, and chloride handling. *Am J Kidney Dis.* 2006;48(4):674–693. doi:10.1053/j.ajkd.2006.06.014

34. Nandagopal R, Vaidyanathan P, Kaplowitz P. Transient pseudohypoaldosteronism due to urinary tract infection in infancy: a report of 4 cases. *Int J Pediatr Endocrinol.* 2009;2009:195728. doi:10.1155/2009/195728

35. Vlachopapadopoulou E, Bonataki M. *Diagnosis of Hypoaldosteronism in Infancy.* Available at: http://dx.doi.org/10.5772/intechopen.97448. Accessed August 11, 2022.

36. Reddy S, Nivedita K. Clinical approach to renal tubular acidosis in children. *Karnataka Paediatr J.* 2020;35(2):88–94. doi:10.25259/KPJ_27_2020

37. Gil-Peña H, Mejía N, Santos F. Renal tubular acidosis. *J Pediatr.* 2014;164(4):691–698.e1. doi:10.1016/j.jpeds.2013.10.085

38. Bagga A, Sinha A. Evaluation of renal tubular acidosis. *Indian J Pediatr.* 2007;74(7):679–686.

39. KDOQI Work Group. KDOQI clinical practice guideline for nutrition in children with CKD: 2008 update. Executive summary. *Am J Kidney Dis.* 2009;53(3 suppl 2):S11–S104. doi:10.1053/j.ajkd.2008.11.017

40. Lopez-Garcia SC, Emma F, Walsh SB, et al. Treatment and long-term outcome in primary distal renal tubular acidosis. *Nephrol Dial Transplant.* 2019;34(6):981–991. doi:10.1093/ndt/gfy409

Chapter 14

Renal Near-Infrared Spectroscopy Use in the Neonate

Valerie Y. Chock, MD, MS Epi

Chapter Outline

As bedside monitoring capabilities continue to advance in the neonatal intensive care unit, renal tissue oxygenation monitoring with near-infrared spectroscopy (NIRS) has emerged as a potentially useful tool for clinicians. Renal perfusion and oxygen utilization by the neonatal kidney is impacted by many factors including gestational age, chronological age, hemodynamic status of the infant, fluid balance, and other underlying conditions. Renal tissue oxygen saturation ($RrSO_2$) can be measured continuously and noninvasively to enhance understanding of kidney health in vulnerable neonatal populations. In addition to providing real-time information, an advantage to monitoring renal saturation is the potential to detect changes earlier than traditional indicators of kidney injury such as alterations in urine output or serum creatinine, allowing time for interventions before permanent kidney injury occurs (Fig. 14.1).

Review of Near-Infrared Spectroscopy

NIRS is a bedside technology that has gained traction as a monitoring tool in the neonatal intensive care unit (NICU).[1] Commercially available NIRS devices all function using the same principles. Near-infrared light with wavelengths between 685 and 880 nm is emitted from a sensor placed on an infant's skin. The light passes through the underlying soft tissue or bone and penetrates to a depth of 1.5–3 cm depending on sensor configuration and number of wavelengths, where it is then partially absorbed by oxygenated and deoxygenated hemoglobin. Remaining light is reflected back to a detector on the sensor, and a tissue saturation level is calculated. Although similar in theory to pulse oximetry, NIRS does not rely on pulsatile blood flow and instead measures a heavily venous-weighted tissue saturation (approximately 75% venous and 25% arterial depending upon machine algorithm). Thus NIRS can be utilized for the simultaneous tissue oxygen

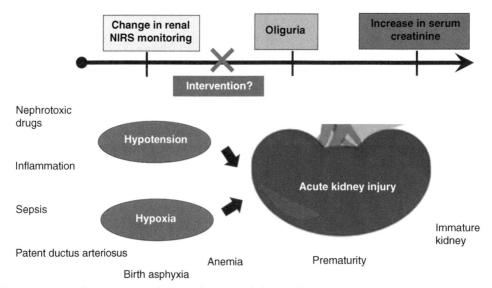

Fig. 14.1 Many factors contribute to poor renal oxygenation and perfusion, leading to the development of neonatal acute kidney injury. Near-infrared spectroscopy (*NIRS*) monitoring will detect these changes before clinical evidence of oliguria or elevation in serum creatinine occurs and potentially allow time for interventions to prevent acute kidney injury.

saturation monitoring of various end organs. Fractional tissue oxygen extraction (fTOE) by the monitored organ can also be calculated with knowledge of overall systemic oxygenation (SpO_2) and regional tissue oxygenation (rSO_2) using the following formula: $fTOE = (SpO_2 - rSO_2)/SpO_2$. Although several studies have demonstrated the utility of cerebral NIRS monitoring in reducing cerebral hypoxia with the potential for improving longer-term neurodevelopmental outcomes,[2,3] much less is known about NIRS monitoring of the kidney.

Renal Near-Infrared Spectroscopy Sensor Placement and Monitoring Techniques

Appropriate placement of a renal NIRS sensor in a neonate has been described in a paravertebral location below the costal margin and above the iliac crest between the T12–L2 location but not crossing the spine.[4,5] Limited research has demonstrated that this placement correlates with ultrasound markers of renal blood flow.[6,7] Ongoing research into renal sensor placement is focused on left versus right differences, specific depth of measurement, simultaneous arterial and venous blood gas sampling, use of point of care ultrasound, and comeasurement of liver or intestinal

oxygenation. At an even more granular level, renal tissue oxygenation may mostly be reflective of perfusion of glomeruli in the renal cortex, although there is less oxygen delivery to more distal segments of the collecting tubules, which are at particular risk for hypoxic injury.[8] Kidney size will certainly be affected by gestational age and maturational processes, with implications for optimal depth of NIRS measurement.

Practical concerns of renal NIRS monitoring in the NICU must be considered. Skin integrity is of particular importance in the preterm infant with a thin stratum corneum. Use of a skin dressing or barrier such as Mepitel (Molnlycke, Gothenburg, Sweden) under an NIRS sensor has been described for preterm skin protection[9] and has not altered the validity of NIRS measures.[10] High-humidity conditions within a NICU isolette may also interfere with sensor adherence, although securing a renal NIRS sensor within the diaper may be feasible. As with any device in direct contact with infant skin, care must be taken to avoid pressure injuries, particularly if the infant is lying on the sensor for prolonged periods of time. Strict adherence to clinical protocols for turning and positioning infants in the NICU should be followed to reduce risk and for monitoring of skin integrity. Optimal duration of maintaining a renal NIRS sensor in one location is also unknown, but rotating sites is another described practice.[9]

Correlation of renal NIRS data with other physiologic variables is also an important consideration. The neonatal kidney is exquisitely sensitive to cardiac output with 10% of cardiac output directed to the kidneys.[11] As the kidney is not as well autoregulated as the brain, factors such as blood pressure and systemic oxygen saturation are likely to have a significant impact on renal NIRS measures. Time-synchronized evaluation of these vital signs may assist with clinician interpretation of renal NIRS. Moreover, simultaneous monitoring of cerebral NIRS values will provide insight into the relative effect of physiologic or pathologic processes on the kidney as compared with the brain. Optimal data capture practices and approach to missing values or artifacts have been described for cerebral or mesenteric NIRS monitoring,[12,13] and application to renal NIRS monitoring may be reasonable.

Normal Renal Saturation Ranges

Several small studies have reported $RrSO_2$ ranges in the neonatal period, although definitive thresholds based on renal sequelae have yet to be established. Literature from term infants describe $RrSO_2$ values as being 10%–15% higher than concurrent cerebral saturation values.[14] In term infants, beginning in the delivery room, $RrSO_2$ has been measured at 40% in the first 2–3 minutes of age with a slow increase to ~85% by 10 minutes.[15] A concomitant decrease in renal fTOE from ~40% down to <10% by 10 minutes after birth was observed in the transitional period and distinctly contrasts with a higher, preserved oxygen extraction by the brain.[15] In a separate study measuring $RrSO_2$ in the first 48 hours of life, $RrSO_2$ peaked at about 92% on the first day and then gradually decreased to 89% on the second day.[16] As the kidney is one of the most metabolically active organs, this finding may reflect increased kidney function and renal oxygen extraction over time.

Preterm infants exhibit a more complex trajectory of renal saturation ranges. Factors including gestational age, chronological age, growth restriction, patency of the ductus arteriosus, and severity of illness may influence $RrSO_2$ values.[4] In general, preterm infants tend to have lower and more variable $RrSO_2$ levels compared with term infants. In a study of 80 preterm infants between 25 and 29 weeks' gestational age, the median $RrSO_2$ was between 63% and 72% in the first 48 hours of age.[17] A two-center study of 109 preterm infants <32 weeks' gestation found a 20% mean decrease in $RrSO_2$ in the first 60 hours of life with a subsequent plateau in values for the remaining first week of life with median $RrSO_2$ at 67% (interquartile range 59%–74%).[18] These findings are similar to a small study of preterm infants <36 weeks' gestation with $RrSO_2$ decreasing from 80% down to mid-60% by 3 weeks after birth.[19] The overall trend of a decrease in $RrSO_2$ in the first few days may coincide with an increased glomerular filtration rate and subsequent increased oxygen utilization by the kidneys. Investigators also found increasing $RrSO_2$ levels with higher gestational ages, with a 2.1% increase in baseline $RrSO_2$ for each week of gestation between 24 and 32 weeks.[18] The additional vascularization found in more mature kidneys may account for the increase in $RrSO_2$ seen with advancing gestational age.

Acute Kidney Injury: At-Risk Populations and Early Detection

As previously described, there are no established thresholds for abnormal renal saturation. Notably, abnormal $RrSO_2$ values have largely been extrapolated from cerebral NIRS studies in which a >20% decline or <40% threshold value has been associated with brain ischemia and injury.[20,21] However, limited data exist about renal thresholds of hypoperfusion and association with acute kidney injury (AKI). Measures appear to be dependent on the neonatal population being monitored, possibly indicating different mechanisms of renal injury. A compilation of abnormal $RrSO_2$ values from studies of various neonatal populations at high risk for AKI is listed in Table 14.1 and described in the following sections. Measuring renal fTOE requires knowledge of simultaneous SpO_2 values, but may potentially be a better marker for AKI risk than $RrSO_2$ alone and deserves further investigation.

PRETERM INFANTS

A premature infant with developing kidneys and lower nephron numbers may be exposed to substantial hemodynamic changes throughout their NICU course, putting them at high risk for AKI. Exposure to nephrotoxic agents, sepsis, fluid shifts, effects of a

TABLE 14.1	Renal NIRS Thresholds for AKI in Various At-Risk Populations			
Authors	**Number of Subjects**	**% With AKI**	**AKI Definition**	**RrSO$_2$ (%) Cutoff for AKI (or Comparison of RrSO$_2$ With non-AKI Group)**
Preterm				
Bonsante et al. 2019[24]	128	9.4	>1.5 mg/dL after day of life 1	Mean 69.7% ± 11.3% vs. 80.4% ± 9.5% on day 1
Harer et al. 2021[9]	35	8.6	Modified neonatal KDIGO	Median 32.4% (27.9%–47.1%) vs. 60% (58.4%–62%) in first week
Postcardiac Surgery				
Adams et al. 2019[34]	70	61	KDIGO	≥30% decline from baseline intraoperatively
Neunhoeffer et al. 2016[35]	50	40	pRIFLE	<64.8% at 24 h postoperatively
Ruf et al. 2015[32]	59	48	pRIFLE	<65% for ≥95 min or >25% decline from baseline for ≥23 min intraoperatively
Hazle et al. 2013[36]	49	86	AKIN or KDIGO	No association with AKI
Owens et al. 2011[33]	40	38	pRIFLE or SCr increase ≥0.4 mg/dL and 50%	<50% for ≥2 h in first 48 h postoperatively
Hypoxic Ischemic Encephalopathy				
Chock et al. 2018[5]	38	39%	Gupta or AKIN	>75% between 24 and 48 h of age

AKI, acute kidney injury; *AKIN*, Acute Kidney Injury Network; *KDIGO*, Kidney Disease: Improving Global Outcomes; *NIRS*, near-infrared spectroscopy; *pRIFLE*, Pediatric risk, injury, failure, loss, and end-stage; *RrSO$_2$*, renal tissue oxygen saturation; *SCr*, serum creatinine.

patent ductus arteriosus (PDA), anemia, suboptimal nutrition, and ongoing hypoxia from immature lung function may also contribute to the increased risk for AKI. A systematic review and metaanalysis found the overall rate of AKI in premature and low birth weight neonates was 25% (95% confidence interval 20%–30%).[22] AKI was also independently associated with increased mortality and length of hospital stay.[23] Renal NIRS monitoring has the potential for early detection of AKI in the preterm infant, allowing time for interventions to improve renal perfusion and ameliorating renal injury. In a study of 128 preterm infants <32 weeks' gestation, lower RrSO$_2$ on the first day of life was associated with developing AKI in the first week (mean RrSO$_2$ 69.7% ± 11.3% in those with AKI vs. 80.4% ± 9.5% in those without AKI).[24] Another prospective study using renal NIRS monitoring found that preterm infants <32 weeks' gestation with AKI based on the modified neonatal Kidney Disease: Improving Global Outcomes definition, had lower median RrSO$_2$ values compared with those without AKI over the first week of age (32.4% vs. 60%, $P < .001$), and decreases in RrSO$_2$ occurred over 48 hours prior

to changes in serum creatinine and urine output.[9] Renal NIRS may detect preterm infants at risk for kidney impairment prior to a traditional diagnosis of AKI. As early detection is the key to prevention, renal NIRS monitoring holds significant promise for future investigations. However, it is important to note that although a statistical association between low renal NIRS values and AKI was found, further investigation from carefully designed studies in larger populations is needed to demonstrate the predictive ability of RrSO$_2$ for identifying AKI. Similar to NIRS studies aimed at decreasing the burden of cerebral hypoxia,[2] targeted interventions to address declines in RrSO$_2$ may be investigated to reduce AKI in the preterm infant.

PATENT DUCTUS ARTERIOSUS

Preterm infants are specifically at higher risk for developing AKI due to the effects of a hemodynamically significant patent ductus arteriosus (hsPDA). Decreased systemic blood flow from left-to-right shunting through an open ductus may lead to poor renal perfusion and ensuing AKI with oliguria and rise in serum creatinine. In an analysis of over 500 very low birth weight neonates, those with a PDA were more likely to have AKI (odds ratio 3.74, 95% confidence interval 2.17–6.44).[25]

Several investigators have explored the utility of NIRS measures to determine the hemodynamic significance of a PDA.[26–30] In a large prospective study of 123 preterm infants <32 weeks' gestation, higher $RrSO_2$ was found in infants without a PDA compared with those with a hsPDA after 72 hours of age. Renal fTOE was also lower in the no PDA group compared with the hsPDA group.[30] Similarly, in a retrospective study of preterm infants <29 weeks' gestation who were routinely monitored with NIRS at a median age of 7 days, an $RrSO_2$ < 66% was associated with a hsPDA by echocardiography with sensitivity of 81% and specificity of 77% (area under the curve = 0.79), positive predictive value 74%, and negative predictive value 83%.[27] The ability of lower $RrSO_2$ values to predict an hsPDA has not been replicated in all studies however, with differences potentially due to definition of a hsPDA, timing of monitoring, and presence of other confounding factors such as pressor support and supplemental oxygen use.[28,29]

Medications to treat an hsPDA also may have detrimental effects on renal blood flow. For example, indomethacin not only constricts ductal tissue but may also transiently decrease renal blood flow and $RrSO_2$ values.[31] Theoretically, early reversal of renal hypoxia may prevent AKI after exposure to indomethacin.

NEONATES AFTER CARDIAC SURGERY

Infants with congenital heart disease undergoing cardiac surgery with cardiopulmonary bypass have also been investigated with renal NIRS monitoring given their high risk for AKI. Significantly lower $RrSO_2$ values were found beginning intraoperatively and extending 48 hours postoperatively for infants undergoing cardiopulmonary bypass who developed AKI compared with those with normal renal function.[32] Other studies have also found an association between prolonged low $RrSO_2$ and AKI.[33–35] The congenital heart disease population with mixing lesions may have lower overall systemic arterial oxygen saturations, which may result in low $RrSO_2$ levels at baseline. In these patients, the degree of change in $RrSO_2$ may be more indicative of renal impairment than the absolute $RrSO_2$ value. For example, although $RrSO_2$ was correlated with serum

creatinine-based Kidney Disease: Improving Global Outcomes criteria for AKI, an intraoperative decline in $RrSO_2$ > 30% was even more closely correlated with urine biomarkers of renal injury such as Tissue inhibitor of metalloproteinases 2 (TIMP2), neutrophil gelatinase-associated lipocalin, and insulin-like growth factor-binding protein 7 (IGFBP-7).[34] A different study found postoperative time spent with $RrSO_2$ < 50% correlated with elevated urine biomarkers but not with AKI.[36] These findings suggest that serum creatinine may not be the best marker to detect kidney injury after cardiac surgery, but $RrSO_2$ may be more sensitive in detecting subclinical AKI.

HYPOXIC ISCHEMIC ENCEPHALOPATHY

Another population of neonates at significant risk for AKI are those with hypoxic ischemic encephalopathy (HIE) after birth asphyxia. Neonates with AKI and HIE have a longer hospital stay, prolonged mechanical ventilation, and greater risk of abnormal brain MRI than infants with HIE but not AKI.[37,38] Although cerebral NIRS monitoring has been found to improve prediction of abnormal brain imaging and long-term neurodevelopmental impairment,[39,40] much less is known about the utility of renal NIRS monitoring in the HIE population. In a study of 38 neonates undergoing therapeutic hypothermia for HIE, $RrSO_2$ was lower than cerebral saturation during the cooling period but increased after rewarming.[5] However, by 24 hours after birth, the 15 infants that developed AKI had higher $RrSO_2$ levels than those without AKI, and an $RrSO_2$ > 75% was associated with AKI with sensitivity of 79% and specificity of 82% (area under the curve = 0.76), positive predictive value 73%, and negative predictive value 86%.[5] Compared with both the preterm and postoperative cardiac populations with lower $RrSO_2$ levels predicting AKI, the neonates with HIE had higher $RrSO_2$ levels and decreased renal fTOE associated with AKI. This difference may indicate a different pathophysiology of renal injury in the HIE population. A potentially neuromediated limitation of oxygen extraction by an injured or hypoxic kidney could result in these abnormally high $RrSO_2$ levels. Therapeutic agents like caffeine or theophylline increase renal perfusion and have been shown to improve urinary output after HIE.[41] NIRS monitoring may aid future investigation into the utility of such drugs for reducing AKI in the HIE population.

Renal Near-Infrared Spectroscopy Monitoring in Other Neonatal Populations

Aside from populations with increased risk of AKI, there are other neonatal settings in which renal NIRS monitoring may be useful as an early sign of poor end-organ perfusion. For example, infants with hemodynamic instability including those with congenital heart disease, sepsis, and shock may exhibit changes in $RrSO_2$ as the first indication of impaired cardiac output and poor somatic perfusion before traditional measures like oliguria, increased lactate, acidosis, or elevated creatinine. Identifying changes in renal tissue oxygenation may facilitate earlier implementation of important therapeutic interventions.

AORTIC COARCTATION

One specific example is the neonate with concern for aortic coarctation. Diagnostic capabilities have improved with fetal echocardiograms identifying cases suspicious for hypoplasia or narrowing of the aortic arch and possible coarctation. However, the severity of presentation and need for initiation of prostaglandin therapy or immediate surgical intervention is often obscured in the presence of an open ductus arteriosus immediately after birth. As the PDA closes, systemic blood flow becomes impaired, resulting in signs of a blood pressure gradient between lower and upper extremities, differences in pre- and postductal oxygen saturation, metabolic acidosis, delayed capillary refill time, and oliguria. NIRS monitoring provides an early, real-time indicator of decreased kidney perfusion in the setting of a closing PDA (Fig. 14.2), typically hours before any of the aforementioned signs become clinically apparent. At least one center has developed a neonatal aortic coarctation clinical pathway for perinatal management that incorporates NIRS monitoring as a routine part of risk-stratified care.[42]

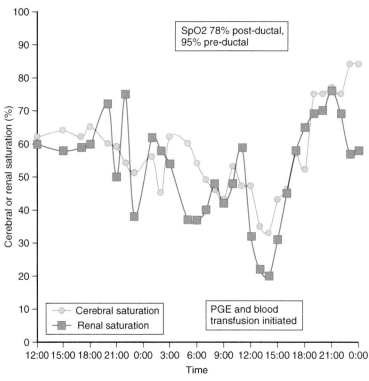

Fig. 14.2 An 8-day old term infant with prenatal suspicion for aortic coarctation had stable lactate levels and normal urine output and was warm and well-perfused. Near-infrared spectroscopy (NIRS) measures steadily decreased over 12 hours, with renal saturations ranging from 20% to 30%. Systemic oxygen saturation only changed minimally. The NIRS changes prompted a follow-up echocardiogram, which revealed juxtaductal coarctation of the aorta. The infant was started on prostaglandin (PGE), received a packed red blood cell transfusion, and was placed on supplemental oxygen with return of NIRS measures back to baseline.

HYPOPLASTIC LEFT HEART SYNDROME

Similar principles have guided management of infants with hypoplastic left heart syndrome in which impaired systemic blood flow may be detected by renal NIRS monitoring before alterations in urine output, serum creatinine, or systemic saturation.[43] In a historical cohort study, Johnson et al. found that routine preoperative cerebral and renal NIRS monitoring in patients with hypoplastic left heart syndrome reduced the need for invasive therapies, including mechanical ventilation and inspired gas administration, with no difference in mortality or duration of hospital stay.[44] Although concern exists for excessive intervention with the availability of additional bedside data, this study demonstrates how NIRS monitoring may also help to reassure clinicians if tissue saturation levels are adequate.

EXTRACORPOREAL LIFE SUPPORT

Extracorporeal life support (ECLS) has been utilized to improve survival in neonates with refractory respiratory or cardiac failure. Close monitoring of these patients on bypass is required due to inherent risks of anticoagulation, thrombosis, and hemodynamic instability with an ECLS circuit. A decline in renal NIRS measures ahead of conventional ECLS monitoring parameters has been reported after hemorrhagic complications.[45] In one case, a decrease in RrSO$_2$ to 21% occurred prior to evidence of abdominal distention, decreased urine output, or anemia and prompted diagnosis of hemoperitoneum and massive subcapsular liver hemorrhage. In a separate case, an abrupt decline in RrSO$_2$ from 57% down to 29% over a 2-hour period was the first clinical indication of a pericardial effusion in an infant on ECLS who otherwise appeared to have stable hemodynamic parameters.[45] Similarly, renal NIRS measures preceded a decline in mean arterial blood pressure and were associated with decreased urine output in a small cohort of six neonates with congenital diaphragmatic hernia on ECLS.[46] Routine renal NIRS monitoring in the ECLS population may be beneficial for early identification of impaired tissue perfusion and potential complications.

SURGICAL PATIENTS

Monitoring of renal saturations may also detect periods of renal hypoxia during neonatal surgery and in the postoperative period and serve as a guide for necessary interventions. Intraoperative monitoring of renal saturations in neonates undergoing noncardiac surgeries found RrSO$_2$ fell below a 40% threshold for 19% of the time, and conventional monitoring of heart rate, blood pressure, and systemic saturation did not detect all episodes of tissue hypoxia.[47] Moreover, renal NIRS detected tissue hypoxia twice as frequently as SpO$_2$ (9% vs. 4.8%). When investigating operative interventions, fluid boluses significantly increased RrSO$_2$ by 25%–35% and epidural analgesia administration decreased RrSO$_2$ by 25%–30%.[47] Gastrointestinal surgeries in particular, where organs are manipulated, may potentially lead to increased intraabdominal pressure, fluid shifts, hemorrhage, and inflammation, contributing to hemodynamic instability and poor renal perfusion in the perioperative period. In a study of 13 patients with esophageal atresia undergoing open surgical repair, a significant reduction in RrSO$_2$ from a median baseline of about 80% down to approximately 60% between 6 and 24 hours postoperatively was then followed by a decrease in urine output and attributed to relative hypovolemia.[48] Infants with gastroschisis undergoing staged closure with bowel reduction in a silo were noted to have a 2.5% decrease in RrSO$_2$ with each episode of bowel reduction.[49] The authors concluded that renal NIRS monitoring correlates well with even minimal increases in intraabdominal pressure and may be useful for detection of abdominal compartment syndrome in these at-risk patients.

CONGENITAL RENAL ANOMALIES AND RENAL REPLACEMENT THERAPY

Although relatively unexplored, the population of neonates with congenital abnormalities of the kidney and urinary tract and those requiring renal replacement therapy may also benefit from monitoring of renal saturations. As infants with congenital abnormalities of the kidney and urinary tract undergo postnatal assessment of renal function, optimization of renal perfusion as measured by RrSO$_2$ could be an important aspect of neonatal management. In the fetal period, a subset of patients with congenital bilateral renal agenesis, cystic kidney disease, or severe lower urinary tract obstruction with early pregnancy renal anhydramnios may be candidates for the ongoing trial of serial amnioinfusions (NCT 03101891).[50] Although prevention of otherwise lethal pulmonary hypoplasia is a goal of fetal intervention, it remains unclear whether longer-term hemodynamic and hypoxic complications may occur in survivors in the neonatal period. However, renal NIRS monitoring (even in the baby without kidneys) may be critical as a marker of somatic perfusion in this population and will still reflect changes in descending aortic blood flow. Similarly, for those neonates with renal failure requiring peritoneal dialysis, ultrafiltration, or continuous renal replacement therapy, renal NIRS monitoring may be of benefit to detect early hemodynamic changes that occur with fluid shifts.[51] These patients are additionally at risk for sepsis, anemia, and hemorrhage, conditions for which renal NIRS monitoring has aided early detection.[43,52] In older infants and children, NIRS monitoring of kidney graft perfusion after renal transplant has also been described.[53]

Future Considerations

The potential for renal NIRS monitoring to improve neonatal kidney health continues to develop as neonatologists gain experience with clinical application and promote clinical investigations in the field. Future research may integrate the added utility of renal saturation measures with other early markers of kidney dysfunction including urine biomarkers, bedside renal imaging modalities, and real-time monitoring of glomerular filtration rate. Algorithms to direct clinician responses based on high or low thresholds of renal oxygen saturation, similar to ongoing efforts with neonatal cerebral hypoxia monitoring,[54] may be developed. Renal NIRS monitoring will be critical for evaluation of interventions to improve kidney perfusion, including distinguishing populations that may benefit from theophylline or caffeine pharmacotherapy. Ultimately, the precise role of renal NIRS monitoring in reducing AKI and preventing long-term chronic kidney disease in the neonatal population must be established.

REFERENCES

1. Hunter CL, Oei JL, Suzuki K, Lui K, Schindler T. Patterns of use of near-infrared spectroscopy in neonatal intensive care units: International usage survey. *Acta Paediatr.* 2018;107:1198–1204. Available at: https://doi.org/10.1111/apa.14271

2. Hyttel-Sorensen S, Pellicer A, Alderliesten T, et al. Cerebral near infrared spectroscopy oximetry in extremely preterm infants: phase II randomised clinical trial. *BMJ.* 2015;350:g7635.
3. Alderliesten T, van Bel F, van der Aa NE, et al. Low cerebral oxygenation in preterm infants is associated with adverse neurodevelopmental outcome. *J Pediatr.* 2019;207:109–116.e2.
4. Harer MW, Chock VY. Renal tissue oxygenation monitoring—an opportunity to improve kidney outcomes in the vulnerable neonatal population. *Front Pediatr.* 2020;8:241.
5. Chock VY, Frymoyer A, Yeh CG, Van Meurs KP. Renal saturation and acute kidney injury in neonates with hypoxic ischemic encephalopathy undergoing therapeutic hypothermia. *J Pediatr.* 2018;200:232–239.e1.
6. Altit G, Bhombal S, Tacy TA, Chock VY. End-organ saturation differences in early neonatal transition for left- versus right-sided congenital heart disease. *Neonatology.* 2018;114:53–61.
7. Ortmann LA, Fontenot EE, Seib PM, Eble BK, Brown R, Bhutta AT. Use of near-infrared spectroscopy for estimation of renal oxygenation in children with heart disease. *Pediatr Cardiol.* 2011;32:748–753.
8. Scholz H, Boivin FJ, Schmidt-Ott KM, et al. Kidney physiology and susceptibility to acute kidney injury: implications for renoprotection. *Nat Rev Nephrol.* 2021;17:335–349.
9. Harer MW, Adegboro CO, Richard LJ, McAdams RM. Non-invasive continuous renal tissue oxygenation monitoring to identify preterm neonates at risk for acute kidney injury. *Pediatr Nephrol.* 2021;36:1617–1625.
10. Cerbo RM, Maragliano R, Pozzi M, et al. Global perfusion assessment and tissue oxygen saturation in preterm infants: where are we? *Early Hum Dev.* 2013;89(suppl 1):S44–S46.
11. Nada A, Bonachea EM, Askenazi DJ. Acute kidney injury in the fetus and neonate. *Semin Fetal Neonatal Med.* 2017;22:90–97.
12. Vesoulis ZA, Mintzer JP, Chock VY. Neonatal NIRS monitoring: recommendations for data capture and review of analytics. *J Perinatol.* 2021;41:675–688.
13. Guo Y, Wang Y, Marin T, Easley K, Patel RM, Josephson CD. Statistical methods for characterizing transfusion-related changes in regional oxygenation using near-infrared spectroscopy (NIRS) in preterm infants. *Stat Methods Med Res.* 2019;28:2710–2723.
14. Bernal NP, Hoffman GM, Ghanayem NS, Arca MJ. Cerebral and somatic near-infrared spectroscopy in normal newborns. *J Pediatr Surg.* 2010;45:1306–1310.
15. Montaldo P, De Leonibus C, Giordano L, De Vivo M, Giliberti P. Cerebral, renal and mesenteric regional oxygen saturation of term infants during transition. *J Pediatr Surg.* 2015;50:1273–1277.
16. Bailey SM, Hendricks-Munoz KD, Mally P. Cerebral, renal, and splanchnic tissue oxygen saturation values in healthy term newborns. *Am J Perinatol.* 2014;31:339–344.
17. Richter AE, Schat TE, Van Braeckel KNJA, Scherjon SA, Bos AF, Kooi EMW. The effect of maternal antihypertensive drugs on the cerebral, renal and splanchnic tissue oxygen extraction of preterm neonates. *Neonatology.* 2016;110:163–171.
18. Harer MW, Condit PE, Chuck JE, Lasarev MR, Chock VY. Renal oxygenation measured by near infrared spectroscopy in preterm neonates in the first week. *Pediatr Res.* 2022;92(6):1744–1748.
19. McNeill S, Gatenby JC, McElroy S, Engelhardt B. Normal cerebral, renal and abdominal regional oxygen saturations using near-infrared spectroscopy in preterm infants. *J Perinatol.* 2011;31:51–57.
20. Hoffman GM, Ghanayem NS, Tweddell JS. Noninvasive assessment of cardiac output. *Semin Thorac Cardiovasc Surg Pediatr Card Surg Annu.* 2005;12–21.

21. Kurth CD, McCann JC, Wu J, Miles L, Loepke AW. Cerebral oxygen saturation-time threshold for hypoxic-ischemic injury in piglets. *Anesth Analg.* 2009;108:1268–1277.
22. Wu Y, Wang H, Pei J, Jiang X, Tang J. Acute kidney injury in premature and low birth weight neonates: a systematic review and meta-analysis. *Pediatr Nephrol.* 2022;37:275–287. Available at: https://doi.org/10.1007/s00467-021-05251-0
23. Jetton JG, Boohaker LJ, Sethi SK, et al. Incidence and outcomes of neonatal acute kidney injury (AWAKEN): a multicentre, multinational, observational cohort study. *Lancet Child Adolesc Health.* 2017;1:184–194.
24. Bonsante F, Ramful D, Binquet C, et al. Low renal oxygen saturation at near-infrared spectroscopy on the first day of life is associated with developing acute kidney injury in very preterm infants. *Neonatology.* 2019;115:198–204.
25. Guillet R, Selewski DT, Griffin R, et al. Relationship of patent ductus arteriosus management with neonatal AKI. *J Perinatol.* 2021;41:1441–1447.
26. Underwood MA, Milstein JM, Sherman MP. Near-infrared spectroscopy as a screening tool for patent ductus arteriosus in extremely low birth weight infants. *Neonatology.* 2007;91:134–139.
27. Chock VY, Rose LA, Mante JV, Punn R. Near-infrared spectroscopy for detection of a significant patent ductus arteriosus. *Pediatr Res.* 2016;80:675–680. Available at: https://doi.org/10.1038/pr.2016.148
28. Petrova A, Bhatt M, Mehta R. Regional tissue oxygenation in preterm born infants in association with echocardiographically significant patent ductus arteriosus. *J Perinatol.* 2011;31:460–464.
29. van der Laan ME, Roofthooft MTR, Fries MWA, et al. A hemodynamically significant patent ductus arteriosus does not affect cerebral or renal tissue oxygenation in preterm infants. *Neonatology.* 2016;110:141–147.
30. Navikiene J, Virsilas E, Vankeviciene R, Liubsys A, Jankauskiene A. Brain and renal oxygenation measured by NIRS related to patent ductus arteriosus in preterm infants: a prospective observational study. *BMC Pediatr.* 2021;21:559.
31. Bhatt M, Petrova A, Mehta R. Does treatment of patent ductus arteriosus with cyclooxygenase inhibitors affect neonatal regional tissue oxygenation? *Pediatr Cardiol.* 2012;33:1307–1314.
32. Ruf B, Bonelli V, Balling G, et al. Intraoperative renal near-infrared spectroscopy indicates developing acute kidney injury in infants undergoing cardiac surgery with cardiopulmonary bypass: a case-control study. *Crit Care.* 2015;19:27.
33. Owens GE, King K, Gurney JG, Charpie JR. Low renal oximetry correlates with acute kidney injury after infant cardiac surgery. *Pediatr Cardiol.* 2011;32:183–188.
34. Adams PS, Vargas D, Baust T, et al. Associations of perioperative renal oximetry via near-infrared spectroscopy, urinary biomarkers, and postoperative acute kidney injury in infants after congenital heart surgery: should creatinine continue to be the gold standard? *Pediatr Crit Care Med.* 2019;20:27–37.
35. Neunhoeffer F, Wiest M, Sandner K, et al. Non-invasive measurement of renal perfusion and oxygen metabolism to predict postoperative acute kidney injury in neonates and infants after cardiopulmonary bypass surgery. *Br J Anaesth.* 2016;117:623–634.
36. Hazle MA, Gajarski RJ, Aiyagari R, et al. Urinary biomarkers and renal near-infrared spectroscopy predict ICU outcomes following cardiac surgery in infants under 6 months of age. *J Thorac Cardiovasc Surg.* 2013;146:861–867.e1.
37. Selewski DT, Jordan BK, Askenazi DJ, Dechert RE, Sarkar S. Acute kidney injury in asphyxiated newborns treated with therapeutic hypothermia. *J Pediatr.* 2013;162:725–729.e1.
38. Sarkar S, Askenazi DJ, Jordan BK, et al. Relationship between acute kidney injury and brain MRI findings in asphyxiated newborns after therapeutic hypothermia. *Pediatr Res.* 2014; 75:431–435.
39. Ancora G, Maranella E, Grandi S, et al. Early predictors of short term neurodevelopmental outcome in asphyxiated cooled infants. A combined brain amplitude integrated electroencephalography and near infrared spectroscopy study. *Brain Dev.* 2013;35:26–31.
40. Goeral K, Urlesberger B, Giordano V, et al. Prediction of outcome in neonates with hypoxic-ischemic encephalopathy II: role of amplitude-integrated electroencephalography and cerebral oxygen saturation measured by near-infrared spectroscopy. *Neonatology.* 2017;112:193–202.
41. Chock VY, Cho SH, Frymoyer A. Aminophylline for renal protection in neonatal hypoxic-ischemic encephalopathy in the era of therapeutic hypothermia. *Pediatr Res.* 2021;89:974–980.
42. Maskatia SA, Kwiatkowski D, Bhombal S, et al. A fetal risk stratification pathway for neonatal aortic coarctation reduces medical exposure. *J Pediatr.* 2021;237:102–108.e3.
43. Chock VY, Variane GFT, Netto A, Van Meurs KP. NIRS improves hemodynamic monitoring and detection of risk for cerebral injury: cases in the neonatal intensive care nursery. *J Matern Fetal Neonatal Med.* 2020;33:1802–1810.
44. Johnson BA, Hoffman GM, Tweddell JS, et al. Near-infrared spectroscopy in neonates before palliation of hypoplastic left heart syndrome. *Ann Thorac Surg.* 2009;87:571–577.
45. Noh C, Van Meurs KP, Danzer E, Chock VY. Near-infrared spectroscopy as a hemodynamic monitoring tool during neonatal extracorporeal life support: a case series. *J Extra Corpor Technol.* 2022;54(1):61–66.
46. Lau PE, Cruz S, Garcia-Prats J, et al. Use of renal near-infrared spectroscopy measurements in congenital diaphragmatic hernia patients on ECMO. *J Pediatr Surg.* 2017;52:689–692.
47. Koch HW, Hansen TG. Perioperative use of cerebral and renal near-infrared spectroscopy in neonates: a 24-h observational study. *Paediatr Anaesth.* 2016;26:190–198.
48. Conforti A, Giliberti P, Mondi V, et al. Near infrared spectroscopy: experience on esophageal atresia infants. *J Pediatr Surg.* 2014;49:1064–1068.
49. Stienstra RM, McHoney M. Near-infrared spectroscopy (NIRS) measured tissue oxygenation in neonates with gastroschisis: a pilot study. *J Matern Fetal Neonatal Med.* 2022;35(25): 5099–5107.
50. O'Hare EM, Jelin AC, Miller JL, et al. Amnioinfusions to treat early onset anhydramnios caused by renal anomalies: background and rationale for the renal anhydramnios fetal therapy trial. *Fetal Diagn Ther.* 2019;45:365–372.
51. Ito K, Ookawara S, Uchida T, et al. Measurement of tissue oxygenation using near-infrared spectroscopy in patients undergoing hemodialysis. *J Vis Exp.* 2020;164:e61721. Available at: https://doi.org/10.3791/61721
52. Variane GFT, Chock VY, Netto A, Pietrobom RFR, Van Meurs KP. Simultaneous near-infrared spectroscopy (NIRS) and amplitude-integrated electroencephalography (aEEG): dual use of brain monitoring techniques improves our understanding of physiology. *Front Pediatr.* 2019;7:560.
53. Maly S, Janousek L, Bortel R, et al. NIRS-based monitoring of kidney graft perfusion. *PLoS One.* 2020;15:e0243154.
54. Hansen ML, Pellicer A, Gluud C, et al. Cerebral near-infrared spectroscopy monitoring versus treatment as usual for extremely preterm infants: a protocol for the SafeBoosC randomised clinical phase III trial. *Trials.* 2019;20:811.

Chapter 15

Urosepsis and Uroprophylaxis

Noa Fleiss, MD, and Melissa Posner, MD

Chapter Outline

Introduction

Late-onset sepsis, defined as sepsis occurring after 72 hours of age, is a significant cause of morbidity and mortality in term and preterm neonates. Most of the research on neonatal sepsis has thus far focused on blood and cerebrospinal fluid (CSF) findings, while comparatively little information exists regarding the prevalence and significance of urosepsis and urinary tract infections (UTIs) in this population. The most recent consensus report by the American Academy of Pediatrics on UTI excluded making recommendations for infants 0–2 months of age due to the ongoing lack of available data.[1] From a clinical standpoint, this has led to significant practice variation and lack of consensus in the approach to managing UTIs in neonates less than 2 months of age, especially in preterm infants.[2,3] Although previous research has shown that the characteristics of UTIs in this population differ from those in older infants and children, inconsistent diagnostic and treatment criteria have made it difficult to determine true prevalence rates, ideal treatment durations, and appropriate prophylaxis and imaging guidelines.

Epidemiology

In general, UTIs in neonates are found in higher prevalence than older populations, have higher rates of associated urosepsis, are more likely to be caused by non–*Escherichia coli* pathogens, and predominantly affect males.[4–7]

OVERALL PREVALENCE

Approximately 5% of children aged 2 to 24 months with unexplained fever are found to have a UTI.[1] Prevalence can range from 0.1% to 1% in all neonates and 9% to 25% when considering just preterm neonates.[6,8,9] Multiple studies have demonstrated that rates of UTIs increase with decreasing gestational age as well as decreasing birth weight.[3,6,10] Levy et al. reported UTI was significantly more common in very low birth weight (VLBW) infants than in infants with a birth weight of >1500 g (3.2% vs. 0.4%),[3] and Drumm et al. noted the rate of UTI in their extremely low birthweight population was 13.8% vs. 8.5% in their VLBW infants.[6] In general, overall prevalence has been difficult to determine due to inconsistent diagnostic criteria, which will be discussed later.

RATES OF UROSEPSIS

Urosepsis is defined as isolation of an identical bacterial pathogen in a concomitant blood culture and urine culture. Rates of urosepsis in term infants can vary from 4% to 12%.[5,11] In preterm neonates, rates of urosepsis have been found to be significantly higher, ranging anywhere from 11% to 38%.[3,12,13] In one of the largest retrospective reviews available, Downey et al. evaluated data from 322 neonatal intensive care units (NICUs) in the Pediatrix Medical Group network over a 13-year period to determine rates of concordance between positive urine cultures and blood or CSF cultures. They found that 13% of neonates with a UTI also had a concomitant blood culture with the same bacterial pathogen, and 3% had a positive CSF culture with the same pathogen. The risk of urosepsis increased with decreasing gestational age and birth weight, specifically in those infants born less than 26 weeks' gestation and weighing less than 1500 g. *Staphylococcus* UTIs were most likely to be concordant (38%), followed by *Candida* (23%). Although gram-negative organisms were the most frequent causative organisms for UTIs in neonates, they were concordant with blood cultures only 6% of the time.[12] Given the high rates of urosepsis in the preterm population as well as the elevated risk of concomitant meningitis, it is recommended that in an infant that appears clinically ill, clinicians obtain accurate and timely blood and CSF cultures whenever a UTI is suspected to ensure this vulnerable population is being treated appropriately.

COMMON PATHOGENS

Escherichia coli is by far the most common causative pathogen in community-acquired UTIs in term infants and neonates and has been shown to account for up

TABLE 15.1 Differences in Incidence of Common Pathogens Isolated in Nosocomial Urinary Tract Infections in Preterm Neonatal Intensive Care Unit Neonates as Compared With Community-Acquired Urinary Tract Infections in Term Infants

Organism	Term Infant Incidence (%)[5,11,14,15]	Preterm Neonate Incidence (%)[6,10,12,16]
Escherichia coli	71–91	4–27
Klebsiella spp.	4–10	21–43
Enterococcus spp.	2–10	13–19
Enterobacter spp.	3–4	12–19
Pseudomonas spp.	1	8
Candida spp.	0	15–39
CoNS	0.3	14–20

CoNS, coagulase-negative staphylococci.

to 90% of infections in prior studies.[14] In hospitalized preterm patients with predominantly nosocomially acquired UTIs, *Klebsiella*, *Enterobacter* spp., *Enterococcus* spp., coagulase-negative staphylococci, and *Candida* spp. are found with much higher frequency (Table 15.1). *E. coli* is less commonly seen in this population, with an average incidence of approximately 18%, though some single-center studies have reported rates as high as 27% in the VLBW population.[3] It is important to note that although coagulase-negative staphylococci is generally considered a contaminant in most term infants and older children, it can in fact be a causative agent for UTI in premature neonates. Downey et al. reported isolation of coagulase-negative staphylococci in 14% of catheterized urine culture samples from infants with suspected infection and 18% concordance with positive blood cultures.[12]

MALE PREDOMINANCE AND THE ROLE OF CIRCUMCISION

Although female sex has previously been identified as a protective clinical factor with regards to neonatal UTI,[13] a clear male predominance has been associated with UTI in both term and preterm infants. In multiple retrospective studies of term infants with community-acquired UTIs, approximately 75%–85% of the affected study population were male.[5,11] The same can be said for premature infants in the NICU, where approximately 65%–75% of positive UTIs are in male infants.[3,6,13]

Male infants who are uncircumcised have significantly higher rates of UTIs than those who have undergone circumcision.[1] A metaanalysis by Shaikh et al. reported that among febrile male infants less than 3 months of age, only 2.4% of the boys who had been circumcised were diagnosed with a UTI and 20.1% of the uncircumcised boys had a UTI.[17] A separate metaanalysis found that the single risk factor of lack of circumcision confers a 23.3% chance of UTI during one's lifetime.[18] Although there are limited data with regards to the effects of circumcision in premature infants on rates of UTIs, the data suggest that there are higher rates of UTI in preterm infants who are not circumcised by the time of discharge, and that circumcision may be beneficial in reducing the risk for recurrent future UTIs in this population.[19] Clinicians should therefore be mindful of such trends when counseling families with preterm male infants on the risks and benefits of undergoing circumcision prior to discharge from a neonatal intensive care unit.

Diagnostic Considerations

PREFERRED SAMPLE COLLECTION

Diagnosing UTIs in the preterm and neonatal population can be challenging for a number of reasons, beginning with the mode of urine sampling. To obtain a urine culture, which is considered the gold standard for diagnosing UTIs, it is important to obtain a sterile, uncontaminated urine sample. The two main techniques for collecting a sterile sample in neonates include suprapubic aspiration or transurethral catheterization. Although both of these techniques are considered invasive, in general noninvasive techniques such as a clean catch or bag urine sample are not considered sufficiently sterile to be able to adequately diagnose a UTI. Research has shown that the risks of contamination with perineal bacteria from a bag specimen are high with false-positive rates of up to 88%.[1]

Suprapubic aspiration has generally been considered the gold standard for detecting bacteria in the urine due to its enhanced sterility,[1] although there are many limitations associated with this technique. Not only does it require a high degree of technical expertise and experience, but it is also viewed as significantly

more invasive than transurethral catheterization by both parents and physicians. Additionally, a prospective, randomized controlled study by Kozer et al. found that in infants younger than 2 months of age, suprapubic aspiration was more painful than transurethral catheterization.[20] These findings were further validated in a follow-up study by El-Naggar et al., which focused specifically on preterm infants. In this prospective, single-blind, randomized clinical trial 48 preterm infants with a mean gestational age of 27 weeks were randomized to either suprapubic aspiration or transurethral catheterization. Pain scores were noted to be significantly higher in those infants who received suprapubic aspiration when compared with infants who underwent transurethral catheterization.[21] Although not statistically significant, it is worth noting that both studies also demonstrated a higher procedure success rate in the transurethral catheterization group when compared with the suprapubic aspiration group.[20,21] Therefore, although both suprapubic aspiration and transurethral catheterization are considered acceptable techniques for urine collection and diagnosing UTI, transurethral catheterization is preferred due to its higher success rates, less invasive nature, and decreased level of pain and discomfort inflicted on the infant.

VARIATIONS IN DIAGNOSTIC CRITERIA

There is a lack of consensus on diagnostic criteria for UTIs in the preterm and neonatal population. NICU patients with UTI often present with nonspecific symptomatology such as apnea and bradycardia, respiratory distress, desaturation events, temperature instability, vomiting, diarrhea, and lethargy, making it difficult to rely on clinical manifestations for diagnosis.[5,13,22] Laboratory indices have also not been found to be particularly sensitive or specific for the diagnosis of UTI. In a study by Foglia et al., maximal white blood cell count and C-reactive protein did not differ significantly between UTI cases and controls in their neonatal intensive care unit population, with poor positive predictive value for both tests.[10] Diagnosis is therefore based on growth of bacteria from a sterilely obtained urine culture. However, much of the current variability in practice centered around what level of growth constitutes a true bacterial infection of the urine as opposed to contamination that does not require treatment. These cutoffs vary both nationally

TABLE 15.2 Variations in Published Urinary Tract Infection Guidelines in Children With Suggested Bacterial Colony Cutoff Values Depending on Urine Sample Collection Method

Guideline (Reference)	Suprapubic Aspiration (CFU/mL)	Transurethral Catheterization (CFU/mL)	Clean Catch (CFU/mL)
CDC 2020[23]	$\geq 10^5$	$\geq 10^5$	Not defined
ESPU 2015[24]	Any growth	$\geq 10^3$–5×10^4	$\geq 10^4$–10^5
AAP 2011[1]	$\geq 5 \times 10^4$	$\geq 5 \times 10^4$	Not defined
Canada 2014[25]	Any growth	$\geq 5 \times 10^4$	$\geq 10^5$
Italy 2020[26]	$\geq 10^4$	$\geq 10^4$	$\geq 10^5$
Germany 2007[27]	Any growth	$> 10^4$	$> 10^5$

AAP, American Academy of Pediatrics; *CDC*, Centers for Disease Control; *CFU*, Colony-forming unit; *ESPU*, European Society for Pediatric Urology.

and internationally depending on the sampling method used to obtain urine (Table 15.2).

To limit treatment of asymptomatic bacteriuria, the American Academy of Pediatrics (AAP) consensus guidelines from 2011 suggest an appropriate threshold to diagnose UTI in infants and children is the presence of at least 50,000 colony-forming unit (CFU)/mL of a single urinary pathogen in conjunction with a urinalysis with evidence of pyuria.[1] This is somewhat different from the 2020 Centers for Disease Control recommendations for children under 1 year of age, which define a UTI as follows: at least one abnormal sign including fever, hypothermia, apnea, bradycardia, lethargy, or feeding intolerance and a positive urine culture in a specimen obtained sterilely containing no more than two species, one of which is a bacterium with $>100,000$ CFU/mL.[23] Similar to the AAP guidelines, the Centers for Disease Control guidelines also suggest that a positive urinalysis can be helpful in differentiating true infections from contamination if colony counts are $<100,000$ CFU/mL. Contamination has generally been defined as the presence of more than two pathogens, colony counts $< 10,000$ CFU/mL on urine culture, or colony counts $<100,000$ CFU/mL on urine culture in conjunction with a negative urinalysis.[23,28]

The diagnostic criteria of $\geq 10,000$ CFU/mL of one or two organisms isolated via catheterization or suprapubic aspiration is one of the more commonly used definitions of UTI in neonates.[3,6,10,13] However, in clinical practice, many institutions follow the AAP recommendations and utilize a cutoff value of $>50,000$ CFU/mL even though this has not been validated in infants less than 2 months of age. Other experts feel that the cutoff value of $>50,000$ CFU/mL is too high.

For example, Clarke et al. noted that 10% of the infants who had a positive urine culture with bacterial counts ranging from 1000 to 10,000 CFU/mL also had a blood culture positive for the same organism, indicating that a stricter cutoff value in this population may have inadvertently missed a significant number of urosepsis cases.[13] Additionally, a Swedish study demonstrated that applying a cutoff level of 50,000 CFU/mL carries a risk of ignoring a significant portion of infants with UTI. Furthermore, these infants have similar risk of vesicoureteral reflux (VUR) and renal damage as those with a high bacterial count.[14] Lower bacterial counts have also been found more frequently in urinary infections caused by non–E. coli species and in preterm populations.[14,29] In general, although no specific guidelines exist regarding appropriate bacterial cutoffs in the neonatal population, the current body of literature seems to support utilizing lower colony counts of $>10,000$ CFU/mL to diagnose UTI in this age group given the unreliability of clinical signs and laboratory indices, the predilection toward non–E. coli infections, and the increased risk of potentially missing an underlying anatomic issue that could lead to further complications later in life.

THE ROLE OF URINALYSIS

Historically, urinalysis alone has been felt to be an unreliable predictor of UTI due to its low sensitivity and specificity, and general consensus is that it should always be performed and interpreted in conjunction with a urine culture when diagnosing a UTI. Although this still holds true, recent studies have suggested that the utility and predictive value of a positive urinalysis may be underutilized. Tzimenatos et al. evaluated the sensitivity and specificity of a positive urinalysis result (defined by the presence of any leukocyte esterase, nitrite, or pyuria with >5 white blood cells per high-power field) in febrile infants less than 60 days old using two different definitions of UTI: urine culture with growth >50,000 or growth >10,000 CFU/mL of a uropathogen. The sensitivity of a positive urinalysis increased with increasing colony counts; with the >50,000 CFU/mL group, the sensitivity was 94%, compared with a sensitivity of 87% in the >10,000 CFU/mL group.[30] This is consistent with other more recent studies that have used a more conservative definition of UTI with a higher colony count[31,32] and perhaps explains why past studies that used much lower colony counts to define UTIs reported significantly lower sensitivities and specificities with regards to urinalysis. This has also been shown to be true in NICU populations, where higher colony counts are associated with increased specificity and sensitivity of positive urinalyses, though the values are generally lower than in older populations likely due to differences in inflammatory responses.[2] Overall, a urinalysis can be a useful adjunct to the urine culture when diagnosing a UTI in the neonatal population, though further management and treatment strategies including appropriate antibiotic choices must ultimately rely on urine culture results.

Treatment

APPROPRIATE ANTIBIOTIC CHOICE

When a UTI is suspected in a neonate, treatment with broad-spectrum antibiotics should be initiated as soon as possible, as early and appropriate treatment has been shown to prevent severe parenchymal involvement and renal damage.[4] Parenteral or IV antibacterial therapy is preferred over oral medications due to the high rates of urosepsis observed in the neonatal population. This is especially true in high-risk populations such as preterm infants in the neonatal intensive care unit where rates of urosepsis are even higher and the bioavailability of most antibiotics is not known.[33] In term infants and older children, combination therapy with ampicillin and an aminoglycoside (i.e., gentamicin) is generally considered appropriate first-line treatment with adequate therapeutic efficacy.[22] This same regimen can also be utilized for preterm NICU infants if UTI is suspected within the first few days of life. However, if UTI is suspected in the context of a late-onset sepsis evaluation, broadening antibiotic coverage should be considered

due to the increased risk of a nosocomial pathogen causing the infection.[34,35] Antibiotic coverage should be narrowed based on the sensitivities and specificities of urine, blood, and CSF culture results. When choosing antibiotic coverage, clinicians should also take into account resistance patterns of common urinary pathogens in both their NICU environment and community as these can vary substantially by both clinical practice setting and geographic location.

LENGTH OF TREATMENT

Neonates with UTI and concomitant bacteremia are usually treated with parenteral antibiotics for 7 to 14 days, as per standard sepsis management recommendations.[1] Management of neonates with isolated UTI without bacteremia varies. Although many centers will preferentially utilize parenteral antibiotics for the duration of treatment, the optimal amount of time for treatment is controversial and can vary widely based on expert opinion and center-specific guidelines. A study by Brady et al. evaluated the effectiveness of "short" (≤3 days) versus "long" (≥4 days) courses of IV antibiotic treatment in more than 12,000 infants less than 6 months of age who were hospitalized for acute UTI or pyelonephritis. The end point of the study was readmission due to UTI recurrence within 30 days (defined as treatment failure). There was no significant difference in treatment failure rates noted between the two patient groups, with a 1.6% failure rate in "short" duration therapy and a 2.2% failure rate with "long" duration therapy.[36] In older infants, Benador found that the risk of renal scarring was no different between infants who received 3 days of IV antibiotic therapy vs. infants who received 10 days of IV antibiotic therapy for treatment of uncomplicated UTI.[37] As increasing numbers of studies have shown the negative effects of prolonged antibiotic exposure in NICU infants, such as increased risk of invasive fungal infections, disruption of the microbiome, and development of antibiotic resistance, more and more clinicians are opting for shorter antibiotic courses when treating uncomplicated UTIs.[38]

Uroprophylaxis

CONGENITAL ANOMALIES OF THE KIDNEY AND URINARY TRACT

Infants with an increased risk for developing recurrent UTIs often have congenital anomalies of the kidney and urinary tract (CAKUT), which account for 20%–30% of all major congenital birth defects.[39] Neonates and infants who are at an increased risk for UTIs may have a form of CAKUT that is associated with an obstructive uropathy, affecting the antegrade flow of urine.[40] The main concern in infants with interference to urinary flow involves the potential risk for dilation of the ureters and kidneys, which can lead to renal parenchymal disease and renal failure. Additionally, there is a risk of recurrent episodes of UTI and pyelonephritis secondary to urinary stasis, which can further exacerbate the development of chronic kidney disease.[41–45] The most common etiologies of obstructive uropathy include ureteropelvic junction obstruction, ureterovesical junction obstruction, posterior urethral valves, duplicated collecting system with ureterocele, urethral atresia or stricture, VUR, and multicystic dysplastic kidney.[40] Obstructive uropathies are detected through radiologic imaging modalities, most commonly during prenatal ultrasound, but often postnatally following a first febrile UTI.

ROLE OF DIAGNOSTIC IMAGING

The AAP guidelines currently recommend that all infants aged 2 to 24 months with a first febrile UTI obtain a renal and bladder ultrasound to assess for any anatomic malformations. A voiding cystourethrogram (VCUG) is then recommended if there is any evidence of hydronephrosis or renal scarring on renal ultrasound, which may be suggestive of an obstructive uropathy, most commonly VUR.[46] VUR refers to the backflow of urine from the bladder to the upper urinary tract and is graded from I to V, indicating severity as determined by the VCUG.[45] Similar to the diagnosis of UTI in the neonatal population, there remains inconsistencies in the literature regarding imaging for the diagnosis of VUR in this population.

In a retrospective study of 197 neonates with fever and culture-proven UTI, Wallace et al. found that the sensitivity of a renal ultrasound detecting grades I–V VUR on a follow-up VCUG was 32.7% (95% confidence interval [CI], 20.0%–47.5%). However, when the authors looked at the sensitivity of renal ultrasound to detect high-grade VUR (IV–V), it was 86.7%.[47] Another study looking at NICU patients with a prior diagnosis of UTI found that renal pelvis dilation detected on renal ultrasound was not predictive of VUR on VCUG.[2] Similarly, Walawender et al.

reviewed 81 NICU patients admitted to Nationwide Children's Hospital system and found that the sensitivity of a renal ultrasound for detection of VUR on a follow-up VCUG was only 60%.[48]

With the variability in the sensitivity and predictive value of diagnostic imaging for infants at risk for recurrent UTIs, the role of antibiotic prophylaxis for UTI prevention is highly debated and controversial.[43] With some etiologies of obstructive uropathy, surgical management is the treatment of choice, and antibiotic prophylaxis is indicated until the obstruction is surgically corrected. Other etiologies can have spontaneous resolution of the anatomic defect over time, and surgery (with or without antibiotic prophylaxis) is not immediately warranted. In these cases, the decision to start antibiotics as prophylaxis is sometimes delayed. Furthermore, with the growing body of literature describing the risks of long-term antibiotic administration, a less aggressive surveillance "watch and wait" approach may be considered.[43,45]

VESICOURETERAL REFLUX

In infants and neonates, with VUR and hydronephrosis, the initiation of uroprophylaxis is controversial. The main clinical concern in infants with persistent VUR is the potential risk for long-term sequelae secondary to recurrent episodes of UTI and pyelonephritis.[41–45] Although current literature on VUR focuses on older infants and children, there is a paucity of data regarding neonates. Although antibiotic prophylaxis remains an option for UTI prevention in children with VUR, a newer observational approach, predicated on frequent renal ultrasounds and surveillance of infants for symptoms consistent with febrile UTIs, has also become a viable option.[43]

The RIVUR trial (Randomized Intervention for Children with Vesicoureteral Reflux)[49] was a landmark study that randomized 607 infants and children with VUR and one or two prior UTIs to either intervention with antibiotic prophylaxis or placebo. The risk of recurrent febrile UTI was reduced by 50% in the intervention group (hazard ratio 0.5; 95% CI 0.34–0.74); however, the authors found no difference in the incidence of new renal scarring between the treatment groups. The children in the RIVUR trial had very close follow-up with high adherence rates, suggesting that close surveillance of infants by their families for early detection of symptomatic UTIs, and short-term antibiotic

TABLE 15.3 Current Recommendations for the Evaluation and Treatment of Vesicoureteral Reflux in Infants Less Than 1 Year of Age

Infants < 1 Year Old	EAU Guidelines[54]	AUA Guidelines[55]
When to obtain VCUG	Prenatally diagnosed hydronephrosis and first febrile UTI Siblings or offspring of VUR patients, if evidence of renal scarring on renal ultrasound and/or hx of UTI Febrile UTI Lower urinary tract dysfunction	Prenatally diagnosed hydronephrosis (high-grade, 3 and 4) Siblings or offspring of VUR patients if evidence of renal scarring on renal ultrasound and/or hx of UTI Febrile UTI Lower urinary tract dysfunction
Antibiotics prophylaxis	First-line treatment if diagnosed with VUR regardless of grade	First-line treatment if diagnosed with VUR (any grade) and febrile UTI or high-grade VUR (III–V) in the absence of febrile UTI
Surveillance option	Not option in first year of life	Option in absence of febrile UTI and VUR grade I–II

AUA, American Urological Association; *EAU*, European Association of Urology; *hx*, history; *UTI*, urinary tract infection; *VCUG*, voiding cystourethrogram; *VUR*, vesicoureteral reflux.

treatment may preclude long-term sequelae regardless of antibiotic prophylaxis. A Swedish reflux study[50] comparing recurrence of febrile UTIs in children with VUR found recurrence to be significantly lower in females randomized to the antibiotic prophylaxis group compared with the placebo observation group (19% vs. 57%, $P = .0002$). Yet, this reduction was not observed in males. Conversely, Pennesi et al. found that the risk of having at least one febrile UTI recurrence was not different between infants randomized to antibiotic prophylaxis versus placebo over a 2-year follow up (relative risk 1.2, 95% CI 0.68–2.11).[51] A Cochrane review from 2019 of 34 studies on this topic found no benefit of antibiotic prophylaxis in the prevention of symptomatic and febrile UTIs in children and infants with VUR.[52] Adherence of parents and caregivers to recommended practices regarding antibiotic administration to infants for prophylaxis must also be considered and may account for some of the variability seen between these studies.[45,53]

The European Association of Urology[54] and the American Urological Association[55] provide expert opinions and guidelines for the diagnosis and management of VUR in infants less than 1 year of age. Both references highlight lack of quality data to elucidate the controversies of this topic, and although they do present recommendations, they do not present a consensus. Nevertheless, both references recommend VCUG for infants with prenatal diagnosis of hydronephrosis and

for infants who have siblings or parents with history of VUR. These recommendations include antibiotic prophylaxis as first-line treatment for all infants with VUR in infancy at less than 1 year of age (Table 15.3).

HYDRONEPHROSIS

Fetal hydronephrosis, or dilation of the renal pelvis, is commonly seen on antenatal ultrasound with a reported occurrence of 1% to 5% of all pregnancies.[56] A significant percentage of antenatal hydronephrosis (AHN) is transient and will spontaneously resolve. Therefore, only a small percentage of infants may have AHN secondary to clinically significant CAKUT and require early diagnosis and intervention. As a result of prenatal ultrasounds, neonates with urologic and renal structural anomalies are being detected in utero, prior to any development of clinical symptoms.[57] The decision of whether or not to start prophylactic antibiotics for AHN after birth largely depends on the grading score for AHN as developed by the Society for Fetal Urology (SFU). The grading system has been widely adapted for reliable classification of severity of AHN and is based on the renal pelvic diameter (RPD).[58] An RPD less than 10 mm is considered mild and grade I; an RPD greater than 15 mm is severe, and these infants often develop significant disease requiring surgical correction. In addition, other risk factors for postnatal renal pathology include oligohydramnios, prematurity, megacystitis,[59,60] parenchymal thinning, ureteral dilatation, increased echogenicity of the pyramids, poor corticomedullary differentiation,[61] presence of renal cysts, and chromosomal anomalies.[56]

A metaanalysis assessing the risk of postnatal pathology in infants with confirmed AHN found that there was a significant correlation with increasing degree of hydronephrosis. The authors noted a 11.9% risk of postnatal pathology or significant renal disease in patients with mild AHN, a 45.1% of significant pathology with moderate hydronephrosis, and 88.3% risk with severe.[62] However, this does not hold true for VUR, as these authors could not demonstrate a significant difference in the incidence of VUR among patients with mild, moderate, and severe AHN. The most common etiologies of AHN were transient dilation of the collecting system, urinary tract obstructive uropathy (commonly at the ureteropelvic junction and vesicoureteral junction), as well as nonobstructive malformations including megaureters and VUR.[56]

The indication for antibiotic prophylaxis is often based on postnatal ultrasound findings, the severity of the hydronephrosis, whether or not it is unilateral vs. bilateral, and the etiology of the hydronephrosis. In a cohort review[63] of 430 infants without VUR, Lee et al. found that 40% of infants with high-grade hydronephrosis developed a UTI, in contrast to 33% with grade III and only 4% of infants with grade I (P < .001). Presence of hydroureter was also associated with increased frequency of UTI. Similarly, another study looked at severe obstructive hydronephrosis secondary to obstruction within the upper urinary tract and found the incidence of UTI to be approximately 34% before surgical correction.[64] Despite a myriad of similar studies[65,66] there has been a paucity of randomized controlled clinical trials evaluating the role of antibiotic prophylaxis in AHN for prevention of UTIs. One systematic review of 21 studies found that for high-grade hydronephrosis (SFU grade III and IV) antibiotic prophylaxis decreased the rates of UTI in those that were treated compared with those not treated (14.6% vs. 28.9%). The authors also found that with low-grade hydronephrosis (SFU grade I and II) there was no significant differences in the pooled UTI rates between those treated with antibiotics and those who were not (2.2% vs. 2.8%).[57] Based on the current evidence, and recommendations from SFU consensus statement for prenatal hydronephrosis, starting prophylactic antibiotic is beneficial in high-risk neonates and infants, including those with higher grades of hydronephrosis.[56]

Antibiotic Regimens for Uroprophylaxis

Once prophylactic antibiotics are decided on by the clinician, the most common options for neonates are amoxicillin and ampicillin and less commonly, cephalosporins. Although these agents are not first-line treatment options in older children, due to a concern regarding their resistance profile among gram-negative bacilli,[67,68] they are currently the safest agents to use in the neonatal population. The more common agents prescribed for UTI prophylaxis in infants older than 2 months of age include trimethoprim in combination with sulfamethoxazole (TMP-SMX) (which was the prophylaxis treatment of choice in the landmark RIVUR trial) or nitrofurantoin.[69] Long-term use of TMP-SMX and nitrofurantoin has been associated with several adverse reactions most commonly nausea, vomiting, and allergic skin reactions.[70] In the neonatal population both TMP-SMX and nitrofurantoin have been shown to increase the risk of bilirubin toxicity and therefore are avoided.[71]

Long-Term Considerations for Antimicrobial Exposure

Neonates and children with prolonged antimicrobial exposure run the risk of developing breakthrough UTIs through uropathogen resistance.[68] A metaanalysis examining randomized controlled trials studying patients with a history of VUR on prolonged antibiotic prophylaxis vs. placebo found that patients with prolonged antimicrobial exposure were more likely to have a multidrug-resistant infection (33% vs. 6%, P < .001) and had 6.4 times the odds of developing a multidrug-resistant infection.[72] As a result, clinicians should weigh the risks and benefits of prophylaxis as a management strategy. Although currently the expert opinions for the neonatal population still favor the use of antibiotic prophylaxis in neonates with VUR and high-grade hydronephrosis, more studies are needed in this age group to assess and compare the potential risks of a "watchful waiting" surveillance approach, as has been described in older children.[73]

REFERENCES

1. Roberts KB, Subcommittee on Urinary Tract Infection, Steering Committee on Quality Improvement and Management. Urinary tract infection: clinical practice guideline for the diagnosis and management of the initial UTI in febrile infants and children 2 to 24 months. *Pediatrics.* 2011;128(3):595–610. doi:10.1542/peds.2011-1330
2. Weems M, Wei D, Ramanathan R, Barton L, Vachon L, Sardesai S. Urinary tract infections in a neonatal intensive care unit. *Am J Perinatol.* 2014;32(7):695–702. doi:10.1055/s-0034-1395474
3. Levy I, Comarsca J, Davidovits M, Klinger G, Sirota L, Linder N. Urinary tract infection in preterm infants: the protective role of breastfeeding. *Pediatr Nephrol.* 2009;24(3):527–531. doi:10.1007/s00467-008-1007-7
4. Beetz R. Evaluation and management of urinary tract infections in the neonate. *Curr Opin Pediatr.* 2012;24(2):205–211. doi:10.1097/MOP.0b013e32834f0423
5. Bonadio W, Maida G. Urinary tract infection in outpatient febrile infants younger than 30 days of age: a 10-year evaluation. *Pediatr Infect Dis J.* 2014;33(4):342–344. doi:10.1097/INF.0000000000000110
6. Drumm CM, Siddiqui JN, Desale S, Ramasethu J. Urinary tract infection is common in VLBW infants. *J Perinatol.* 2019;39(1):80–85. doi:10.1038/s41372-018-0226-4
7. Ruangkit C, Satpute A, Vogt BA, Hoyen C, Viswanathan S. Incidence and risk factors of urinary tract infection in very low birth weight infants. *J Neonatal Perinatal Med.* 2016;9(1):83–90. doi:10.3233/NPM-16915055
8. Mohseny AB, van Velze V, Steggerda SJ, Smits-Wintjens VEHJ, Bekker V, Lopriore E. Late-onset sepsis due to urinary tract infection in very preterm neonates is not uncommon. *Eur J Pediatr.* 2018;177(1):33–38. doi:10.1007/s00431-017-3030-9
9. Bauer S, Eliakim A, Pomeranz A, et al. Urinary tract infection in very low birth weight preterm infants. *Pediatr Infect Dis J.* 2003;22(5):426–430. doi:10.1097/01.inf.0000065690.64686.c9
10. Foglia EE, Lorch SA. Clinical predictors of urinary tract infection in the neonatal intensive care unit. *J Neonatal Perinatal Med.* 2012;5(4):327–333. doi:10.3233/NPM-1262812
11. Magin EC, Garcia-Garcia JJ, Sert SZ, Giralt AG, Cubells CL. Efficacy of short-term intravenous antibiotic in neonates with urinary tract infection. *Pediatr Emerg Care.* 2007;23(2):83–86. doi:10.1097/PEC.0b013e3180302c47
12. Downey LC, Benjamin DK, Clark RH, et al. Urinary tract infection concordance with positive blood and cerebrospinal fluid cultures in the neonatal intensive care unit. *J Perinatol.* 2013;33(4):302–306. doi:10.1038/jp.2012.111
13. Clarke D, Gowrishankar M, Etches P, Lee BE, Robinson JL. Management and outcome of positive urine cultures in a neonatal intensive care unit. *J Infect Public Health.* 2010;3(4):152–158. doi:10.1016/j.jiph.2010.09.003
14. Swerkersson S, Jodal U, Åhrén C, Sixt R, Stokland E, Hansson S. Urinary tract infection in infants: the significance of low bacterial count. *Pediatr Nephrol.* 2016;31(2):239–245. doi:10.1007/s00467-015-3199-y
15. Grupo de Hospitales Castrillo, López Sastre JB, Ramos Aparicio A, Coto Cotallo GD, Fernández Colomer B, Crespo Hernández M. Urinary tract infection in the newborn: clinical and radio imaging studies. *Pediatr Nephrol.* 2007;22(10):1735–1741. doi:10.1007/s00467-007-0556-5
16. Tamim MM, Alesseh H, Aziz H. Analysis of the efficacy of urine culture as part of sepsis evaluation in the premature infant. *Pediatr Infect Dis J.* 2003;22(9):805–808. doi:10.1097/01.inf.0000083822.31857.43
17. Shaikh N, Morone NE, Bost JE, Farrell MH. Prevalence of urinary tract infection in childhood: a meta-analysis. *Pediatr Infect Dis J.* 2008;27(4):302–308. doi:10.1097/INF.0b013e31815e4122
18. Morris BJ, Wiswell TE. Circumcision and lifetime risk of urinary tract infection: a systematic review and meta-analysis. *J Urol.* 2013;189(6):2118–2124. doi:10.1016/j.juro.2012.11.114
19. Cason DL, Carter BS, Bhatia J. Can circumcision prevent recurrent urinary tract infections in hospitalized infants? *Clin Pediatr (Phila).* 2000;39(12):699–703. doi:10.1177/000992280003901203
20. Kozer E, Rosenbloom E, Goldman D, Lavy G, Rosenfeld N, Goldman M. Pain in infants who are younger than 2 months during suprapubic aspiration and transurethral bladder catheterization: a randomized, controlled study. *Pediatrics.* 2006;118(1):e51–e56. doi:10.1542/peds.2005-2326
21. El-Naggar W, Yiu A, Mohamed A, et al. Comparison of pain during two methods of urine collection in preterm infants. *Pediatrics.* 2010;125(6):1224–1229. doi:10.1542/peds.2009-3284
22. Kanellopoulos TA, Salakos C, Spiliopoulou I, Ellina A, Nikolakopoulou NM, Papanastasiou DA. First urinary tract infection in neonates, infants and young children: a comparative study. *Pediatr Nephrol.* 2006;21(8):1131–1137. doi:10.1007/s00467-006-0158-7
23. Centers for Disease Control and Prevention. Device Associated Module: UTI. Urinary Tract Infection (*Catheter-Associated Urinary Tract Infection [CAUTI] and Non-Catheter-Associated Urinary Tract Infection [UTI]) Events.*; Jan 2023. URL: https://www.cdc.gov/nhsn/pdfs/pscmanual/7psccauticurrent.pdf
24. Stein R, Dogan HS, Hoebeke P, et al. Urinary tract infections in children: EAU/ESPU guidelines. *Eur Urol.* 2015;67(3):546–558. doi:10.1016/j.eururo.2014.11.007
25. Robinson JL, Finlay JC, Lang ME, Bortolussi R, Canadian Paediatric Society, Infectious Diseases and Immunization Committee, Community Paediatrics Committee. Urinary tract infections in infants and children: diagnosis and management. *Paediatr Child Health.* 2014;19(6):315–325. doi:10.1093/pch/19.6.315
26. Ammenti A, Alberici I, Brugnara M, et al. Updated Italian recommendations for the diagnosis, treatment and follow up of the first febrile urinary tract infection in young children. *Acta Paediatr.* 2020;109(2):236–247. doi:10.1111/apa.14988
27. Beetz R, Bachmann H, Gatermann S, et al. Harnwegsinfektionen im Säuglings- und Kindesalter: Konsensusempfehlungen zu Diagnostik, Therapie und Prophylaxe. *Urologe.* 2007;46(2):112–123. doi:10.1007/s00120-006-1254-9
28. Wingerter S, Bachur R. Risk factors for contamination of catheterized urine specimens in febrile children. *Pediatr Emerg Care.* 2011;27(1):1–4. doi:10.1097/PEC.0b013e3182037c20
29. Kanellopoulos TA, Vassilakos PJ, Kantzis M, Ellina A, Kolonitsiou F, Papanastasiou DA. Low bacterial count urinary tract infections in infants and young children. *Eur J Pediatr.* 2005;164(6):355–361. doi:10.1007/s00431-005-1632-0
30. Tzimenatos L, Mahajan P, Dayan PS, et al. Accuracy of the urinalysis for urinary tract infections in febrile infants 60 days and younger. *Pediatrics.* 2018;141(2):e20173068. doi:10.1542/peds.2017-3068
31. Glissmeyer EW, Korgenski EK, Wilkes J, et al. Dipstick screening for urinary tract infection in febrile infants. *Pediatrics.* 2014;133(5):e1121–e1127. doi:10.1542/peds.2013-3291
32. Velasco R, Benito H, Mozun R, et al. Using a urine dipstick to identify a positive urine culture in young febrile infants is as effective as in older patients. *Acta Paediatr.* 2015;104(1):e39–e44. doi:10.1111/apa.12789

33. Arshad M, Seed PC. Urinary tract infections in the infant. *Clin Perinatol.* 2015;42(1):17–28. doi:10.1016/j.clp.2014.10.003

34. Shane A, Stoll B. Recent developments and current issues in the epidemiology, diagnosis, and management of bacterial and fungal neonatal sepsis. *Am J Perinatol.* 2013;30(2):131–142. doi:10.1055/s-0032-1333413

35. Wagstaff JS, Durrant RJ, Newman MG, et al. Antibiotic treatment of suspected and confirmed neonatal sepsis within 28 days of birth: a retrospective analysis. *Front Pharmacol.* 2019;10: 1191. doi:10.3389/fphar.2019.01191

36. Brady PW, Conway PH, Goudie A. Length of intravenous antibiotic therapy and treatment failure in infants with urinary tract infections. *Pediatrics.* 2010;126(2):196–203. doi:10.1542/peds. 2009-2948

37. Benador D. Randomised controlled trial of three day versus 10 day intravenous antibiotics in acute pyelonephritis: effect on renal scarring. *Arch Dis Child.* 2001;84(3):241–246. doi: 10.1136/adc.84.3.241

38. Gorski DP, Bauer AS, Menda NS, Harer MW. Treatment of positive urine cultures in the neonatal intensive care unit: a guideline to reduce antibiotic utilization. *J Perinatol.* 2021; 41(6):1474–1479. doi:10.1038/s41372-021-01079-6

39. Rosenblum S, Pal A, Reidy K. Renal development in the fetus and premature infant. *Semin Fetal Neonatal Med.* 2017; 22(2):58–66. doi:10.1016/j.siny.2017.01.001

40. Becker A, Baum M. Obstructive uropathy. *Early Hum Dev.* 2006;82(1):15–22. doi:10.1016/j.earlhumdev.2005.11.002

41. Shaikh N, Ewing AL, Bhatnagar S, Hoberman A. Risk of renal scarring in children with a first urinary tract infection: a systematic review. *Pediatrics.* 2010;126(6):1084–1091. doi:10.1542/peds.2010-0685

42. Swerkersson S, Jodal U, Sixt R, Stokland E, Hansson S. Relationship among vesicoureteral reflux, urinary tract infection and renal damage in children. *J Urol.* 2007;178(2):647–651; discussion 650-651. doi:10.1016/j.juro.2007.04.004

43. Agostiniani R, Mariotti P. The natural history of vesicoureteral reflux. *J Matern Fetal Neonatal Med.* 2011;24(suppl 1):2–3. doi :10.3109/14767058.2011.607557

44. Lee LC, Lorenzo AJ, Koyle MA. The role of voiding cystourethrography in the investigation of children with urinary tract infections. *Can Urol Assoc J.* 2016;10(5-6):210–214. doi:10.5489/cuaj.3610

45. Läckgren G, Cooper CS, Neveus T, Kirsch AJ. Management of vesicoureteral reflux: what have we learned over the last 20 years? *Front Pediatr.* 2021;9:650326. doi:10.3389/fped.2021.650326

46. Subcommittee on Urinary Tract Infection. Reaffirmation of AAP Clinical Practice Guideline: the diagnosis and management of the initial urinary tract infection in febrile infants and young children 2-24 months of age. *Pediatrics.* 2016;138(6):e20163026. doi:10.1542/peds.2016-3026

47. Wallace SS, Zhang W, Mahmood NF, et al. Renal ultrasound for infants younger than 2 months with a febrile urinary tract infection. *AJR Am J Roentgenol.* 2015;205(4):894–898. doi:10.2214/AJR.15.14424

48. Walawender L, Hains DS, Schwaderer AL. Diagnosis and imaging of neonatal UTIs. *Pediatr Neonatol.* 2020;61(2):195–200. doi:10.1016/j.pedneo.2019.10.003

49. RIVUR Trial Investigators, Hoberman A, Greenfield SP, et al. Antimicrobial prophylaxis for children with vesicoureteral reflux. *N Engl J Med.* 2014;370(25):2367–2376. doi:10.1056/NEJMoa1401811

50. Brandström P, Esbjörner E, Herthelius M, Swerkersson S, Jodal U, Hansson S. The Swedish reflux trial in children: III. Urinary tract infection pattern. *J Urol.* 2010;184(1):286–291. doi:10.1016/j.juro.2010.01.061

51. Pennesi M, Travan L, Peratoner L, et al. Is antibiotic prophylaxis in children with vesicoureteral reflux effective in preventing pyelonephritis and renal scars? A randomized, controlled trial. *Pediatrics.* 2008;121(6):e1489–e1494. doi:10.1542/peds.2007-2652

52. Williams G, Hodson EM, Craig JC. Interventions for primary vesicoureteric reflux. *Cochrane Database Syst Rev.* 2019;2: CD001532. doi:10.1002/14651858.CD001532.pub5

53. Hensle TW, Hyun G, Grogg AL, Eaddy M. Part 2: Examining pediatric vesicoureteral reflux: a real-world evaluation of treatment patterns and outcomes. *Curr Med Res Opin.* 2007; 23(suppl 4):S7–S13. doi:10.1185/030079907X226221

54. Tekgül S, Riedmiller H, Hoebeke P, et al. EAU guidelines on vesicoureteral reflux in children. *Eur Urol.* 2012;62(3): 534–542. doi:10.1016/j.eururo.2012.05.059

55. Peters C, Skoog S, Arant B, et al. *Management and Screening of Primary Vesicoureteral Reflux in Children.* (2010, Amended 2017). Available at: https://www.auanet.org/guidelines/guidelines/vesicoureteral-reflux-guideline. Accessed January 13, 2022.

56. Nguyen HT, Herndon CDA, Cooper C, et al. The Society for Fetal Urology consensus statement on the evaluation and management of antenatal hydronephrosis. *J Pediatr Urol.* 2010; 6(3):212–231. doi:10.1016/j.jpurol.2010.02.205

57. Braga LH, Mijovic H, Farrokhyar F, Pemberton J, DeMaria J, Lorenzo AJ. Antibiotic prophylaxis for urinary tract infections in antenatal hydronephrosis. *Pediatrics.* 2013;131(1):e251–e261. doi:10.1542/peds.2012-1870

58. Keays MA, Guerra LA, Mihill J, et al. Reliability assessment of Society for Fetal Urology ultrasound grading system for hydronephrosis. *J Urol.* 2008;180(suppl 4):1680–1682; discussion 1682-1683. doi:10.1016/j.juro.2008.03.107

59. Oliveira EA, Diniz JS, Cabral AC, et al. Prognostic factors in fetal hydronephrosis: a multivariate analysis. *Pediatr Nephrol.* 1999;13(9):859–864. doi:10.1007/s004670050716

60. Oliveira EA, Diniz JS, Cabral AC, et al. Predictive factors of fetal urethral obstruction: a multivariate analysis. *Fetal Diagn Ther.* 2000;15(3):180–186. doi:10.1159/000021002

61. Chavhan G, Daneman A, Moineddin R, Lim R, Langlois V, Traubici J. Renal pyramid echogenicity in ureteropelvic junction obstruction: correlation between altered echogenicity and differential renal function. *Pediatr Radiol.* 2008;38(10): 1068–1073. doi:10.1007/s00247-008-0943-5

62. Lee RS, Cendron M, Kinnamon DD, Nguyen HT. Antenatal hydronephrosis as a predictor of postnatal outcome: a meta-analysis. *Pediatrics.* 2006;118(2):586–593. doi:10.1542/peds.2006-0120

63. Lee JH, Choi HS, Kim JK, et al. Nonrefluxing neonatal hydronephrosis and the risk of urinary tract infection. *J Urol.* 2008;179(4):1524–1528. doi:10.1016/j.juro.2007.11.090

64. Song SH, Lee SB, Park YS, Kim KS. Is antibiotic prophylaxis necessary in infants with obstructive hydronephrosis? *J Urol.* 2007;177(3):1098–1101; discussion 1101. doi:10.1016/j.juro.2006.11.002

65. van Eerde AM, Meutgeert MH, de Jong TPVM, Giltay JC. Vesico-ureteral reflux in children with prenatally detected hydronephrosis: a systematic review. *Ultrasound Obstet Gynecol.* 2007;29(4):463–469. doi:10.1002/uog.3975

66. Estrada CR, Peters CA, Retik AB, Nguyen HT. Vesicoureteral reflux and urinary tract infection in children with a history of

prenatal hydronephrosis—should voiding cystourethrography be performed in cases of postnatally persistent grade II hydronephrosis? *J Urol.* 2009;181(2):801–806; discussion 806-807. doi:10.1016/j.juro.2008.10.057

67. Cheng CH, Tsai MH, Huang YC, et al. Antibiotic resistance patterns of community-acquired urinary tract infections in children with vesicoureteral reflux receiving prophylactic antibiotic therapy. *Pediatrics.* 2008;122(6):1212–1217. doi:10.1542/peds.2007-2926

68. Wald ER. Vesicoureteral reflux: the role of antibiotic prophylaxis. *Pediatrics.* 2006;117(3):919–922. doi:10.1542/peds.2005-2139

69. Practice parameter: the diagnosis, treatment, and evaluation of the initial urinary tract infection in febrile infants and young children. American Academy of Pediatrics. Committee on Quality Improvement. Subcommittee on Urinary Tract Infection. *Pediatrics.* 1999;103(4 Pt 1):843–852. doi:10.1542/peds.103.4.843

70. Uhari M, Nuutinen M, Turtinen J. Adverse reactions in children during long-term antimicrobial therapy. *Pediatr Infect Dis J.* 1996;15(5):404–408. doi:10.1097/00006454-199605000-00005

71. Mattoo T, Greenfield S. Management of vesicoureteral reflux. In *UpToDate.* 2021. Available at: https://www.uptodate.com/contents/management-of-vesicoureteral-reflux. Accessed January 13, 2022.

72. Selekman RE, Shapiro DJ, Boscardin J, et al. Uropathogen resistance and antibiotic prophylaxis: a meta-analysis. *Pediatrics.* 2018;142(1):e20180119. doi:10.1542/peds.2018-0119

73. Nagler EV, Williams G, Hodson EM, Craig JC. Interventions for primary vesicoureteric reflux. *Cochrane Database Syst Rev.* 2011;(6):CD001532. doi:10.1002/14651858.CD001532.pub4

Chapter 16

Neonatal Hypertension

Joseph T. Flynn, MD, MS

Chapter Outline

Introduction

First described in the 1970s, awareness of neonatal hypertension has increased over the past several decades. Despite this, there is still uncertainty over which neonates require treatment for hypertension, primarily because of conflicting data on normative blood pressure (BP) values in neonates, and also because few reliable outcome data are available. This chapter will review the existing data on normal neonatal BP and will present a reasonable approach to evaluation and management based upon likely causes and pathophysiology. Finally, research needs, especially those related to late-onset hypertension and long-term outcome, will be reviewed.

Normative Values for Neonatal Blood Pressure

FACTORS AFFECTING BLOOD PRESSURE AT BIRTH

There are many complexities to the changing patterns of BPs in the newborn period. Infant characteristics such as gestational age at birth, postnatal and postmenstrual age, as well as appropriateness of size for gestational age all influence BP. Maternal illnesses such as diabetes and other prenatal factors may also affect BP levels following delivery. As in older children, BP values in neonates may vary according to the method of BP assessment (e.g., intraarterial, Doppler, oscillometric) and also according to the infant's state (e.g., sleeping, crying, feeding). All these factors need to be taken into account when reviewing the literature on BP standards, as well as when interpreting BP values in clinical practice. Even though neonatal BPs have been measured for decades, we are still in the early phase of identifying the normal patterns of infant BPs, and there are still many physiologic changes that need further investigation.[1]

Data on BP from 329 infants on the first day of life were published in 1995 by Zubrow et al.[2] They were able to define the mean BP plus upper and lower 95% confidence limits; their data clearly demonstrated increases in BP with increasing gestational age and birth weight (Fig. 16.1). A more recent study by Pejovic et al.,[3] limiting their analysis to hemodynamically stable premature and term infants admitted to the neonatal intensive care unit (NICU), also showed that BPs on day 1 of life correlated with gestational age and birth

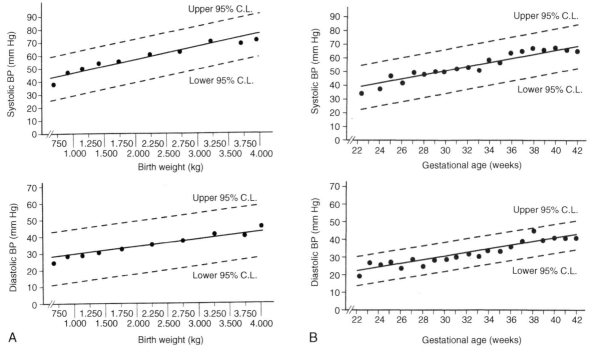

Fig. 16.1 Linear regression of systolic and diastolic blood pressures (BP) by birth weight (A) and gestational age (B), with 95% confidence limits (C.L.) (upper and lower dashed lines). (Reproduced with permission from Zubrow AB, Hulman S, Kushner H, et al. Determinants of blood pressure in infants admitted to neonatal intensive care units: a prospective multicenter study. *J Perinatol.* 1995;15:470–479.)

weight. Healthy term infants do not seem to demonstrate this same pattern.[4]

After the first day of life, it appears that BPs in premature newborns increase more rapidly over the first week or two of life, followed by a slowing of the rate of increase. The previously mentioned Philadelphia study categorized over 600 infants in the NICU into gestational age groups and showed a similar rate of BP increase over the first 5 days of life, regardless of gestational age.[2] The more recent study by Pejovic and colleagues on stable NICU infants showed a similar pattern, with BPs in each gestational age category of premature infants increasing at a faster rate over the first week of life with subsequent slowing.[3] In these infants, they determined that the rate of rise was more rapid in the preterm than full-term infants (Fig. 16.2). As premature neonates mature, it appears that the strongest predictor of BP is postmenstrual age, as seen in Fig. 16.3 from Zubrow et al.[2]

In term infants, appropriateness for gestational age seems to be an important influence on BP. In an Australian study of healthy term infants,[4] BPs were higher on day 2 of life compared with day 1 but not thereafter. A correlation between birth weight and BP on day 3 of life was demonstrated in a large Japanese study of term infants[5]; this study also showed an increase in BP from days 2 through 4 of life, consistent with studies mentioned earlier. A Spanish study demonstrated that small for gestational age infants had the lowest BP at birth but subsequently the fastest rate of rise, so that by 1 month of age, all term infants had similar BPs.[6] Fig. 16.4 summarizes the pattern of change in BP among the various subgroups of infants mentioned previously.[1]

Genetic factors likely also play a role in determining BP, although limited studies have been completed to date. One study identified cytochrome P450 (CYP2D6) CC genotype as being associated with higher BPs in preterm infants during hospitalization and at neonatal follow-up.[7] A more recent study of term infants in Poland demonstrated an association between the 1936A → G AKAP10 genotype and BP,

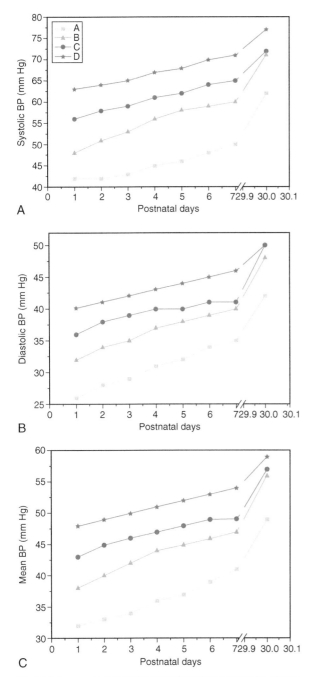

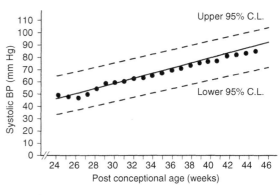

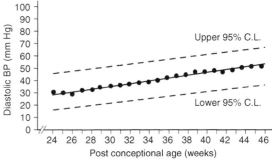

Fig. 16.3 Linear regression of mean systolic (A) and diastolic (B) blood pressures (BP) by postmenstrual (postconceptual) age in weeks, with 95% confidence limits (*C.L.*) (upper and lower dashed lines). (Reproduced with permission from Zubrow AB, Hulman S, Kushner H, et al. Determinants of blood pressure in infants admitted to neonatal intensive care units: a prospective multicenter study. *J Perinatol.* 1995;15:470–479.)

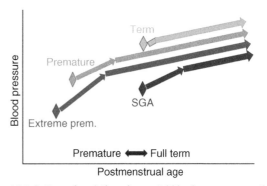

Fig. 16.2 Increase in systolic (a), diastolic (b), and mean (c) blood pressure (BP) during the first month of life in infants classified by estimated gestational age: (A) ≤28 weeks, (B) 29–32 weeks, (C) 33–36 weeks, (D) ≥37 weeks. (Reproduced with permission from Pejovic B, Peco-Antic A, Marinkovic-Eric J. Blood pressure in non-critically ill preterm and full-term neonates. *Pediatr Nephrol.* 2007;22:249–257.)

Fig. 16.4 Pattern of evolution of neonatal blood pressure over the first days and weeks of life. *Prem.*, prematurity; *SGA*, small for gestational age. (Reprinted with permission from Dionne JM. Neonatal and infant hypertension. In: Flynn JT, Ingelfinger JR, Redwine K, eds. *Pediatric Hypertension.* 4th ed. Springer International Publishing; 2018:1–26.)

with heterozygous and homozygous carriers of the 1936G variant having higher mean and diastolic BP than infants homozygous for 1936A.[8] It is likely that additional genetic mutations with an effect on neonatal BP will be identified in the future.

Maternal factors, including medications, underlying illnesses, and adequacy of nutrition during pregnancy, can also influence a neonate's BP.[9] Higher infant BPs have correlated with maternal body mass index > 30 kg/m² and low socioeconomic status in Nigerian infants[10] and in an Australian study to premature infants born to mothers with diabetes or neonates with abnormal uteroplacental perfusion by placental pathology.[11] There is some suggestion in the literature that chorioamnionitis and HELLP (hemolysis, elevated liver enzymes, low platelets) syndrome may be related to lower infant BPs. A recent

systematic review of the maternal factors that can influence BP in newborns came to the conclusion that not enough is known to draw definitive conclusions about the relative impact that each of these processes may have—although it is likely that neonatal BP is impacted by maternal factors, further study is required.[12]

Normal BPs in infants older than 1 month have not been extensively studied recently. The percentile curves reported by the Second Task Force of the National High Blood Pressure Education Program[13] (Fig. 16.5) remain the most widely available reference values. These curves allow BP to be characterized as normal or high not only by age and gender, but also by length (provided in the legend below the curves). Unfortunately, these BP values were determined by a single measurement on awake infants by the Doppler

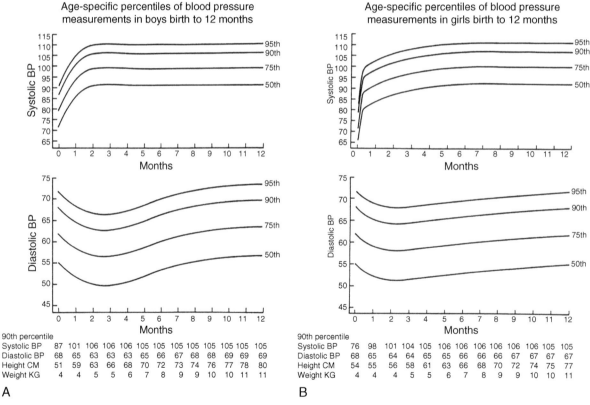

A

90th percentile													
Systolic BP	87	101	106	106	106	105	105	105	105	105	105	105	105
Diastolic BP	68	65	63	63	63	65	66	67	68	68	69	69	69
Height CM	51	59	63	66	68	70	72	73	74	76	77	78	80
Weight KG	4	4	5	5	6	7	8	9	9	10	10	11	11

B

90th percentile													
Systolic BP	76	98	101	104	105	106	106	106	106	106	106	105	105
Diastolic BP	68	65	64	64	65	65	66	66	66	67	67	67	67
Height CM	54	55	56	58	61	63	66	68	70	72	74	75	77
Weight KG	4	4	4	5	5	6	7	8	9	9	10	10	11

Fig. 16.5 Age-specific percentiles for blood pressure in boys (A) and girls (B) from birth to 12 months of age. *BP,* blood pressure. (Reprinted from National Heart Lung, and Blood Institute Task Force on Blood Pressure Control in Children. *Report of the Second Task Force on Blood Pressure Control in Children – 1987.* Bethesda, MD: U. S. Department of Health and Human Services, National High Blood Pressure Education Program.)

method, which reduced the number of diastolic BP readings by more than half. Additionally, several more recent publications suggest that these BP values may be inaccurate. A study of 406 healthy term infants with BPs measured by the oscillometric method on day 2 of life and then at 6 and 12 months of age demonstrated BPs that are slightly higher than the Task Force values.[14] Comparison with the more recently published values for 1-year-olds in the 2017 American of Academy of Pediatrics (AAP) guideline on childhood hypertension[15] reveals significant differences that further call into question the validity of the 1987 curves. These issues highlight that there is clearly a pressing need for new normative BP data on infants during the first year of life.

WHAT LEVEL OF BLOOD PRESSURE SHOULD BE CONSIDERED HYPERTENSIVE?

In older children, the definition of hypertension is persistent systolic and/or diastolic BP equal to or greater than the 95th percentile for age, sex, and height.[15] As can be deduced from the preceding discussion, there is considerable variation in neonatal BP, and no generally agreed upon reference values are available. For term infants and infants between 1 and 12 months of age, the best available reference data, even despite the potential flaws noted earlier, would be those from the Second Task Force Report[13] (see Fig. 16.5). In this age group, one could diagnose hypertension if the infant's BP is repeatedly greater than or equal to the 95th percentile for an infant of comparable age (also note that weight and length are given below the curves and could also be used to help determine if an infant's BP is normal or high).

The major unresolved question is what BP values to use in diagnosing hypertension in preterm infants. Dionne and colleagues[16] combined published data (including from the studies mentioned previously) to derive a table of reference data for infants from 26 to 44 weeks' postmenstrual ages (Table 16.1) that contain reference values for the 50th, 95th, and 99th percentiles of mean arterial pressure and systolic and diastolic BP. Use of this table was endorsed in the 2017 AAP guideline. Using these data, our recommendation is that infants with BP values persistently at or above the 95th percentile warrant closer monitoring, and those with BP values above the 99th percentile would clearly

TABLE 16.1 Neonatal Blood Pressure Percentiles

Postmenstrual Age	50th Percentile	95th Percentile	99th Percentile
44 Weeks			
SBP	88	105	110
DBP	50	68	73
MAP	63	80	85
42 Weeks			
SBP	85	98	102
DBP	50	65	70
MAP	62	76	81
40 Weeks			
SBP	80	95	100
DBP	50	65	70
MAP	60	75	80
38 Weeks			
SBP	75	90	95
DBP	45	60	65
MAP	55	70	75
36 Weeks			
SBP	70	85	90
DBP	40	55	60
MAP	50	65	70
34 Weeks			
SBP	68	83	88
DBP	40	55	60
MAP	48	62	69
32 Weeks			
SBP	65	80	85
DBP	40	55	60
MAP	48	65	68
30 Weeks			
SBP	60	75	80
DBP	38	50	54
MAP	45	58	63
28 Weeks			
SBP	55	72	77
DBP	30	50	56
MAP	38	57	63
26 Weeks			
SBP	50	70	76
DBP	30	48	53
MAP	38	55	61

DBP, diastolic blood pressure; *MAP*, mean arterial pressure; *SBP*, systolic blood pressure.
Adapted from Dionne JM, Abitbol CL, Flynn JT. Hypertension in infancy: diagnosis, management and outcome. *Pediatr Nephrol*. 2012;27:17–32.

merit investigation and possibly initiation of antihypertensive drug therapy. These decisions need to be tempered by clinical circumstances and personal experience.

Incidence

Hypertension is so unusual in otherwise healthy term infants that routine BP determination is not advocated for this group. For preterm and otherwise high-risk neonates admitted to modern NICUs, reported incidences of hypertension in published case series range from 0.2% to 3%. In an Australian study of approximately 2500 infants followed for over 4 years, the prevalence of hypertension was 1.3%.[17] Antenatal steroids, maternal hypertension, umbilical arterial catheter placement, postnatal acute renal failure, and chronic lung disease were among the most common concurrent conditions in the infants with hypertension. A more recent single-center case series from Texas demonstrated a nearly identical incidence of hypertension, although the focus was on treated patients.[18] Prenatal factors such as antenatal steroid administration, maternal hypertension, and maternal substance abuse were associated with the diagnosis of hypertension in that study.

Larger, multicenter studies examining neonatal hypertension have been rare. An incidence of around 1% was found in a study using administrative data from a consortium of pediatric hospitals.[19] The most common factors associated with hypertension in that study were extracorporeal membrane oxygenation (ECMO) treatment and either congenital or acquired kidney disease. The Assessment of Worldwide Acute Kidney Injury Epidemiology in Neonates investigators described an incidence of diagnosed hypertension of 1.8% in the 24 centers participating in that consortium.[20] Using their own internally generated set of "normative" neonatal BP data, they also found that another 3.7% of neonates had undiagnosed hypertension. These data need to be replicated and confirmed using the more widely accepted BP percentiles published by Dionne and colleagues.[16]

Hypertension may also be detected long after discharge from the NICU. In a retrospective review of over 650 infants seen in follow-up after discharge from a tertiary level NICU, Friedman and Hustead found an incidence of hypertension (defined as systolic BP of > 113 mm Hg on three consecutive visits over 6 weeks) of 2.6%.[21] Hypertension in this study was detected at a mean age of approximately 2 months postterm when corrected for prematurity. Infants in this study who developed hypertension tended to have lower initial Apgar scores and slightly longer NICU stays than infants who remained normotensive, indicating a somewhat greater likelihood of developing hypertension in sicker babies. Unfortunately, this study has not been replicated, so the current prevalence of hypertension in high-risk infants remains unclear. However, these data do support routine BP monitoring following NICU discharge, as recommended in the 2017 AAP guideline.[15]

Differential Diagnosis

As in older infants and children, the potential causes of hypertension in neonates are numerous (Table 16.2), with the most common diagnosis probably umbilical artery catheter-associated thromboembolism affecting either the aorta and/or the renal arteries. This was first demonstrated in the early 1970s. Hypertension was reported to develop in infants who had undergone umbilical arterial catheterization even when thrombi were unable to be demonstrated in the renal arteries.

Although there have been several studies that have examined duration of line placement and line position as factors involved in thrombus formation, these data have not been conclusive. Longer duration of umbilical catheter placement has been associated with higher rates of thrombus formation.[22] A Cochrane review comparing "low" versus "high" umbilical artery catheters determined that the "high" catheter placement was associated with fewer ischemic events such as necrotizing enterocolitis, but that hypertension occurred at equal frequency with either position.[23] Thus, it is assumed that catheter-related hypertension is related to thrombus formation at the time of line placement because of disruption of the vascular endothelium of the umbilical artery, particularly in preterm infants.

Fibromuscular dysplasia leading to renal artery stenosis is a rare but extremely important cause of renovascular hypertension in the neonate. Many of these infants may have main renal arteries that appear normal on angiography but demonstrate significant

TABLE 16.2 Causes of Neonatal Hypertension

Renovascular	**Cardiac**
Thromboembolism	Aortic coarctation
Renal artery stenosis	**Medications/intoxications**
Midaortic coarctation	Infant
Renal venous thrombosis	Dexamethasone
Compression of renal artery	Adrenergic agents
Idiopathic arterial calcification	Vitamin D intoxication
Congenital rubella syndrome	Theophylline
Renal parenchymal disease	Caffeine
Congenital	Pancuronium
Polycystic kidney disease	Phenylephrine
Multicystic-dysplastic kidney disease	Maternal
Tuberous sclerosis	Cocaine
Ureteropelvic junction obstruction	Heroin
Unilateral renal hypoplasia	Antenatal steroids
Congenital nephrotic syndrome	**Neoplasia**
ACE inhibitor fetopathy	Wilms tumor
Acquired	Mesoblastic nephroma
Acute kidney injury	Neuroblastoma
Cortical necrosis	Pheochromocytoma
Interstitial nephritis	**Neurologic**
Hemolytic-uremic syndrome	Pain
Obstruction (stones, tumors)	Intracranial hypertension
Pulmonary	Seizures
Bronchopulmonary dysplasia	Familial dysautonomia
Pneumothorax	Subdural hematoma
Endocrine	**Miscellaneous**
Congenital adrenal hyperplasia	Adrenal hemorrhage
11-β-hydroxylase deficiency	Birth asphyxia
17-hydroxylase deficiency	Closure of abdominal wall defect
Hyperaldosteronism	Extracorporeal membrane oxygenation
Hyperthyroidism	Hypercalcemia
Pseudohypoaldosteronism type II	Phthalate exposure?
Glucocorticoid remediable	Traction
aldosteronism	Volume overload

ACE, angiotensin-converting enzyme.

branch vessel disease that can cause severe hypertension.[24] In addition, renal artery stenosis may also be accompanied by midaortic coarctation and cerebral vascular stenoses.[24,25] Several other vascular problems may also lead to neonatal hypertension, including renal venous or arterial thrombosis, idiopathic arterial calcification, and compression of the renal arteries by tumors.

After renovascular causes, the next largest group of infants with hypertension are those with congenital kidney disease. Although both autosomal dominant and autosomal recessive polycystic kidney disease (PKD) may present in the newborn period with severe

nephromegaly and hypertension, recessive PKD more commonly leads to hypertension early, sometimes in the first month of life.[26] Hypertension has also been reported in infants with unilateral multicystic dysplastic kidneys (MCDK),[27] possibly due to renin production by the MCDK itself.[28,29] Kidney obstruction may be accompanied by hypertension, for example, in infants with congenital ureteropelvic-junction obstruction. The importance of congenital urologic malformations as a cause of neonatal hypertension was demonstrated in a referral series from Brazil,[30] in which 13 of 15 hypertensive infants had urologic causes. Median age at diagnosis of hypertension was 20 days (range

5–70 days), emphasizing the need for regular BP measurement in infants with urologic malformations to detect hypertension.

The other important group of hypertensive neonates are those with bronchopulmonary dysplasia (BPD). BPD-associated hypertension was first described in the mid-1980s by Abman and colleagues,[31] who found the incidence of hypertension in infants with BPD was 43%, versus an incidence of 4.5% in infants without BPD. Over half of the infants with BPD who developed hypertension did not display it until after discharge from the NICU, again highlighting the need for measurement of BP in NICU "graduates."

Other studies have subsequently confirmed that hypertension occurs more commonly in infants with BPD compared with infants of similar gestational age or birth weight without BPD. Factors such as hypoxemia and increased severity of BPD appear to be correlated with the development of hypertension.[32] Alterations in aortic wall thickness and vasomotor functioning in infants with BPD were seen in one recent study,[33] suggesting another potential mechanism for the higher incidence of hypertension in this group. An alternative view is that since many of these infants will have had umbilical lines placed, it is also possible that BPD is actually a comorbidity for line-associated thromboembolic disease (see previous discussion). Although updated studies are sorely needed, these observations reinforce the impression that infants with severe BPD are clearly at increased risk and need close monitoring for the development of hypertension. This is especially true in infants who require ongoing treatment with oxygen, diuretics, and/or corticosteroids.

Hypertension may also be secondary to disorders of several other organ systems or may develop because of treatment with various pharmacologic agents (see Table 16.2). An important association is hypertension associated with ECMO,[18,19] which in one case series affected over 90% of infants receiving venovenous ECMO.[34] The pathogenesis of ECMO-associated hypertension appears to be multifactorial and may be due to fluid overload and impaired water and sodium handling by the kidney, and it does not appear to be related to alterations in renin activity. A novel cause of hypertension recently reported is exposure to phthalates, which are ubiquitous in intravenous tubing and respiratory equipment used in the NICU; the proposed mechanism of hypertension is activation of the mineralocorticoid receptor through inhibition of 11 beta hydroxysteroid dehydrogenase type 2.[35] This is provocative and requires further confirmation.

Clinical Presentation

Except in critically ill infants with severe hypertension, in many infants in the NICU, high BP will be detected on routine monitoring of vital signs, making it difficult to identify infants with true hypertension that warrants further evaluation and/or treatment. This is primarily a consequence of the changing nature of BP in neonates and the difficulty in knowing what BP level should be considered high (see preceding sections). However, some classic presentations of neonatal hypertension have been described, including congestive heart failure and cardiogenic shock.[36,37] In the less acutely ill infant, feeding difficulties, unexplained tachypnea, apnea, lethargy, irritability, or seizures may constitute symptoms of unsuspected hypertension. In older infants who have been discharged from the nursery, unexplained irritability or failure to thrive may be the only manifestations of hypertension.

Diagnostic Evaluation

BLOOD PRESSURE MEASUREMENT

As in older children, accurate BP measurement is crucial so that hypertension will be correctly identified. The gold standard for BP measurement in neonates remains direct intraarterial measurement.[38] There is reasonable correlation between umbilical artery and peripheral artery catheter BPs in neonates, so no specific site is preferred. Indirect methods of measuring the BP such as palpation and auscultation are not practical in neonates, especially in the NICU setting, and ultrasonic Doppler assessment has largely been replaced by oscillometric devices. Methods of BP measurement in neonates have recently been comprehensively reviewed.[38]

Oscillometric devices are easy to use and provide the ability to follow BP trends over time. Studies have shown reasonably good correlation between oscillometric and umbilical or radial artery BP in neonates and young children.[16,38] They are especially useful for infants who require BP monitoring after discharge from the NICU. However, not all oscillometric devices are equal. A few studies have compared different oscillometric BP monitors to direct arterial measurements in neonates and have shown that accuracy varied depending on the size of the infant,[38] with a higher likelihood of oscillometric methods to overread BP compared with direct measurement.[39] Oscillometry appears to be less accurate in neonates with mean arterial pressure <30 mm Hg; in such infants, direct/intraarterial measurement of BP is preferable.[38]

Many factors can influence the accuracy of BP measurements in neonates. BP will obviously be higher in infants who are crying vs. those who are resting (Fig. 16.6), and even in a quiet infant, activities such as feeding or sucking on a pacifier may increase the BP.[5,40,41] Given this, consistent measurement technique becomes of paramount importance in obtaining accurate BP values. A standard protocol as suggested by Nwankwo and colleagues[42] may result in decreased variability of BP readings, ensuring that accurate BP values will be available to guide clinical decision-making. Elements of this protocol include:

- Infant should be either prone or supine, and resting quietly.
- Delay BP measurements until ≥1.5 hours after a medical procedure or feeding.

- Use appropriately sized cuff and measure BP in right upper arm.
- Obtain several BP measurements in succession using an oscillometric device.

As in patients of any age, correct cuff size is essential in obtaining accurate BP measurements in neonates. A cuff width–to–arm circumference ratio of 0.5 appears to ensure the most accurate readings.[38] Finally, it is important to recognize that calf BP values may be equivalent to BP values obtained in the upper arm until about 6 months of age,[43] so it is acceptable to measure BP in the lower extremity during the first few months of life. Efforts should be made to use the same extremity for sequential measurements.

DIAGNOSTIC APPROACH

Diagnosing the cause of the high BP should be straightforward in most neonates. A relatively focused history should be obtained, paying attention to determining whether there were any pertinent prenatal exposures, as well as to the details of the infant's clinical course and any concurrent conditions. The procedures that the infant has undergone (e.g., umbilical catheter placement) should be reviewed, and the

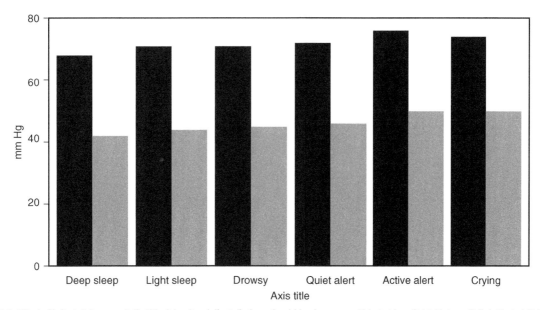

Fig. 16.6 Effect of infant state on systolic (*black bars*) and diastolic (*gray bars*) blood pressure. (Adapted from Satoh M, Inoue R, Tada H, et al. Reference values and associated factors for Japanese newborns' blood pressure and pulse rate: the babies' and their parents' longitudinal observation in Suzuki Memorial Hospital on intrauterine period (BOSHI) study. *J Hypertens.* 2016;34:1578–1585.)

infant's current medication list should be scrutinized for substances that can increase BP.

The physical examination should be focused on obtaining information to assist in narrowing the differential diagnosis. BP readings should be obtained in all four extremities at least once to rule out aortic coarctation. However, as mentioned previously, since lower extremity BP readings may be similar to upper extremity readings, an echocardiogram is required to confirm this diagnosis.[43] The general appearance of the infant should be assessed, with particular attention paid to the presence of any dysmorphic features that may indicate an obvious diagnosis such as congenital adrenal hyperplasia. Careful cardiac and abdominal examinations should be performed. The presence of a flank mass or of an epigastric bruit may point the clinician toward diagnosis of either ureteropelvic junction obstruction or renal artery stenosis, respectively.

Since the correct diagnosis is usually suggested by the history and physical examination, and since there is typically ample prior laboratory data available for review, few additional studies will be needed in most instances. It is important to assess kidney function, as well as to examine a specimen of the urine to ascertain the presence of kidney disease. Chest x-ray may be useful in infants with signs of congestive heart failure or in those with a murmur on physical examination. Other diagnostic studies, such as hormone levels, should be obtained when there is pertinent history (Table 16.3). Plasma renin activity is typically quite high in infancy, particularly in premature infants,[44] making renin values difficult to interpret. Given this, assessment of plasma renin activity in the initial evaluation of hypertension in infants may be deferred. An exception to this would be infants with hypokalemia that might suggest a monogenic form of hypertension.[45]

Selected imaging studies may help to establish an etiology of the hypertension. Kidney ultrasound with Doppler should be obtained in almost all hypertensive infants, as it can help uncover potentially correctable causes of hypertension such as renal venous thrombosis,[46] may detect aortic and/or renal arterial thrombi, and can identify anatomic abnormalities or other congenital kidney diseases. Nuclear scanning in our experience has had little role in the assessment of hypertensive infants, primarily due to the immaturity of kidney function in this age group, which makes it difficult to obtain accurate

TABLE 16.3   Diagnostic Testing in Neonatal Hypertension

Generally Useful	Useful in Selected Infants
Urinalysis (±culture)	Thyroid studies
CBC and platelet count	Urine VMA/HVA
Electrolytes	Plasma renin activity
BUN, creatinine	Aldosterone
Calcium	Cortisol
Chest x-ray	Echocardiogram
Kidney ultrasound with Doppler	Abdominal/pelvic ultrasound
	VCUG
	Aortography
	Renal angiography
	Nuclear scan (DTPA/Mag3)

BUN, blood urea nitrogen; *CBC*, complete blood count; *DTPA*, vanillylmandelic acid; *HVA*, homovanillic acid; *Mag3*, mercaptoacetyltriglycine; *VCUG*; voiding cystourethrogram; *VMA*, vanillylmandelic acid.

studies. Other specific studies, including echocardiograms and voiding cystourethrograms, should be obtained as indicated.

For infants with extremely severe hypertension, renal artery stenosis rises to the top of the differential, making vascular imaging necessary. In neonates, although formal arteriograms utilizing the traditional femoral approach are feasible, most centers lack both the equipment and expertise to perform this safely. CT or MRI can be performed as noninvasive screening studies, but neither has sufficient resolution to detect branch vessel stenosis, which is common in pediatric renovascular hypertension. Given these considerations, in most neonates with suspected renal artery stenosis angiography should be deferred, and the hypertension should be managed medically until the infant is large enough for an arteriogram to be performed safely.

Treatment

The first step in treatment should be correction of any iatrogenic causes of hypertension, such as excessive or unnecessary inotrope administration, dexamethasone or other corticosteroids, hypercalcemia, volume overload, or pain. Hypoxemia should be treated in infants with BPD, and appropriate hormonal replacement should be initiated in those with confirmed endocrine disorders.

Surgery is indicated for treatment of neonatal hypertension in a limited set of circumstances, most notably in infants with obstructive lesions or aortic coarctation. For infants with renal artery stenosis, it may be necessary to manage the infant medically until it has grown sufficiently to undergo definitive repair of the vascular abnormalities. However, unilateral nephrectomy may be needed in rare cases.[47] Infants with hypertension secondary to Wilms tumor or neuroblastoma will require surgical tumor removal, possibly following chemotherapy. Hypertensive infants with MCDK may also benefit from nephrectomy.[48] Infants with malignant hypertension secondary to autosomal recessive PKD may require bilateral nephrectomy. Fortunately, such severely affected infants are rare.

At some point, a decision will need to be made as to whether antihypertensive medications are indicated. Except in severely hypertensive infants with obvious end-organ manifestations (for example, congestive heart failure or seizures), this can be a difficult decision. No data exist on the adverse effects of chronic hypertension in infancy, and few if any antihypertensive medications have ever been studied in neonates. Additionally, as noted earlier, determining what BP threshold at which to consider treatment can be difficult due to the lack of robust normative BP data. Therefore, clinical expertise and expert opinion must be relied upon to guide decision-making.

Oral antihypertensive agents (Table 16.4) are best reserved for infants with less severe hypertension or infants whose acute hypertension has been controlled with intravenous infusions and are ready to be transitioned to chronic therapy. We typically start with the calcium channel blocker isradipine[49] as it can be compounded into a stable 1 mg/mL suspension, facilitating dosing in small infants. Amlodipine may also be used, but its slow onset of action and prolonged duration of effect may be problematic in the acute setting. Other potentially useful vasodilators include hydralazine and minoxidil. Beta blockers may need to be avoided in infants with chronic lung disease. In such infants, diuretics may have a beneficial effect not only in controlling BP but also in improving pulmonary function.[50] On the other hand, it should be noted that propranolol is available commercially as a suspension, which makes it convenient to use when beta blockade is not contraindicated.

Use of angiotensin-converting enzyme inhibitors (ACEIs) in neonates is controversial. Captopril is one of the only antihypertensive agents that has actually been demonstrated to be effective in infants,[51] but it is well known to cause an exaggerated fall in BP in premature infants.[52] Hyperkalemia, acute kidney injury, and severe hypotension have also been reported in infants treated with enalapril.[53,54] These effects are related to the activation of the renin-angiotensin-aldosterone system in neonates, which is a reflection of the importance of the renin-angiotensin-aldosterone system in kidney development.[55,56] Although few data exist on this topic, the concern over use of ACEIs in infants is that they may impair the final stages of kidney maturation. Based on this concern, we typically avoid use of captopril (and other ACEIs) until the preterm infant has reached a corrected postmenstrual age of 44 weeks.

Intermittently administered intravenous agents have a role in therapy in selected hypertensive infants. Hydralazine and labetalol in particular may be useful in infants with mild to moderate hypertension that are not yet candidates for oral therapy because of necrotizing enterocolitis or other forms of gastrointestinal dysfunction. Enalaprilat, the intravenous ACEI, has also been used in the treatment of neonatal renovascular hypertension.[57,58] However, even doses at the lower end of published ranges may lead to significant, prolonged hypotension and oliguric acute kidney injury. It should also be noted that all available pediatric dosing recommendations for enalaprilat are based on one uncontrolled case series.[57] For these reasons, I do not recommend its use in hypertensive neonates.

In infants with acute severe hypertension, continuous intravenous infusions of antihypertensive agents should be utilized.[59] The advantages of intravenous infusions are numerous, most importantly including the ability to quickly titrate the infusion rate to achieve the desired level of BP control. As in patients of any age with acute severe hypertension, care should be taken to avoid too rapid a reduction in BP to avoid cerebral ischemia and hemorrhage,[60] a problem that premature infants in particular are already at increased risk of due to the immaturity of their periventricular circulation. Here again, continuous infusions of intravenous antihypertensives offer a distinct advantage. Published experience[61,62] suggests that the calcium

TABLE 16.4   Recommended Doses for Selected Antihypertensive Agents for Treatment of Hypertensive Infants

Class	Drug	Route	Dose	Interval	Comments
ACE inhibitors[a]	Captopril	Oral	<3 months: 0.01–0.5 mg/kg Max 2 mg/kg per day >3 months: 0.15–0.3 mg/kg Max 6 mg/kg per day	TID	1. First dose may cause rapid drop in BP, especially if receiving diuretics 2. Monitor serum creatinine and K+ 3. Intravenous enalaprilat *not* recommended—see text 4. Limited experience with lisinopril in infants
	Enalapril[a]	Oral	0.08–0.6 mg/kg per day	QD or BID	
	Lisinopril[a]	Oral	0.07–0.6 mg/kg per day	QD	
α and β antagonists	Labetalol	Oral	0.5–1.0 mg/kg Max 10 mg/kg per day	BID or TID	Heart failure, BPD relative contraindications
		IV	0.20–1.0 mg/kg 0.25–3.0 mg/kg per h	Q 4–6 h, infusion	
	Carvedilol	Oral	0.1 mg/kg, up to 0.5 mg/kg	BID	May be useful in heart failure
β-antagonists	Esmolol	IV	100–500 μg/kg per min	Infusion	Very short acting; constant infusion necessary
	Propranolol[a]	Oral	0.5–1.0 mg/kg Max 8–10 mg/kg per day	TID	Monitor heart rate; avoid in BPD
Calcium channel blockers	Amlodipine[a]	Oral	0.05–0.3 mg/kg Max 0.6 mg/kg per day	QD or BID	All may cause reflex tachycardia
	Isradipine	Oral	0.05–0.15 mg/kg Max 0.8 mg/kg per day	QID	
	Nicardipine	IV	1–4 μg/kg per min	Infusion	
Central α-agonist	Clonidine	Oral	5–10 μg/kg per day Max 25 μg/kg per day	TID	May cause mild sedation
Diuretics	Chlorothiazide	Oral	5–15 mg/kg	BID	Monitor electrolytes
	Hydrochlorothiazide	Oral	1–3 mg/kg	QD	
	Spironolactone	Oral	0.5–1.5 mg/kg	BID	
Direct vasodilators	Hydralazine	Oral	0.25–1.0 mg/kg Max 7.5 mg/kg per day	TID or QID	Tachycardia and fluid retention are common side effects
	Minoxidil	IV	0.15–0.6 mg/kg	Q 4 h	
		Oral	0.1–0.2 mg/kg	BID or TID	Tachycardia and fluid retention common side effects; prolonged use causes hypertrichosis
	Sodium nitroprusside	IV	0.5–10 μg/kg per min	Infusion	Thiocyanate toxicity can occur with prolonged (>72 h) use or in renal failure

ACE, angiotensin-converting enzyme; *BID*, twice daily; *BP*, blood pressure; *BPD*, bronchopulmonary dysplasia; *Max*, maximum; *QD*, once daily; *QID*, four times daily; *TID*, three times daily.
[a]Commercially marketed suspension available.

channel blocker nicardipine may be particularly useful in infants with acute severe hypertension. Other drugs that have been successfully used in neonates include esmolol, labetalol, and nitroprusside. Oral agents in general are probably not appropriate given their variable onset and duration of effect and unpredictable antihypertensive response. Whatever agent is used, BP should be monitored continuously via an indwelling arterial catheter or else by frequently repeated (every 10–15 minutes) cuff readings with an oscillometric device so that the dose can be titrated to achieve the desired degree of BP control.

Outcome

Although the underlying cause of hypertension clearly plays a role in determining long-term outcome, for most hypertensive infants, the long-term prognosis should be good. For infants with hypertension related to an umbilical artery catheter, available information suggests that the hypertension will usually resolve over time.[18,63] These infants may require increases in their antihypertensive medications over the first several months following discharge from the nursery as they undergo rapid growth. Following this, it is usually possible to wean their antihypertensives by making no further dose increases as the infant continues to grow. Reliable long-term follow-up data on hypertensive neonates are sparse. In a single-center study, most infants were off medication by 6 months of age.[18] However, in a more recent multicenter study, some neonates who had been discharged from the NICU on antihypertensive medications were still on treatment at 1 year after discharge.[64]

For infants discharged on antihypertensive medications, some method of following home BPs and adjusting medication doses between office visits can be useful. This could include BP monitoring by the primary care provider or use of home BP equipment. In our center, we arrange for rental of hospital-grade oscillometric devices for neonates that require ongoing antihypertensive medication. Use of Doppler devices for home BP monitoring in neonates has also been anecdotally reported.

Some forms of neonatal hypertension may persist beyond infancy, usually hypertension related to parenchymal kidney disease. Infants with renal venous thrombosis may also remain hypertensive,[65] and some of these children will ultimately benefit from removal of the affected kidney. Persistent or late hypertension may also be seen in children who have undergone repair of renal artery stenosis or thoracic aortic coarctation. Reappearance of hypertension in these situations should prompt a search for restenosis by the appropriate imaging studies.

Better long-term outcome studies of infants with neonatal hypertension are needed. Since many of these infants are delivered prior to the completion of nephron development, it is possible that they may not develop the full complement of glomeruli normally seen in term infants.[66] Reduced nephron mass is hypothesized to be a risk factor for the development of adult hypertension.[66–68] Thus, it may be possible that hypertensive neonates (and possibly also normotensive premature neonates) are at increased risk compared with term infants for the development of hypertension in late adolescence or early adulthood.[69] A high incidence of prematurity in children and adolescents with otherwise unexplained hypertension was recently demonstrated in a single-center case series.[70] When studied at the age of 19 years, adolescents with a history of extreme prematurity (gestational age < 26 weeks) had higher central BP than term-born controls.[71] Given the improvements in survival of the most premature infants, is imperative that appropriately designed studies be conducted to address these questions.

Conclusions

Although there are many areas in which better data are needed, particularly with respect to pathophysiology, diagnostic thresholds, and antihypertensive medications, much has been learned about neonatal hypertension over the past decades. Normal BP in neonates is influenced by a variety of factors, including birth weight, gestational age, postnatal age, and maternal factors. Hypertension is more often seen in infants with concurrent conditions such as BPD or in those that have undergone umbilical arterial catheterization. A careful diagnostic evaluation should lead to determination of the underlying cause of hypertension in most infants. Treatment decisions should be tailored to the severity of the hypertension and may include intravenous and/or oral therapy. Most infants will resolve their hypertension over time, although a small number may have persistent BP elevation throughout childhood.

REFERENCES

1. Dionne JM. Determinants of blood pressure in neonates and infants. *Hypertension.* 2021;77:781–787.
2. Zubrow AB, Hulman S, Kushner H, et al. Determinants of blood pressure in infants admitted to neonatal intensive care

units: a prospective multicenter study. *J Perinatol*. 1995;15: 470–479.

3. Pejovic B, Peco-Antic A, Marinkovic-Eric J. Blood pressure in non-critically ill preterm and full-term neonates. *Pediatr Nephrol*. 2007;22:249–257.

4. Kent A, Kecskes Z, Shadbolt B, et al. Normative blood pressure data in the early neonatal period. *Pediatr Nephrol*. 2007; 22:1335–1341.

5. Satoh M, Inoue R, Tada H, et al. Reference values and associated factors for Japanese newborns' blood pressure and pulse rate: the babies' and their parents' longitudinal observation in Suzuki Memorial Hospital on intrauterine period (BOSHI) study. *J Hypertens*. 2016;34:1578–1585.

6. Lurbe E, Garcia-Vicent C, Torro I, et al. First-year blood pressure increase steepest in low birthweight newborns. *J Hypertens*. 2007;25:81–86.

7. Dagle JM, Fisher TJ, Haynes SE, et al. Cytochrome P450 (CYP2D6) genotype is associated with elevated systolic blood pressure in preterm infants after discharge from the neonatal intensive care unit. *J Pediatr*. 2011;159:104–109.

8. Łoniewska B, Kaczmarczyk M, Clark JS, et al. Association of 1936A > G in AKAP10 (A-kinase anchoring protein 10) and blood pressure in Polish full-term newborns. *Blood Press*. 2013;22:51–56.

9. Kent AL, Chaudhari T. Determinants of neonatal blood pressure. *Curr Hypertens Rep*. 2013;15:426–432.

10. Sadoh WE, Ibhanesehbor SE, Monguno AM, Gubler DJ. Predictors of newborn systolic blood pressure. *West Afr J Med*. 2010;29:86–90.

11. Kent AL, Shadbolt B, Hu E, et al. Do maternal- or pregnancy-associated disease states affect blood pressure in the early neonatal period? *Aust N Z J Obstet Gynaecol*. 2009;49:364–370.

12. Rabe H, Bhatt-Mehta V, Bremner SA, et al. Antenatal and perinatal factors influencing neonatal blood pressure: a systematic review. *J Perinatol*. 2021;41:2317–2329.

13. National Heart, Lung, and Blood Institute Task Force on Blood Pressure Control in Children. *Report of the Second Task Force on Blood Pressure Control in Children – 1987*. Bethesda, MD: U. S. Department of Health and Human Services, National High Blood Pressure Education Program.

14. Kent A, Kecskes Z, Shadbolt B, et al. Blood pressure in the first year of life in healthy infants born at term. *Pediatr Nephrol*. 2007;22:1743–1749.

15. Flynn JT, Kaelber DC, Baker-Smith CM, et al. Clinical practice guideline for screening and management of high blood pressure in children and adolescents. *Pediatrics*. 2017;140(2):e20171904.

16. Dionne JM, Abitbol CL, Flynn JT. Hypertension in infancy: diagnosis, management and outcome. *Pediatr Nephrol*. 2012; 27:17–32. Erratum in: *Pediatr Nephrol*. 2012;27:159–160.

17. Seliem WA, Falk MC, Shadbolt B, et al. Antenatal and postnatal risk factors for neonatal hypertension and infant follow-up. *Pediatr Nephrol*. 2007;22:2081–2087.

18. Sahu R, Pannu H, Yu R, et al. Systemic hypertension requiring treatment in the neonatal intensive care unit. *J Pediatr*. 2013;163:84–88.

19. Blowey DL, Duda PJ, Stokes P, Hall M. Incidence and treatment of hypertension in the neonatal intensive care unit. *J Am Soc Hypertens*. 2011;5:478–483.

20. Kraut EJ, Boohaker LJ, Askenazi DJ, et al. Incidence of neonatal hypertension from a large multicenter study [Assessment of Worldwide Acute Kidney Injury Epidemiology in Neonates-AWAKEN]. *Pediatr Res*. 2018;84:279–289. Erratum in: *Pediatr Res*. 2018;84:314.

21. Friedman AL, Hustead VA. Hypertension in babies following discharge from a neonatal intensive care unit. *Pediatr Nephrol*. 1987;1:30–34.

22. Seibert JJ, Taylor BJ, Williamson SL, Williams BJ, Szabo JS, Corbitt SL. Sonographic detection of neonatal umbilical-artery thrombosis: clinical correlation. *Am J Radiol*. 1987;148:965–968.

23. Boo NY, Wong NC, Zulkifli SS, et al. Risk factors associated with umbilical vascular catheter-associated thrombosis in newborn infants. *J Paediatr Child Health*. 1999;35:460–465.

24. Barrington KJ. Umbilical artery catheters in the newborn: effects of position of the catheter tip. *Cochrane Database Syst Rev*. 2009;1:CD000505. doi:10.1002/14651858.CD000505

25. Tullus K, Brennan E, Hamilton G, et al. Renovascular hypertension in children. *Lancet*. 2008;371:1453–1463.

26. Das BB, Recto M, Shoemaker L, et al. Midaortic syndrome presenting as neonatal hypertension. *Pediatr Cardiol*. 2008; 29:1000–1001.

27. Dell KM. The spectrum of polycystic kidney disease in children. *Adv Chronic Kidney Dis*. 2011;18:339–347.

28. Moralıoğlu S, Celayir AC, Bosnalı O, et al. Single center experience in patients with unilateral multicystic dysplastic kidney. *J Pediatr Urol*. 2014;10:763–768.

29. Konda R, Sato H, Ito S, et al. Renin containing cells are present predominantly in scarred areas but not in dysplastic regions in multicystic dysplastic kidney. *J Urol*. 2001;166:1910–1914.

30. Lanzarini VV, Furusawa EA, Sadeck L, et al. Neonatal arterial hypertension in nephro-urological malformations in a tertiary care hospital. *J Hum Hypertens*. 2006;20:679–683.

31. Abman SH, Warady BA, Lum GM, et al. Systemic hypertension in infants with bronchopulmonary dysplasia. *J Pediatr*. 1984; 104:929–931.

32. Anderson AH, Warady BA, Daily DK, et al. Systemic hypertension in infants with severe bronchopulmonary dysplasia: associated clinical factors. *Am J Perinatol*. 1993;10:190–193.

33. Sehgal A, Malikiwi A, Paul E, Tan K, Menahem S. Systemic arterial stiffness in infants with bronchopulmonary dysplasia: potential cause of systemic hypertension. *J Perinatol*. 2016; 36:564–569.

34. Heggen JA, Fortenberry JD, Tanner AJ, et al. Systemic hypertension associated with venovenous extracorporeal membrane oxygenation for pediatric respiratory failure. *J Pediatr Surg*. 2004;39:1626–1631.

35. Jenkins R, Tackitt S, Gievers L, et al. Phthalate-associated hypertension in premature infants: a prospective mechanistic cohort study. *Pediatr Nephrol*. 2019;34:1413–1424.

36. Hawkins KC, Watson AR, Rutter N. Neonatal hypertension and cardiac failure. *Eur J Pediatr*. 1995;154:148–149.

37. Xiao N, Tandon A, Goldstein S, Lorts A. Cardiogenic shock as the initial presentation of neonatal systemic hypertension. *J Neonatal Perinatal Med*. 2013;6:267–272.

38. Dionne JM, Bremner SA, Baygani SK, et al. Method of blood pressure measurement in neonates and infants: a systematic review and analysis. *J Pediatr*. 2020;221:23–31.e5.

39. Dannevig I, Dale H, Liestol K, et al. Blood pressure in the neonate: three non-invasive oscillometric pressure monitors compared with invasively measure blood pressure. *Acta Pediatrica*. 2005;94:191–196.

40. O'Shea J, Dempsey E. A comparison of blood pressure measurements in newborns. *Am J Perinatol*. 2009;26:113–116.

41. Yiallourou SR, Poole H, Prathivadi P, et al. The effects of dummy/pacifier use on infant blood pressure and autonomic activity during sleep. *Sleep Med*. 2014;15:1508–1516.

42. Nwankwo M, Lorenz J, Gardiner J. A standard protocol for blood pressure measurement in the newborn. *Pediatrics.* 1997;99:E10.

43. Crossland DS, Furness JC, Abu-Harb M, et al. Variability of four limb blood pressure in normal neonates. *Arch Dis Child Fetal Neonatal Ed.* 2004;89:F325–F327.

44. Richer C, Hornych H, Amiel-Tison C, et al. Plasma renin activity and its postnatal development in preterm infants. Preliminary report. *Biol Neonate.* 1977;31:301–304.

45. Khandelwal P, Deinum J. Monogenic forms of low-renin hypertension: clinical and molecular insights. *Pediatr Nephrol.* 2022;37(7):1495–1509. doi:10.1007/s00467-021-05246-x

46. Elsaify WM. Neonatal renal vein thrombosis: grey-scale and Doppler ultrasonic features. *Abdom Imaging.* 2009;34:413–418.

47. Kiessling SG, Wadhwa N, Kriss VM, et al. An unusual case of severe therapy-resistant hypertension in a newborn. *Pediatrics.* 2007;119:e301–e304.

48. Kumar B, Upadhyaya VD, Gupta MK, et al. Early nephrectomy in unilateral multicystic dysplastic kidney in children cures hypertension early: an observation. *Eur J Pediatr Surg.* 2017;27:533–537.

49. Miyashita Y, Peterson D, Rees JM, et al. Isradipine treatment of acute hypertension in hospitalized children and adolescents. *J Clin Hypertens (Greenwich).* 2010;12:850–855.

50. Kao LC, Durand DJ, McCrea RC, et al. Randomized trial of long-term diuretic therapy for infants with oxygen-dependent bronchopulmonary dysplasia. *J Pediatr.* 1994;124(5 Pt 1):772–781.

51. O'Dea RF, Mirkin BL, Alward CT, et al. Treatment of neonatal hypertension with captopril. *J Pediatr.* 1988;113:403–406.

52. Tack ED, Perlman JM. Renal failure in sick hypertensive premature infants receiving captopril therapy. *J Pediatr.* 1988;112:805–810.

53. Ku LC, Zimmerman K, Benjamin DK, et al. Safety of enalapril in infants admitted to the neonatal intensive care unit. *Pediatr Cardiol.* 2017;38:155–161.

54. Kanic Z, Kanic V, Hojnik T. Enalapril and acute kidney injury in a hypertensive premature newborn—should it be used or not? *J Pediatr Pharmacol Ther.* 2021;26(6):638–642.

55. Guron G, Friberg P. An intact renin-angiotensin system is a prerequisite for normal renal development. *J Hypertens.* 2000;18:123–137.

56. Bertagnolli M. Preterm birth and renin-angiotensin-aldosterone system: evidences of activation and impact on chronic cardiovascular disease risks. *Protein Pept Lett.* 2017;24:793–798.

57. Wells TG, Bunchman TE, Kearns GL. Treatment of neonatal hypertension with enalaprilat. *J Pediatr.* 1990;117:664–667.

58. Mason T, Polak MJ, Pyles L, et al. Treatment of neonatal renovascular hypertension with intravenous enalapril. *Am J Perinatol.* 1992;9:254–257.

59. Dionne JM, Flynn JT. Management of severe hypertension in the newborn. *Arch Dis Child.* 2017;102:1176–1179.

60. Seeman T, Hamdani G, Mitsnefes M. Hypertensive crisis in children and adolescents. *Pediatr Nephrol.* 2019;34:2523–2537.

61. Gouyon JB, Geneste B, Semama DS, et al. Intravenous nicardipine in hypertensive preterm infants. *Arch Dis Child Fetal Neonatal Ed.* 1997;76:F126–F127.

62. Liviskie CJ, DeAvilla KM, Zeller BN, Najaf T, McPherson CC. Nicardipine for the treatment of neonatal hypertension during extracorporeal membrane oxygenation. *Pediatr Cardiol.* 2019;40:1041–1045.

63. Caplan MS, Cohn RA, Langman CB, et al. Favorable outcome of neonatal aortic thrombosis and renovascular hypertension. *J Pediatr.* 1989;115:291–295.

64. Xiao N, Hamdani G, Starr M, et al. Blood pressure outcomes in neonatal intensive care unit graduates with idiopathic hypertension (abstract). *Kidney Int Rep.* 2019;4:S141.

65. Mocan H, Beattie TJ, Murphy AV. Renal venous thrombosis in infancy: long-term follow-up. *Pediatr Nephrol.* 1991;5:45–49.

66. Abitbol CL, Rodriguez MM. The long-term renal and cardiovascular consequences of prematurity. *Nat Rev Nephrol.* 2012;8:265–274.

67. Keller G, Zimmer G, Mall G, et al. Nephron number in patients with primary hypertension. *N Engl J Med.* 2003;348:101–108.

68. Mackenzie HS, Lawler EV, Brenner BM. Congenital oligonephropathy: the fetal flaw in essential hypertension? *Kidney Int.* 2006;55:S30–S34.

69. Shankaran S, Das A, Bauer CR, et al. Fetal origin of childhood disease: intrauterine growth restriction in term infants and risk for hypertension at 6 years of age. *Arch Pediatr Adolesc Med.* 2006;160:977–981.

70. Gupta-Malhotra M, Banker A, Shete S, et al. Essential hypertension vs. secondary hypertension among children. *Am J Hypertens.* 2015;28:73–80.

71. Hurst JR, Beckmann J, Ni Y, et al. Respiratory and cardiovascular outcomes in survivors of extremely preterm birth at 19 years. *Am J Respir Crit Care Med.* 2020;202:422–432.

Index

Page numbers followed by *b* indicate boxes; *f,* figures; and *t,* tables.

A

Accelerated aging of kidney, after preterm birth, 130
ACEIs. *see* Angiotensin-converting enzyme inhibitors
Acetazolamide. *see* Carbonic anhydrase inhibitors
Acidification process, in nephron, 173, 174f
Acquired pseudohypoaldosteronism, 179
Active transport of sodium, 75
Acute kidney injury (AKI), 14, 120, 126, 185–187
  assessment of, 30–32
  clinical outcomes of, 30
  definition of, 28
  diagnosis of, 28–37
  epidemiology of, 29–30
  hypoxic ischemic encephalopathy, 187
  kidney replacement therapy, 157
    challenges and advancement in, 34–35t
  limitations in, 32
  long-term complications, 34–35
  management of, 33–34
  neonates after cardiac surgery, 187
  patent ductus arteriosus, 186–187
  preterm infants, 185–186
  preventative measures, 32–33
  risk factors of, 29–30, 31t
  in various at-risk populations, 186t
ADH. *see* Antidiuretic hormone
β_2 adrenergic blockers, 57
AKI. *see* Acute kidney injury
Albuterol, 58
Aldosterone, 57, 79–80, 179
Aldosterone deficiency, 84–86
Aldosterone-sensitive distal nephron, 56
Amiloride, 57, 121
Amlodipine, for neonatal hypertension, 213
Ammonia, 173–175, 174f
Amnioinfusions, serial, 48
Amniotic fluid, 42–44
Amniotic fluid homeostasis, 1–2
Amoxicillin, 149–150
Anemia, 166
Aneuploidy, 98–99
Angiotensin-converting enzyme inhibitors (ACEIs), 57, 213
Antenatal hydronephrosis (AHN), 198–199
Antenatal predictors of postnatal renal function, 4–9, 8t
Anterior-posterior renal pelvis diameter (APD), 138
Antibiotic regimens, for uroprophylaxis, 199
Antidiuretic hormone (ADH), 66, 80, 81, 86–87
Aortic coarctation, 188, 188f
Aquaporin 1 (AQP1), 78
Aquaporin 2 (AQP2), 80
Aquaporins 3 (AQP3), 89
Autosomal dominant polycystic kidney disease (ADPKD), 101–102
Autosomal recessive polycystic kidney disease (ARPKD), 102

B

Band-3 protein, 173–175
Bartter syndrome, 86, 89
BEEC. *see* Bladder exstrophy-epispadias complex
Best Pharmaceuticals for Children Act (BPCA), 114–115
Beta blockers, for neonatal hypertension, 213
11 Beta hydroxy-steroid dehydrogenase (11BHSD), 80
Beta trace protein (BTC), 19–20
Bilateral renal agenesis, 100
Bilateral renal hypoplasia, 103
Bladder, anomalies of, 104
Bladder exstrophy-epispadias complex (BEEC), 104
Bladder outlet obstruction, in postnatal UTD, 147–148
Blood pressure (BP)
  diastolic
    high. *see* Hypertension
  factors affecting, at birth, 203–207, 204f, 205f, 206f
  measurement in neonatal hypertension, 210–211, 211f
  normative neonatal values for
    high. *see* Hypertension
  premature newborns, 204
  systolic
    high. *see* Hypertension
Blood urea nitrogen (BUN), 83
Body surface area (BSA), 128–129
BPD. *see* Bronchopulmonary dysplasia
BPD-associated hypertension, 210
Brenner hypothesis, 127
Bronchopulmonary dysplasia (BPD), 114, 117–118, 210
BSA. *see* Body surface area
Bumetanide, 116. *see also* Loop diuretics
BUN. *see* Blood urea nitrogen

C

CAH. *see* Congenital adrenal hyperplasia
CAKUT. *see* Congenital anomalies of the kidneys and urinary tract
Calcium disorders, neonatal. *see specific disorders*
Carbonic anhydrase inhibitors, 121
Cardiovascular disease
  developmental programming of, 127–128
  dialysis in infancy, 166
Caroli disease, 102
Carperitide, 121–122
CDI. *see* Central diabetes insipidus
Central diabetes insipidus (CDI), 88
CF. *see* Cystic fibrosis
Chlorothiazide, 117, 118. *see also* Thiazide diuretics
Chronic dialysis, 157–158
Chronic kidney disease (CKD), 14. *see also* Kidney injury
  kidney replacement therapy and, 157–158
  multiple hit pathways from prematurity to, 130–132, 131f
  neonatal populations at risk for, 133f